T0336563

Glossary of Dental Implantology

Glossary of Dental Implantology

Khalid Almas
West Hartford, CT, USA

Fawad Javed
Rochester, NY, USA

Steph Smith
Limpopo Province, South Africa

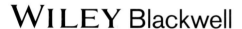

This edition first published 2018
© 2018 John Wiley & Sons, Inc.

All rights reserved. No part of this publication may be reproduced, stored in a retrieval system, or transmitted, in any form or by any means, electronic, mechanical, photocopying, recording or otherwise, except as permitted by law. Advice on how to obtain permission to reuse material from this title is available at http://www.wiley.com/go/permissions.

The right of Khalid Almas, Fawad Javed and Steph Smith to be identified as the authors of this work has been asserted in accordance with law.

Registered Office
John Wiley & Sons, Inc., 111 River Street, Hoboken, NJ 07030, USA

Editorial Office
111 River Street, Hoboken, NJ 07030, USA

For details of our global editorial offices, customer services, and more information about Wiley products visit us at www.wiley.com.

Wiley also publishes its books in a variety of electronic formats and by print-on-demand. Some content that appears in standard print versions of this book may not be available in other formats.

Limit of Liability/Disclaimer of Warranty
The contents of this work are intended to further general scientific research, understanding, and discussion only and are not intended and should not be relied upon as recommending or promoting scientific method, diagnosis, or treatment by physicians for any particular patient. In view of ongoing research, equipment modifications, changes in governmental regulations, and the constant flow of information relating to the use of medicines, equipment, and devices, the reader is urged to review and evaluate the information provided in the package insert or instructions for each medicine, equipment, or device for, among other things, any changes in the instructions or indication of usage and for added warnings and precautions. While the publisher and authors have used their best efforts in preparing this work, they make no representations or warranties with respect to the accuracy or completeness of the contents of this work and specifically disclaim all warranties, including without limitation any implied warranties of merchantability or fitness for a particular purpose. No warranty may be created or extended by sales representatives, written sales materials or promotional statements for this work. The fact that an organization, website, or product is referred to in this work as a citation and/or potential source of further information does not mean that the publisher and authors endorse the information or services the organization, website, or product may provide or recommendations it may make. This work is sold with the understanding that the publisher is not engaged in rendering professional services. The advice and strategies contained herein may not be suitable for your situation. You should consult with a specialist where appropriate. Further, readers should be aware that websites listed in this work may have changed or disappeared between when this work was written and when it is read. Neither the publisher nor authors shall be liable for any loss of profit or any other commercial damages, including but not limited to special, incidental, consequential, or other damages.

Library of Congress Cataloging-in-Publication Data

Names: Almas, Khalid, 1958– author.
Title: Glossary of dental implantology / by Khalid Almas, Fawad Javed, Steph Smith.
Description: Hoboken, NJ : Wiley, [2018] | Includes bibliographical references and index. |
Identifiers: LCCN 2017057634 (print) | LCCN 2017058924 (ebook) | ISBN 9781118985366 (pdf) |
    ISBN 9781118985342 (epub) | ISBN 9781118626887 (cloth)
Subjects: LCSH: Dental implants–Dictionaries.
Classification: LCC RK667.I45 (ebook) | LCC RK667.I45 A46 2018 (print) | DDC 617.6/9303–dc23
LC record available at https://lccn.loc.gov/2017057634

Cover Design: Wiley
Cover Image: (Background) © Pinghung Chen / EyeEm/Gettyimages; (Dental Implant) Courtesy of Esra Khalil

Set in 10/12pt Warnock by SPi Global, Pondicherry, India

Printed in Singapore by C.O.S. Printers Pte Ltd

10 9 8 7 6 5 4 3 2 1

Khalid Almas

This work is dedicated to my wife, Pakeeza Waheed, and children, Arooba, Areej, and Muhammad Nabeel, for their immeasurable love, unconditional support, and unwavering perseverance.

Fawad Javed

I dedicate this work to my family for their endless support and love.

Steph Smith

This work is dedicated to my wife, Sandra, for her enduring and steadfast love. To my children, Raymond and Lauren, for their love and dedication, who always inspire me to cherish the immense beauty of life.

"To acquire knowledge, one must study; but to acquire wisdom, one must observe" (Marilyn vos Savant)

Contents

Foreword   *ix*

Preface   *xi*

A   *1*

B   *21*

C   *35*

D   *59*

E   *71*

F   *83*

G   *93*

H   *101*

I   *109*

J   *123*

K   *125*

L   *127*

M   *135*

N   *151*

O   *157*

P   *167*

Q   *189*

R   *191*

S   *203*

T   *221*

U   *233*

V   *235*

W   *239*

X   *241*

Y   *243*

Z   *245*

Appendix A   Digital Dental Terms   *247*

Appendix B   Useful Websites   *251*

Appendix C   Recommended Reading   *257*

Foreword

I am pleased to write the foreword for *Glossary of Dental Implantology*. Dental implantology has evolved over recent decades to become one of the most important aspects of clinical dentistry around the globe. There are many dictionaries and glossaries involving various specialties in the medical and dental sciences, including dental implantology. The current compilation is a unified effort to provide a consensual and evidence-based global platform for orodental implant terminology for effective communication among dental professionals, clinicians, researchers, and scientists. Comprehensive in scope, the glossary defines terms for all aspects of dental implantology, compiled in one book.

The authors are experienced academicians, clinicians, and educators. Their experience and dedication in the fundamental and clinical aspects of dental implantology have given them a unique vantage point to succeed in this endeavor. Their choice of terminologies, based on classic and current literature, makes this compilation a must-read for all who practice dental implantology. I commend the authors for this unified and outstanding current effort to serve the profession.

Georgios Romanos, DDS, PhD,
Prof. Dr. med. dent.
Professor of Periodontology
Stony Brook University, Stony Brook,
New York, USA
and
Professor of Oral Surgery and
Implant Dentistry
University of Frankfurt, Frankfurt, Germany
October 2017

Preface

Implantology is the most rapidly expanding discipline in dentistry. The successes achieved in both professional development and awareness amongst the general population, together with the industrial growth of dental implantology, have led to the unprecedented yield in patient care and comfort over the past three decades.

This glossary provides a unified, consensual, and evidence-based source of definitions and terminologies used in implant dentistry. The terminology applicable to daily dental implant practice is envisaged to promote effective communication among various dental team members, including surgeons, restorative practitioners, and laboratory technicians, the composition thereof becoming an integral part of dental implantology. The careful selection and verification of various definitions and related terms in the ever-expanding field of implant dentistry informs the glossary, encompassing a unique and contemporary standard enriched with classic and currently accepted terminology pertinent to the interdisciplinary practice of implant dentistry. The inclusion of recent advances in 3D imaging, navigational and guided surgical approaches, biomechanics, regenerative materials, and digital workflow has produced a holistic, comprehensive, and very contemporary text.

For successful diagnosis and treatment planning in implant dentistry, which is to be rendered in a comprehensive manner, encompassing a multidisciplinary team approach for a predictable outcome, meaningful communication is needed among the various team members. This is provided for in the glossary by means of an effective common language to be utilized by various dental team members, incorporating biological and biomechanical viewpoints. The team that functions effectively due to the absence of technical language barriers can confidently overcome and master the challenging situations encountered in the diagnosis, treatment, and long-term maintenance of dental implants.

We would like to thank Dr G.P. Schincaglia, the former Program Director of Advanced Periodontics, at the University of Connecticut, School of Dental Medicine, USA (currently at West Virginia University, School of Dentistry, USA), for his insightful discussions on classic and current literature concerning implant terminology. Special thanks are also due to Ms Jessica Kilham, from the University of Connecticut Health Center Library (currently the Research and Instruction Librarian at Quinnipiac University, USA), for her help in obtaining resources and literature searches. We also thank Professor Khalid Mahmood, the former Head of Information, Learning and Research Commons (ILRC) at the University of Dammam, Saudi Arabia (currently at the University of Punjab, Lahore, Pakistan), for his help in information management. The above mentioned are thanked for their contributions including their exquisite technical knowhow and skills in the library sciences required for the compilation of this glossary.

Due to limitations of space, not all reference materials have been included. However, the editors would like to acknowledge and thank each and every author, professional organization and interest group whose scientific publications have had an impact on this glossary for the common good of the dental profession.

Special thanks are due to Rick Blanchette, the Commissioning Editor of Wiley-Blackwell for North America, who advised on the approval process of the glossary proposal. The staff at Wiley Publishing Company in USA, Europe, and Asia are thanked for their continuous support, expertise, and patience over the years in the preparation of this glossary.

In summary, this consensual and evidence-based glossary provides a descriptive source to clinicians and academicians, to supplement their efforts in providing high standards of care in dental implant therapy, including predictable outcomes. Researchers are also provided with a useful knowledge tool to further the frontiers of research so as to improve the quality of life of the global population in need of implant therapy.

Autumn 2017   *KA, FJ, SS*

A

ABBM (abbrev.): Anorganic bovine bone matrix.

ABM (abbrev.): Anorganic bone matrix.

aberrant: Varying or deviating from the usual or normal course, form, or location.

abfraction: The hypothetical process leading to the loss of cervical tooth structure due to a combination of abrasion, erosion, and/or occlusal forces; data supporting this term as a discrete clinical entity is equivocal. See: Abrasion, Erosion.

abrasion: The wearing away of tooth structure or restorative material through an abnormal mechanical process.

abscess (Latin: *abscessus*): An immunologically contained and controlled lesion that is an accumulation of pus (neutrophils) in a pocket found in tissue. Caused by inflammation induced by either (1) a localized infection caused by bacteria or parasites or (2) foreign materials lodged in the tissue. It is a defensive mechanism to prevent the dissemination of the infection to other parts of the body.

abscess: **Acute a.**: An abscess of relative short duration, typically producing pain and local inflammation. **Apical a.**: Inflammatory condition characterized by formation of purulent exudate involving the dental pulp or pulpal remnants and the tissues surrounding the apex of a tooth. **Chronic a.**: 1. Abscess of comparatively slow development with little evidence of inflammation. There may be an intermittent discharge of purulent matter. 2. Long-standing collection of purulent exudate. It may follow an acute abscess. See: Abscess, Residual. **Gingival a.**: A localized purulent infection that involves the marginal gingiva or interdental papilla. **Pericoronal a.**: A localized purulent infection within the tissue surrounding the crown of a partially erupted tooth. **Periodontal a.** (Parietal a.): Localized purulent inflammation in the periodontal tissues, also called lateral periodontal abscess. **Pulpal a.**: Inflammation of the dental pulp characterized by the formation of purulent exudate. **Residual a.**: Abscess produced by the residues of a previous inflammatory process. **Wandering a.**: Abscess in which purulent material flows along a course of decreased resistance and discharges at a distant point.

absorbable: See: Bioabsorbable material.

absorbed radiation dose (also known as *total ionizing dose*, TID): The quantity of ionizing radiation (measured in joules [unit of energy] per kilogram or gray [GY] units) that a patient absorbs during diagnostic or therapeutic radiation. The absorbed dose is dependent upon (1) the incident radiation and (2) the absorbing material (i.e., an X-ray beam may deposit four times the radiation dose in bone as that deposited in air, or none may be deposited in a vacuum).

absorption: 1. Passage of a substance into the interior of another substance. 2. Passage of fluids or substances through tissues. 3. Attenuation of radiation energy by the substance through which it passes.

abutment: 1. The component that interfaces with the implant fixture (implant body) and the prosthetic entity. It may be constructed to accept screw- or cement-retained prosthetics and be made of

Glossary of Dental Implantology, First Edition. Khalid Almas, Fawad Javed and Steph Smith.
© 2018 John Wiley & Sons, Inc. Published 2018 by John Wiley & Sons, Inc.

titanium, alloyed metals, ceramic, zirconia; be custom made; or be uniformly produced by manufacturers. The abutment may have one or multiple pieces and can be straight or angled. **Pier a.**: An abutment positioned between adjacent abutments. 2. Tooth, tooth root, or implant component that serves as support and/or retention for a dental prosthesis. **Screw design of a.**: Prosthetic implant component manufactured with threads at the apical portion of the element. This term refers to the manufacture of a specific thread pattern unique to a particular implant company. **Tightness of a.**: Amount of clamping force present within the body of an abutment screw following placement. See: Preload.

abutment analog: A replica of the dental implant abutment that is used when making an impression for the laboratory fabrication of the definitive implant abutment. The implant abutment may be made of brass, aluminum, steel, or plastic.

abutment clamp: Forceps used to assist in the positioning of an abutment on a dental implant platform, or any device used for positioning a dental implant abutment upon the dental implant body.

abutment connection: The act of fastening an abutment to a dental implant, or of connecting an abutment to an endosseous implant.

abutment driver: Instrument or device used to assist in the delivery and tightening of an abutment to a dental implant.

abutment healing cap: Any temporary cover used to provide a seal over the superior portion of a dental implant; most such covers are metallic and are intended for interim usage following exposure of the dental implant's superior surface.

abutment holder: Instrument that provides abutment retention for extraoral preparation and polishing procedures.

abutment–implant interface: Common contact surface area between an implant abutment and the supporting implant.

abutment impression coping: See: Impression coping.

abutment-level impression: The impression of an abutment either directly, using conventional impression techniques, or indirectly, using an abutment impression coping. See: Implant-level impression.

abutment mount: Prefabricated device, usually packaged with an abutment, used for the transfer of an abutment to a dental implant intraorally.

abutment post: That component of a dental implant abutment which extends into the internal structure of a dental implant and is used to provide retention and/or stability to the dental implant abutment.

abutment screw: A threaded fastener used to connect an abutment to a dental implant. It is usually torqued to a final seating position, or single-piece implant component with a threaded apical portion that can be connected directly to the implant. No additional screw is required to connect and secure the abutment component, or that component which secures the dental implant abutment to the dental implant body.

abutment selection: A step in the prosthodontic treatment whereby a decision is made regarding the type of abutment to be used for the restoration based on dental implant angulation, interarch space, soft tissue (mucosal) height, planned prosthesis, occlusal factors (e.g., opposing dentition, parafunction), esthetics, and phonetic considerations.

abutment swapping: See: Platform switching.

abutment transfer device: See: Orientation jig.

access hole: Opening in a replacement tooth's occlusal or lingual surface of an implant-retained prosthesis that provides entrance for abutment or prosthesis screw placement or removal.

accessory ostium: Occasional opening of the maxillary sinus either into the infundibulum or directly in the wall of the middle meatus. See: Ostium (maxillary sinus).

accretion: An accumulation of plaque, calculus, or material alba on teeth or dental implants.

acellular: Devoid of cells.

acellular dermal allograft: Allogenic skin graft, derived from a human cadaver, consisting of a thin split-thickness of dermis, devoid of cellular content following a tissue preparation process.

acetaminophen: Amide of acetic acid and p-aminophenol, a nonopioid analgesic and antipyretic drug, which may be administered orally or rectally.

acid-etched implant: External surface of an implant body that has been modified by the chemical action of an acidic medium. The subtractive surface is intended to enhance osseointegration.

acid-etched surface: Treatment of a surface with an acid in order to increase its surface area by subtraction. See: Subtractive surface treatment.

acid etching: Act of modifying an implant surface by exposure to an acidic medium with the intention of enhancing osseointegration.

acquired centric: See: Occlusion, centric.

acquired immunity: Specialized form of immunity involving antibodies and lymphocytes. Active immunity develops after exposure to a suitable agent (e.g., by an attack of a disease or by injection of antigens), and passive immunity occurs with transfer of antibody or lymphocytes from an immune donor.

acquired immunodeficiency syndrome: See: AIDS.

acrylic crown: See: Acrylic restoration.

acrylic resin: Any of a group of thermoplastic resins made by polymerizing esters of acrylic or methyl methacrylate acids.

acrylic resin veneer: Usually referring to fixed dental prosthesis, the veneering or lamination of the facial and/or buccal surfaces of a crown or fixed dental prosthesis using acrylic resin. The intention of such veneering is to provide a natural tooth color to the viewable portions of the restoration.

acrylic restoration: Tooth or other prosthetic restoration fabricated from acrylic resin, such as an acrylic crown.

Actinobacillus actinomycetemcomitans: Gram-negative, fermentative, nonmotile, coccoid or rod-shaped bacterium of the family Pasteurellaceae, part of the normal mammalian microflora. This bacterium has been associated with periodontal infections and, in particular, early-onset, aggressive forms of periodontal disease. See: *Aggregatibacter actinomycetemcomitans*.

Actinomyces israelii: A gram-positive, nonmotile, facultatively anaerobic, pleomorphic bacterium. It is commonly found in the soil but can also be found in dental plaque and the intestinal tract of mammals. It is typically a commensal bacterium.

Actinomyces naeslundii: A gram-positive, nonmotile, facultatively anaerobic, pleomorphic bacterium found in marginal and interproximal plaque of healthy individuals. Cell morphology is often curved or branching rods. An early colonizer of the tooth surface.

Actinomyces viscosus: A pathogenic bacterial species that is catalase positive, gram positive, facultative anaerobic, nonmotile, filamentous, and pleomorphic. It is an indigenous microflora that colonizes the mouth of humans and is often affiliated with gingivitis, periodontitis, and root caries.

actinomycosis: A subacute to chronic bacterial infection caused by *Actinomyces*. A common form is cervicofacial (i.e., lumpy jaw).

activating tool: Instrument used to increase or reduce the retention of an attachment. See: Attachment.

active eruption: See: Eruption, dental.

actual implant length/diameter: The exact measurement of the length and diameter of a dental implant. See: Nominal implant length/diameter.

acute: 1. Sharp, severe. 2. Denoting the swift onset and course of a disease.

acute abscess: Abscess of relatively short duration, typically producing local swelling, inflammation, and pain.

acute infection: Infection with a rapid onset and usually a severe course.

acyclovir: A synthetic acyclic purine nucleoside that may be used systemically. Drug of choice in simple mucocutaneous herpes simplex, in immunocompromised patients with initial herpes genitalis. Also active against herpes virus including *H. zoster* and *H. varicella*.

adaptation: 1. The act or process of adapting; the state of being adapted. 2. The act of purposefully adapting two surfaces to provide intimate contact. 3. The progressive adjusted changes in sensitivity that regularly accompany continuous sensory stimulation or lack of stimulation. 4. In dentistry, (1) the degree of fit between a prosthesis and supporting structures, (2) the degree of proximity of a restorative material to a tooth preparation, (3) the adjustment of orthodontic bands to teeth.

adaptation syndrome: The body's short- and long-term response to accommodate stress.

added surface: See: Additive surface treatment.

additive fabrication: See: Solid freeform fabrication (SFF).

additive manufacturing (AM): The "process of joining materials to make objects from 3D model data, usually layer upon layer, as opposed to subtractive manufacturing methodologies, such as traditional machining," as defined by the American Society for Testing Materials (ASTM).

additive manufacturing file (AMF): An open standard file format for describing objects for additive manufacturing processes such as 3D printing. The official ISO/ASTM 52915:2013 standard is an XML-based format designed to allow any computer-aided design software to describe the shape and composition of any 3D object to be fabricated on any 3D printer. Unlike its predecessor STL format, AMF has native support for color, materials, lattices, and constellations.

additive surface treatment: Added surface. Alteration of the surface of a dental implant by addition of material. See: Subtractive surface treatment, textured surface.

adenitis: Inflammation of a lymph node or gland.

adenopathy: Pathologic enlargement of glands, especially lymphatic glands.

adenovirus: A DNA virus 80–90 nanometers in size. It can cause respiratory illness and conjunctivitis in humans. Human adenoviruses comprise at least 31 serotypes that can be divided into three groups on the basis of oncogenicity.

adherence: The act or quality of uniting two or more surfaces or parts.

adhesion: Physical process of attachment of a substance to the surface of another substance, usually due to a molecular attraction that exists between the surfaces.

adhesive: Intervening substance used to unite adjoining surfaces. In maxillofacial prosthetics, adhesives are used for border adaptation, marginal seal, and the retention of facial, auricular, nasal, or orbital prostheses. Systems commonly used include biphasic adhesive tape and medical-grade adhesives.

adiadochokinesia: Inability to make opposing movements in quick succession, such as jaw opening and closing.

adipose atrophy: Loss of fat tissue.

adjunctive treatment: Supplemental or additional therapeutic treatments used in conjunction with the primary treatment. In periodontics, it generally refers to procedures other than scaling and root planing and surgical therapy, such as chemotherapy, occlusal therapy, and restorative care.

adjustable anterior guidance: The anterior guide portion on a dental articulator that allows for variable (individualized) settings that provide guidance for the occlusion in protrusive and lateral protrusive movements.

adjustable articulator: A dental articulator that is adjustable in the sagittal and horizontal planes to duplicate or simulate recorded mandibular jaw movements.

adjustable attachment system: Stud-shaped attachment in which the stud (easily replaced) serves as the patrix and the matrix consists of a metal housing. The base of the patrix can be cast to or soldered as part of a coping, and the matrix can be incorporated into the dental prosthesis. The patrix is adjustable using a special tool to modify the spread of the patrix width.

adjustment: Modification of a tooth or prosthetic restoration to improve its appearance, fit, or function.

adjustment, occlusal: See: Occlusal adjustment.

ADO (abbrev.): See: Algorithmic dental occlusion.

adsorption: The attachment of a substance to the surface of another.

adult periodontitis: See: Periodontitis.

aerobe: A microorganism that can live and grow in the presence of molecular oxygen.

aerobic: Environmental conditions that contain atmospheric levels of oxygen. Used in reference to microorganisms that grow optimally under these conditions. See: Facultative.

age atrophy: A wasting or decrease in size or physiological activity of the body related to the normal aging process.

agenesis: Failure of a body part to form.

Aggregatibacter actinomycetemcomitans: A gram-negative, nonmotile, facultatively anaerobic, rod-shaped bacterium found in subgingival and marginal plaque of healthy and periodontally diseased individuals.

aggressive periodontitis: See: Periodontitis.

agnathia: A growth-related defect characterized by a severely undersized mandible or no mandible.

agranulocytosis: Neutropenia; can be acute or chronic depending on the duration of the illness.

AIDS: Acronym for acquired immunodeficiency syndrome, caused by HIV (human immunodeficiency virus), that leaves the body vulnerable to a host of life-threatening illnesses. There is no cure for AIDS, but treatment with antiviral medication can suppress symptoms.

ailing implant: General term for a dental implant affected by periimplant mucositis, without bone loss. For some authors, an ailing dental implant is an implant with a history of bone loss that is not progressing. See: Periimplant mucositis, Periimplantitis.

air abrasion: A wearing away of a material's surface due to particulate material carried by an air current.

Akers' clasp: The archetypal direct retainer for removable partial dentures that comprises a rest, guide plate, retentive arm, and reciprocal arm. Akers' clasps are customarily directed away from the area that is edentulous. If they are directed toward the edentulous area, they are called reverse Akers' clasps. This clasp was named after its inventor, Polk E. Akers.

ala nasi: The expanded outer wall of cartilage on the lateral aspect of the nose.

ala-tragus line: A line that runs from the inferior border of the ala of the nose to a point on the tragus (usually the tip) of the ear. It is often correlated with the tragus of the opposite ear. It is used in determining the ala-tragus plane. The ala-tragus and occlusal planes should be parallel.

albicans: Candidiasis attributable to *C. tropicalis*, *C. parapsilosis*, *C. pseudotropicalis*, and *C. stellatoidea* have also been cultivated from the oral cavity.

alendronate sodium: Oral nitrogen-containing bisphosphonate used for the treatment of osteoporosis. It acts as a specific inhibitor of osteoclast-mediated bone resorption. See: Bisphosphonate.

algae: See: Calcified algae.

alginate: An impression material derived from seaweed that sets in an irreversible rubbery mass.

algipore: See: Calcified algae, Porous marine-derived coralline hydroxyapatite.

algorithm: An instance of logic written into software by software developers to be effective for computer(s) to produce output from given input. An algorithm is a procedure or formula for solving a problem in a finite, logical manner. Algorithms are self-contained, step-by-step sets of operations to be performed by the software program. They are widely used in 3D digital designing and manufacturing.

algorithmic dental occlusion (ADO): Computer algorithms used to establish virtual occlusion and movements. The algorithms encode physical motions and responses for each tooth and its respective antagonists and neighboring teeth. The advantage of ADO is that it allows for pursuing the goal of optimal occlusion, as defined by clinical standards, with the untiring effort of a computer.

alkaline phosphatase: Enzyme found in high concentrations in osteoblasts; commonly located on cytoplasmic processes extending into the osteoid. The level of alkaline phosphatase in serum is a systemic indicator for bone formation.

allele: One of two or more different genes that may occupy the same locus on a specific chromosome.

allergen: A substance capable of producing allergy or specific hypersensitivity.

allergy: The altered reactivity of a sensitized individual on exposure to an allergen.

allodynia: Pain resulting from a nonnoxious stimulus to normal skin or mucosa that does not normally provoke pain.

allogeneic: Antigenically distinct individuals or tissues from the same genetic species. In transplantation biology, denoting individuals (or tissues) that are of the same species however antigenically distinct; also called homologous allogeneic graft. See: Homograft.

allogeneic bone graft: Graft between genetically dissimilar members of the same species. Iliac cancellous bone and marrow, freeze-dried bone allograft (FDBA), and demineralized freeze-dried bone allograft (DFDBA) are available commercially from tissue banks.

allogenic graft: See: Allograft.

allograft: 1. See: Graft, Allograft. 2. A graft material used to augment a tissue that is from the same species but genetically dissimilar individuals.

allograft: (syn): Allogenic graft. Graft tissue from genetically dissimilar members of the same species. Four types exist: frozen, freeze-dried bone allograft (FDBA), demineralized freeze-dried bone allograft (DFDBA), and solvent-dehydrated mineralized allograft.

alloplast: 1. An inert foreign body used for implantation within tissue. 2. A material originating from a nonliving source that surgically replaces missing tissue or augments that which remains.

alloplastic graft: 1. See: Alloplast. 2. Graft material consisting of an inert material such as hydroxyapatite (HA), tricalcium phosphate (TCP), polymethylmethacrylate (PMMA) and hydroxyethylmethacrylate (HEMA) polymer, or bioactive glass that is derived either synthetically or from a foreign, inert source.

alloplastic material: Any nonbiologic material suitable for implantation as an alloplast.

alloy: A mixture of two or more metals or metalloids that are mutually soluble in the molten state; distinguished as binary, ternary, quaternary, etc., depending on the number of metals within the mixture. Alloying elements are added to alter the hardness, strength, and toughness of a metallic element, thus obtaining properties not found in a pure metal. Alloys may also be classified on the basis of their behavior when solidified.

alloying element: Metallic or nonmetallic elements added to or retained by a pure metal for the purpose of giving that metal special properties.

all-polymer prosthesis: A nonmetallic or nonceramic removable or fixed dental prosthesis composed of a glass fiber-reinforced composite framework with a particulate composite resin covering or overlay.

altered cast: A technique in which a removable partial denture frame is related to the existing dentition by sectioning the cast on which the frame was constructed. A new overimpression is made and pieced together with the existing cast.

aluminous porcelain: A ceramic material with >35% aluminum oxide (by volume) glass matrix phase.

aluminum oxide: 1. A metallic oxide constituent of dental porcelain that increases hardness and viscosity. 2. A high-strength ceramic crystal dispersed throughout a glassy phase to increase its strength, as in aluminous dental porcelain used to fabricate aluminous porcelain crowns. 3. A finely ground ceramic particle (frequently 50 μm) often used in conjunction with air-borne particle abrasion of metal castings before the application of porcelain as with metal ceramic restorations. Aluminum oxide has been replaced by titanium as the material of choice for implants.

alveolar: 1. Pertaining to an alveolus. See: Alveolus. 2. The portion of jaw bones that support teeth or that supported teeth at one time. 3. Related to the alveolar process, the maxillary or mandibular ridge of bone that supports the roots of teeth.

alveolar atrophy: Decrease in the volume of the alveolar process occurring after tooth loss, decreased function, and/or localized overloading from an improperly fitting removable partial or complete denture.

alveolar augmentation: 1. See: Augmentation. 2. Surgical placement of bone augmentation material(s) to increase or alter the volume of the alveolar bone. 3. Any surgical procedure employed to alter the contour of the residual alveolar ridge.

alveolar bone: 1. See: Bone, alveolar. 2. That part of the maxilla or mandible comprising the tooth-bearing and/or supporting part of the jawbones. It consists of cortical plates, the vestibular plate being the thinnest, and trabecular bone. **Quantity of a. b.:** Of major importance to the outcome of implant placement, bone volume at a given implant site ideally should be at least 10 mm in vertical dimension and 6 mm in horizontal dimension. 3. The bony portion of the mandible or maxillae in which the roots of the teeth are held by fibers of the periodontal ligament; also called dental alveolus.

alveolar bone proper: The bone lining the alveoli; also called cribriform plate due to the numerous perforating channels (Volkmann's canals), lamina dura due to the radiographic appearance, fibrous endosteum due to the fibers of the periodontal ligament, bundle bone due to the large quantity of Sharpey's fibers. See: Buccal plate, Lingual plate.

alveolar crest: The most coronal portion of the alveolar process.

alveolar defect: A deficiency in the contour of the alveolar ridge in the vertical (apicocoronal) and/or horizontal (buccolingual, mesiodistal) direction.

alveolar distraction osteogenesis: 1. See: Distraction osteogenesis. 2. Augmentation procedure involving the surgical mobilization, transport, and fixation of an alveolar bone segment. A mechanical distraction device allows a gradual, controlled displacement of the mobile bone segment at an ideal rate of 0.4 mm a day. Following the desired augmentation, the device is left in place for 3–4 weeks for consolidation of the newly formed bone.

alveolar mucosa: 1. See: Mucosa, alveolar. 2. Lining mucosa. The lining mucosa that covers the alveolar process apical to the mucogingival junction. It consists of a non-keratinized epithelium lining a connective tissue that is loosely attached to the periosteum and is movable. See: Oral mucosa.

alveolar nerve: Either of the superior alveolar nerve branches of the maxillary nerve of the second division of the trigeminal nerve (rami alveolares superiores posteriores, ramus alveolaris superior medius, and ramus alveolaris superior anteriores). Supplies sensory innervation to the maxillary molars, the premolars, or the canine and incisors, respectively. The inferior alveolar nerve (nervus alveolaris inferior) is the largest branch of the mandibular nerve of the third division of the trigeminal nerve or cranial nerve V, which supplies sensory innervation to the mandibular teeth, lower lip, and chin.

alveolar preservation: See: Ridge preservation.

alveolar process: 1. See: Alveolar ridge, Alveolar process, Residual ridge, Ridge. 2. The (alveolar) portion of jaw bones comprising the compact and cancellous portion of bone surrounding and supporting the teeth, or that supported teeth at one time.

alveolar recess: A cavity in the maxillary sinus floor formed by a septum.

alveolar reconstruction: Any surgical procedure employed to recreate a severely resorbed residual alveolar ridge, or surgical reconstruction of an atrophic alveolar ridge that does not allow for simultaneous implant placement because of the extent of bone deficiency.

alveolar resorption: See: Residual ridge resorption.

alveolar ridge: 1. See: Residual ridge. 2. The ridge portion of the jaw bone that supports teeth or that supported teeth at one time.

3. The bony ridge of the maxilla or mandible that contains the alveoli, or the osseous part of the mandible and maxilla remaining after removal of teeth, i.e., alveolar process. See: Alveolus, Residual ridge, Ridge.

alveolar ridge augmentation: 1. See: Augmentation. 2. Surgical augmentation of the alveolar ridge in a horizontal and/or vertical direction using one of several approaches based on the size and/or location of the defect.

alveolar ridge defect: 1. See: Alveolar defect, Ridge defect. 2. Circumscribed absence of tissue in a residual alveolar ridge. **Implant placement in a. r. d.**: Requires simultaneous guided bone regeneration (GBR). Prerequisites for a simultaneous approach are: (1) implant placement in a correct prosthetic position, (2) good primary stability of the placed implant, and (3) an appropriate defect morphology that allows for a predictable regenerative treatment outcome. Vertical defects are more demanding than horizontal defects, as are one-wall, two-wall, and three-wall defects. **Morphology of a. r. d.**: Classified as horizontal and/or vertical deficiencies. Classification is important for determining the prognosis of bone augmentation procedures.

alveolar ridge resorption: See: Ridge resorption.

alveolar septum: See: Interalveolar septum.

alveolectomy: 1. See: Osteotomy. 2. Surgical removal of all or a portion of the alveolar process of the jaw bone(s), usually performed to achieve acceptable ridge contour in preparation for construction of a denture or placement of an implant.

alveoloplasty: 1. See: Osteoplasty. 2. The surgical procedure of altering the alveolar ridge or its surrounding bony structures by cutting, smoothing, or reshaping to correct the alveolar ridge external contour in preparation for prosthetic rehabilitation.

alveolus (plural: alveoli): The socket in the bone into which a tooth is attached by means of the periodontal ligament, or one of the cavities or sockets within the alveolar process of the maxillae or mandible in which the attachment complex held the root of a tooth after the tooth's removal.

AM (abbrev.): Additive manufacturing.

AMF (abbrev.): Additive manufacturing file.

aminoglycosides: A group of antibiotics (streptomycin, gentamycin, tobramycin) commonly combined synergistically with penicillins.

amorphous: Having no rigid shape or organized structure, without crystalline structure; having random arrangement of atoms in space.

amoxicillin: Broad-spectrum antibiotic, a semi-synthetic derivative of ampicillin, with a superior absorption and a bioavailability of 70–80% with very low toxicity. It is effective against gram-positive and gram-negative bacteria and may be combined with clavulanic acid to counteract the beta-lactamase destruction of penicillin by resistant bacteria. This antibiotic is often used in the treatment of infections caused by susceptible strains of *Haemophilus influenzae, Escherichia coli, Proteus mirabilis, Neisseria gonorrhoeae*, streptococci (including *Streptococcus faecalis and S. pneumoniae*), and nonpenicillinase-producing staphylococci of the oral cavity. It is the primary drug for antibiotic prophylaxis. See: Clavulanic acid.

amputate: The intentional surgical removal of diseased tissue; relating to dentistry, may be amputating a root from a multirooted tooth or the removal of a portion of a root.

anachoresis: A process through which circulating bacteria, pigments, metallic substances, foreign proteins, and other materials are fixated to areas of inflammation.

anaerobe: A microorganism that can survive in partial or complete absence of molecular oxygen.

anaerobic: Used in reference to microorganisms that can survive and grow in the absence of molecular oxygen.

analgesia: Absence of sensibility to pain, designating particularly the relief of pain without loss of consciousness.

analgesic: 1. An agent that alleviates pain without causing loss of consciousness.

Two general categories exist: opioid and nonopioid. See: Blocking agent, Diagnostic block. 2. (adj): Relieving pain.

analgesic blocking agent: Any analgesic that blocks or prohibits sensory perception.

analgesic diagnostic block: the selective use of a local anesthetic injection or application of a topical anesthetic to identify a pain source.

analog/analogue: Prosthetic component or element, the working surface of which is an exact duplicate of a specific surgical and/or prosthetic component. Typically, it is made of brass, aluminum, steel, or plastic and is used in the fabrication of the dental prosthesis. This element is typically incorporated in dental laboratory procedures to facilitate fabrication of an accurate master cast and/or prosthesis and can be incorporated into a model for patient education purposes. See: Replica.

analog workflow: Process of performing a task using physical means and materials, usually carried out by hand as opposed to using digital technology.

analysis of variance (ANOVA): 1. Test assessing the statistical significance of the differences among the obtained means of two or more random samples from a given population. 2. Statistical test to compare three or more groups on the mean value of a continuous response variable.

anamnesis: 1. A recalling to mind; a reminiscence. 2. The past history of disease or injury based on the patient's memory or recall at the time of interview and examination. 3. A preliminary past medical history of a medical or psychiatric patient.

anaphoresis: In electrophoresis, the movement of anions (negatively charged particles) in a solution or suspension toward the anode.

anaphylactic shock: A severe, sometimes fatal, immediate allergic reaction, usually occurring seconds to minutes after exposure to an antigen and mediated via histamine.

anaphylaxis: Immediate hypersensitivity response to antigenic challenge, mediated by IgE and mast cells; typically life-threatening.

anatomic crown: The portion of a natural tooth that extends coronal from the cementoenamel junction; also called anatomical crown. See: Crown.

anatomic crown exposure: A surgical procedure designed to expose the anatomic crown by removal of soft tissue and, when necessary, supporting alveolar bone. See: Crown lengthening.

anatomic healing abutment: Prosthetic implant component that may be cylindrical in cross-section but widens in diameter towards the coronal surface. The three-dimensional design of a healing abutment is intended to guide healing of the periimplant sulcus for a cross-sectional shape that simulates a soft tissue emergence profile. See: Healing abutment.

anatomic landmark: A significant anatomic structure that is used as a reference point or orientation guide.

anatomic occlusion: An occlusal arrangement for dental prostheses wherein the posterior artificial teeth have masticatory surfaces that closely resemble those of the natural healthy dentition and articulate with similar natural or artificial surfaces; also called anatomical occlusion.

anatomic teeth: 1. Teeth that have prominent cusps on the masticating surfaces and are designed to articulate with the teeth of the opposing natural or prosthetic dentition. 2. Anatomic teeth with cuspal inclinations greater than 0° that tend to replica natural tooth anatomy; usage cusp teeth (30–45°) are considered anatomic teeth. Modified occlusal forms are those with a 20° cusp incline or less.

anatomy: 1. A branch of morphology that involves the structures of organs. 2. The structural make-up esp. of an organ or any of its parts. 3. Separating or dividing into parts for examination, anatomic or anatomical.

ANB angle: The angle formed by the anatomic landmarks nasion A line and nasion B line. The lines and angle are determined with a cephalometric analysis.

anchorage area: That area which, by its situation, configuration and/or preparation, is suitable for the retention of a prosthesis anchorage component. See: Endosteal dental implant body.

anchorage, bicortical implant: See: Bicortical stabilization.

anchorage component: A part or device that provides resistance to an imparted force.

anchorage element: See: Endosteal dental implant abutment element(s).

anchor pin: Device used to stabilize a surgical or stereolithographic guide. It engages the underlying bone through a sleeve incorporated in the guide.

ancillary prosthesis: A prosthesis that aids in treatment and is intended for short-term or special usage. It is not the definitive prosthesis.

ancillary prostheses: One of the three main categories of dental prostheses made by those in the field of prosthodontics; any prosthesis not able to be described as either a dental prosthesis or a maxillofacial prosthesis. Examples may include guides, stents, splints, conformers, carriers and the like. Most such prostheses are intended for short-term or special usage.

anesthesia: 1. Absence of all sensation. 2. Loss of feeling or sensation caused by an anesthetic agent to permit diagnostic and treatment procedures; also spelled anaesthesia. **Block a.**: Local anesthesia of a nerve trunk. **General a.**: Depression of the central nervous system caused by anesthetic agents and characterized by simultaneous hypnosis, analgesia, and varying degrees of muscular relaxation, including, typically, the loss of protective laryngeal reflexes. **Infiltration a.**: Local anesthesia of terminal nerves. **Local a.**: Loss of sensation in a localized area of the body, but without central effect. **Regional a.**: Local anesthesia of a regional body area. **Topical a.**: Anesthetic effect produced by the application of an anesthetic agent to a surface area.

anesthetic: Capable of producing anesthesia.

angina pectoris: Paroxysmal thoracic pain with feeling of suffocation and impending death; usually due to anoxia of the myocardium and precipitated by effort or excitement.

angiogenesis: The physiologic process of growth and proliferation of new blood vessels from preexisting vasculature. The process occurs throughout life, in both health and disease, and plays a vital role in growth, development, and wound healing. See: Vascularization.

angiogenic: That which promotes or develops blood vessels, or promotes an increase in vascularization.

Angle's classification of malocclusion: A categorization of malocclusions according to the anteroposterior relationship of the dental arches.

- **Class I malocclusion** (neutroocclusion): Characterized by a normal relationship between the dental arches where the mesiobuccal cusp of the maxillary first permanent molar occludes into the buccal groove of the mandibular first permanent molar. A Class I malocclusion is presented as an internal derangement (e.g., crowding) in one of the arches.
- **Class II malocclusion** (distoocclusion): Characterized by an interarch relationship where the mandibular dental arch is positioned posterior to the maxillary arch. The mandibular first molar is distal to the position seen in neutrocclusion.
- **Class II, Division 1 malocclusion**: The maxillary incisor teeth are in labioversion.
- **Class II, Division 2 malocclusion**: The maxillary central incisors are in linguoversion.
- **Class III malocclusion** (mesioocclusion): The mandibular dental arch is positioned anterior to the maxillary arch. The mandibular first molar is located mesial to the position seen in neutroocclusion.

angle of gingival convergence: According to Schneider, the angle of gingival convergence is located apical to the height of contour on the abutment tooth. It can be identified by viewing the angle formed by the tooth surface gingival to the survey line and the analyzing rod or undercut gauge in a surveyor as it contacts the height of contour.

angled abutment: 1. See: Angulated abutment. 2. A dental implant abutment that diverges away from the long axis of the implant fixture.

angled/angulated abutment: Prosthetic implant component designed to change direction from parallel along the long axis of the implant to a specified angle from parallel.

angled/angulated implant: Relative position of an implant to other adjacent implants or natural dentition.

angular cheilitis: 1. See: Cheilitis, angular. 2. Inflammation of the angles of the mouth causing redness and the production of fissures, also called perleche.

angulated abutment: Any endosteal dental implant abutment which alters the long axis angulation between the dental implant and the angulated dental implant abutment.

angulated abutment: (syn): Angled abutment. Abutment with a body not parallel with the long axis of the dental implant. It is used when the implant is at a different inclination in relation to the proposed prosthesis. See: Nonangulated abutment.

animal model: Use of animals in biomedical research for conducting experiments. The quality, species, and breeding of the animal can help establish the type of animal to be used in the experiment.

anisotropic implant surface: Implant surface that is not isotropic and may have different characteristics when measured or loaded in a different direction.

anisotropic surface: Surface with a directional pattern. See: Isotropic surface.

ankyloglossia: Partial or complete fusion of the tongue with the floor of the mouth or the lingual gingiva due to an abnormally short, midline lingual frenulum, resulting in restricted tongue movement and speech impediments; may be complete or partial. Also known as adherent tongue, lingua frenata, and tongue-tie.

ankylosis: 1. Joint: fibrous or bony fixation. 2. Tooth: fusion of the tooth and the alveolar bone. 3. Union or fusion between two joint components or between a tooth and the alveolar bone, often resulting from traumatic destruction of the periodontal membrane. When ankylosis is established, the tooth will gradually be replaced by bone replacement resorption. See: Functional ankylosis. 4. Immobility, fixation, consolidation and/or joining of a joint or tooth due to injury, disease, or a surgical procedure. Also spelled anchylosis.

anneal: 1. To heat a material followed by cooling in a controlled fashion to improve the material's physical properties. The process results in (1) degassing; (2) removal of internal stresses, providing the required amount of toughness, temper, or softness; and (3) driving impurities from the surface of the material. 2. To heat a material, such as gold foil, to volatilize and drive off impurities from its surface, thus increasing its cohesive properties. 3. To homogenize an amalgam alloy by heating in an oven.

anodization: Electrolytic passivation process used to increase the thickness of the natural oxide layer on the surface of a metal (e.g., titanium). During the process, a dye may be used to color a dental implant component to facilitate its recognition.

anodizing surface treatment: Surfaces of various implant-related components (e.g., abutments, screws) may be anodized to produce coloration, which assists with recognition by the clinician. Anodizing titanium with a yellow or golden color is thought to reduce the tendency for gray show-through of abutments when placed beneath thin tissues.

anodontia: Rare dental condition characterized by congenital absence of all teeth (both deciduous and permanent). Compare: Hypodontia, Oligodontia.

anomaly: A deviation from the usual form, location, or arrangement of a structure.

anorganic bone matrix (ABM): Xenogenic or allogenic bone substitute derived from the mineral portion of bone and used for intraoral grafting procedures. By chemical and physical processes, sterilized osteoconductive deproteinized particles are obtained with a porous, crystalline structure, and chemical composition is similar to normal bone.

anorganic bovine bone matrix (ABBM): Xenogenic bone substitute derived from the mineral portion of bovine bone and used for intraoral grafting procedures. By chemical and physical processes, sterilized osteoconductive deproteinized particles are obtained with a porous, crystalline structure, and chemical composition is similar to normal bone.

ANOVA (abbrev.): Analysis of variance.

antagonist: 1. A tooth in one jaw that articulates with a tooth in the opposing jaw, also called dental antagonist. 2. A substance that tends to nullify the actions of another, such as a drug that binds to cell receptors without eliciting a biologic response. 3. A muscle whose action is the direct opposite of another muscle.

anterior: 1. In front of or the front part; situated in front of. 2. The forward or ventral position. 3. A term used to denote the incisor or canine teeth or the forward region of the mouth.

anterior guidance: 1. The influence of the contacting surfaces of anterior teeth on tooth limiting mandibular movements. 2. The influence of the contacting surfaces of the guide pin and anterior guide table on articulator movements. For usage see: Anterior guide table. 3. The fabrication of a relationship of the anterior teeth preventing posterior tooth contact in all eccentric mandibular movements. See: Anterior protected articulation, Group function, Mutually protected articulation.

anterior guide: See: Anterior guide table.

anterior guide pin: The rigid part of an articulator that is attached to one member and contacts the anterior guide table found on the opposing member. It is used to (1) establish the predetermined vertical dimension, (2) prevent wear and fracture of mounted cast's teeth, and (3) provide guidance (in conjunction with the guide table and condylar elements of the articulator) for the horizontal movements of the articulator's separate members.

anterior guide table: A flat adjustable device in one member of the dental articulator that receives the guide pin of the other member and establishes a base for recreating anterior guidance.

anterior loop: Anatomic phenomenon of the mental nerve that is a continuation of an anterior loop beyond the mental foramen. Attention should be paid to this potential anatomic variation during implant treatment planning. Often anterior loops cannot be identified by radiographic examination. A distance of 4–5 mm anterior to the mental foramen has been recommended.

anterior nasal spine: Triangular pointed projection at the anterior extremity of the intermaxillary suture. It may serve as a source of autogenous bone for intraoral grafting procedures.

anterior open bite: See: Anterior open occlusal relationship.

anterior open occlusal relationship: The lack of anterior tooth contact in any occluding position of the posterior teeth.

anterior open occlusion: An absence of contact of opposing anterior teeth or their substitutes in any jaw positions.

anterior programming device: A custom-made device placed between the opposing anterior teeth to separate them and eliminate their influence on the naturally programmed jaw muscles with the intent of deprogramming the muscles and, therefore, changing the habitual jaw position to a more physiological position. See: Deprogrammer.

anterior protected articulation: A form of mutually protected articulation in which the vertical and horizontal overlap of the anterior teeth disengages the posterior teeth in all mandibular excursive movements. See: Canine protected articulation.

anterior reference point: Any point located on the midface that, together with two posterior reference points, establishes a reference plane.

anterior superior alveolar nerve: Branch of the infraorbital nerve arising within the infraorbital canal. It initially runs laterally within the sinus wall and then curves medially to exit the infraorbital foramen. It supplies the maxillary anterior teeth.

anterior teeth: The maxillary and mandibular incisors and canines.

anteroposterior curve: The anatomic curve established by the occlusal alignment of the teeth, as projected onto the median plane, beginning with the cusp tip of the mandibular canine and following the buccal cusp tips of the premolar and molar teeth, continuing through the anterior border of the mandibular ramus, ending with the anterior most portion of the mandibular condyle.

anteroposterior (AP) spread: Distance from a line drawn between the posterior edges of the two most distal implants in an arch and the midpoint of the most anterior implant in the arch. This measurement is used to calculate the maximum posterior cantilever length of the prosthesis, which is usually 1.5 times the AP spread.

Ante's Law (Irwin H. Ante): Eponymous term that postulates that the in-bone root surface of the supporting teeth for a fixed partial denture should be equal to or greater than the in-bone surface area of the missing tooth or teeth being replaced. Additionally, the in-bone root surface of a removable partial denture abutment tooth or teeth plus the mucosal area of the supporting soft tissue should equal the in-bone surface area of the teeth being replaced.

antibacterial spectrum: The range of bacterial species that is susceptible to a drug (natural, semi-synthetic, or synthetic), resulting in bacterial cell death or inhibition of bacterial growth.

antibiotic: Molecules or agents produced by microorganisms that have the capacity to kill or inhibit the growth of other microorganisms.

antibiotic prophylaxis: Administration of an antibiotic prior to a surgical procedure (e.g., sinus graft) in order to prevent or reduce the incidence of postoperative infection. In patients with a risk of endocarditis, a standard protocol is recommended for certain dental procedures. See: Antibiotic.

antibody: Serum proteins that are induced following interaction with an antigen. They bind specifically to the antigen that induced their formation thereby causing or facilitating the antigen's neutralization. See: Immunoglobulin.

anticoagulant: Any substance or agent that inhibits or prevents the coagulation of blood.

antigen: Any substance recognized by the immune system that induces antibody formation.

antiinflammatory: The property of a substance or treatment that reduces inflammation. See: Corticosteroids, Nonsteroidal antiinflammatory drug.

antimicrobial therapy: The use of specific agents for the control or destruction of microorganisms, either systemically or at specific sites.

antiplaque agent(s): Chemical compounds that alter plaque formation by either directly killing bacteria within biofilms or by modulating pathways associated with biofilm formation.

antirotation: A structural feature of some endosteal dental implant components that prevents relative rotation of fastened parts. This feature may exist between a dental implant body and the dental implant abutment, and/or the dental implant abutment and dental implant abutment element(s). See: Stack.

antiseptic: An agent that inhibits the growth and development of microorganisms.

antral floor: Inferior bony wall of the maxillary sinus cavity. See: Maxillary sinus floor.

antral floor grafting: See: Maxillary sinus floor elevation.

antral mucosa: See: Schneiderian membrane, Maxillary sinus membrane.

antral polyp: Multilocular, pendulous, irregularly shaped edematous space usually associated with rhinosinusitis.

antral septum: See: Septum (maxillary sinus).

antrolith: Calcified mass found in the maxillary sinus, resulting from the complete or partial encrustation of a foreign body (e.g., retained root).

antroscope: An instrument for illuminating and examining the maxillary sinus.

antroscopy: Inspection of an antrum using an antroscope.

antrostomy: The surgical opening of an antrum for purposes of drainage or grafting. See: Sinus graft.

antrum: Based on Greek *antron* meaning "cave," a cavity or chamber in the body, often within bone. See: Sinus: Maxillary cavity of Highmore.

antrum of Highmore: See: Maxillary sinus.

apatite: Calcium phosphate of the composition $Ca_5(PO_4)_3OH$; one of the mineral constituents of teeth and bones (with $CaCO_3$).

apertognathia: An occlusal relationship where opposing teeth are not in contact (i.e., an anterior open bite).

aperture: An opening or orifice.

apex: Anatomic end of a tooth root or root-form implant.

aphagia: Inability to swallow; abstention from eating.

aphasia: Defect or loss of the power of expression by writing, speech or signs, or of comprehending written or spoken language due to disease of or injury to the brain.

aphonia: Loss or absence of voice as a result of the failure of the vocal cords to vibrate properly.

aphtha (plural: aphthae): An ulcer of the oral mucous membrane occurring exclusively on movable tissue.

apical: Referring to, or in the direction of, a root apex. See: Apex.

apical (retrograde) periimplantitis: See: Implant periapical lesion.

apical abscess: A localized collection of pus and inflamed tissue located at or around the apical end of a tooth.

apical curettage: See: Curettage.

apically positioned flap: A flap sutured in a direction apical to its original presurgical position. See: Coronally positioned flap.

apicoectomy: Intentional surgical excision of the apical end of a tooth root.

aplasia: Incomplete development of an organ or tissue. Congenital absence may be characteristic.

aplastic: Without development; not forming.

apoptosis: Morphologic pattern of cell death affecting single cells and marked by shrinkage of the cell, condensation of chromatin, formation of cytoplasmic blebs, and fragmentation of the cell into membrane-bound apoptotic bodies that are eliminated by phagocytosis.

appliance: See: Device, Restoration, Prosthesis.

appositional bone growth: See: Bone modeling.

approximation: The state of being near or close together, as in root approximation.

AP spread (abbrev.): Anteroposterior spread.

arachidonic acid: A 20-carbon essential fatty acid that contains four double bonds (5, 8, II, 14- eicosatetraenoic acid); the precursor of prostaglandins, prostacyclins, thromboxanes, and leukotrienes.

arch: Bony arc formed by the maxillary or mandibular teeth or residual ridge when viewed occlusally.

arch bar: A rigid bar or wire used to stabilize teeth and implants and used for intraarch fixation in the treatment of fractures of the maxilla or mandible.

arch, dental: The curved composite structure of the natural dentition and the alveolar ridge, or the residual bone after the loss of some or all of the natural teeth.

arch form: The outline of the dental arch as viewed from a horizontal plane (i.e., ovoid, square, or tapered).

arch length discrepancy: An incongruent relationship between the arch size of the maxilla or mandible and the teeth present as viewed from the occlusal plane.

architecture: A term with an appropriate modifier, commonly used in periodontics to describe gingival and/or bony form. **Physiologic a.**: A concept of soft tissue or bony form that includes positive architecture in a vertical dimension, buccal-lingual contours devoid of ledges and exostoses, and interradicular grooves. **Positive a.**: When the crest of the interdental gingiva or bone is located coronal to its midfacial midlingual margins. **Reverse a.**: When the crest of the interdental gingiva or bone is located apical to its midfacial and midlingual margins.

archwire: Wire attached to two or more teeth or implants, generally used to guide or retain teeth during orthodontic therapy.

arc of closure: An elliptical or circular arc representing the mandibular path of closure.

arcon: Term derived from the words "articulator" and "condyle" describing a type of articulator that simulates temporomandibular anatomy.

arm prosthesis: Artificial replacement for part or all of the human arm. See: Somatoprosthesis.

arrow point tracer: A device that traces the pattern of mandibular movement typically parallel to the occlusal plane.

artery: Blood vessel that carries oxygenated blood from the heart to tissues and organs.

arthralgia: Pain in one or more joints.

arthritis: Inflammation of a joint or joints.

arthrodial joint: A joint that allows for a sliding motion between surfaces.

arthrodial movement: Gliding joint movement.

arthrography: 1. Roentgenography of a joint after injection of an opaque contrast material. 2. In dentistry, a diagnostic technique that entails filling the lower, upper, or both joint spaces of the temporomandibular joint with a contrast agent to enable radiographic evaluation of the joint and surrounding structures; used to diagnose or confirm disk displacements and perforations.

arthropathy: A disease of a joint.

arthroplasty: Surgical formation or restoration of a joint.

arthrosis: A degenerative disease of a joint.

articular capsule: The fibrous ligament that encloses a joint and limits its motion. It is lined with synovial membrane.

articular cartilage: A thin layer of hyaline cartilage located on the joint surfaces of some bones, not found on the articular surfaces of the temporomandibular joints which is covered with an avascular fibrous tissue.

articular disk: A ring of fibrocartilage that separates the articular surfaces of a joint.

articulating paper: Ink-coated paper strips used to locate and mark occlusal contacts.

articulating tape: Ink-impregnated paper or silk ribbon used to identify contacting occlusal or incisal surfaces.

articulation: 1. The contact relationships of mandibular teeth with maxillary teeth in excursive movements of the mandible. 2. A junction or union between two or more bones. 3. A skeletal joint.

articulator: Apparatus designed to mechanically orient the essential elements of mastication (i.e., temporomandibular joints, jaws, and teeth) in their simulated spatial relationship outside the mouth. The design is based on the degree of mandibular movement simulation desired for the development of an occlusal scheme. **Fully adjustable a.**: Articulating instrument permitting the simulation of three-dimensional mandibular movement and capable of accepting three-dimensional jaw registration records. **Nonadjustable a.**: Hinge-type instrument capable of retaining maxillary and mandibular jaw casts in an established vertical relationship while providing possible vertical motion in an arcing pattern. **Semi-adjustable a.**: Instrument capable of simulating vertical and horizontal movement with or without temporomandibular joint orientation. Joint articular references are commonly reversed with condylar guidance developed according to mechanical equivalents based on anatomic averages. Some semi-adjustable articulators provide for temporomandibular joint orientation and may be either non-Arcon (condylar elements in the upper member) or Arcon (condylar elements in the lower member, as in the human situation).

artifact (imaging): Any feature not present in the original imaged object but that appears in a displayed image. An image artifact is sometimes the result of incorrect operation of the imager, and other times a consequence of natural processes or properties of the human body. It is important to be familiar with the appearance of artifacts because they can obscure, and be mistaken for, pathology. Artifacts may also result in a misfitted prosthesis. Therefore, image artifacts can result in false negatives and false positives.

artificial crown: A metal, plastic, or ceramic restoration that covers three or more axial surfaces and the occlusal surface or incisal edge of a tooth artificial denture: See: Complete denture.

artificial limb: Artificial replacement for part or all of a human arm or leg. See: Somatoprosthesis.

asaccharolytic: The inability of an organism to catabolize carbohydrates. Generally relates to sugar metabolism.

asepsis: 1: Free from infection. 2: The prevention of contact with microorganisms.

aseptic: Free from infection or septic material; sterile, free from pathogenic microorganisms.

asleep: See: Sleeper implant.

Aspergillus: Fungus responsible for maxillary sinus fungal infections (aspergillosis).

astringent: An agent that causes contraction of the tissues, arrests secretion, or controls bleeding.

asymmetrical: Characterized by or pertaining to asymmetry.

asymmetry: Absence or lack of symmetry or balance; dissimilarity in corresponding parts or organs on opposite sides of the body.

atherosclerosis: Form of arteriosclerosis characterized by the deposition of atheromatous plaques containing cholesterol and lipids on the innermost layer of the walls of large- and medium-sized arteries.

atraumatic: Not inflicting or causing damage or injury.

atraumatic extraction: The extraction of a tooth with minimal damage or injury to the surrounding hard and soft tissues.

atresia: Absence or closure of a natural body passage. May also refer to loss of a body part through degeneration. See: Congenital atresia.

atrophic: Reduced both in volume and substance. Bone loss in volume can be a reduction both in width and height, and loss of substance can mean reduction in thickness of cortical bone and width and number of trabeculae.

atrophic alveolar bone: Alveolar bone characterized by resorption after tooth removal. When functional stimulus disappears, the alveolar bone will atrophy.

atrophy: 1. A wasting away. 2. Decrease in size of a cell, organ, tissue or part, a loss of tissue from an anatomic site due to nonuse,

nonstimulation, pressure, or nutrients. See: Atrophic, Disuse atrophy, Ridge atrophy.

attached gingiva: Firm, dense, and often stippled soft tissue that is tightly bound to underlying periosteum, bone, or a natural tooth. See: Gingiva, attached.

attachment: 1. A mechanical device used for fixing, retaining, and stabilizing a dental prosthesis. 2. A retainer that is made of a metal receptacle and a part that fits precisely. The former (the female [matrix] component) is most often contained inside the normal or extended crown contours of the abutment tooth and the latter (the male [patrix] component) is attached to the denture framework or a pontic. Consists of one or more parts, made of titanium, gold, or plastic.

attachment activating tool: See: Activating tool.

attachment apparatus: The anatomic complex around a tooth consisting of the cementum, alveolar bone, and periodontal ligament.

attachment element: Part of the prosthetic component made as a separate unit fitting onto the transmucosal element. "If there is no separate attachment element, the restoration is part of and fabricated with the retentive element." It is the element onto which the restoration is fabricated as cast-to, cemented, or screwed into position.

attachment level: Relative distance from a fixed reference point on a tooth or dental implant to the tip of the periodontal probe during soft tissue diagnostic probing. Health of the attachment apparatus can affect the measurement. See: Clinical attachment level.

attachment level, clinical: When a clinician is performing a periodontal diagnostic probing, it is the distance measured from the end of a periodontal probe to the cementoenamel junction of the tooth being examined. The measurement is an indicator of the health of the supporting soft tissue attachment apparatus. The health of the attachment apparatus can affect the measurement. See: Attachment level, relative.

attachment level, relative: When a clinician is performing periodontal diagnostic probing, it is the distance measured between the end of the periodontal probe and a set reference point on the tooth of interest or a stent. The measurement is an indicator of the health of the supporting soft tissue attachment. The health of the attachment apparatus can affect the measurement. See: Attachment level, clinical.

attachment, new: The union of connective tissue or epithelium with a root surface that has been deprived of its original attachment apparatus. This new attachment may be epithelial adhesion and/or connective adaptation or attachment and may include new cementum.

attachment-retained: Use of a mechanical device for the retention of a prosthesis to an abutment or transmucosal portion of a one-part implant. See: Attachment, Cement-retained, Friction-retained, Screw-retained.

attachment screw: Any component used to secure a fixed dental prosthesis to the dental implant abutment(s), an element directly relating to the specific prosthetic component to which it attaches. Typically, the prosthetic component is seated, and the attachment screw is threaded through the prosthetic component into another component in the implant system, such as the implant. It can be manufactured of various materials, such as gold alloy or titanium. See: Abutment screw.

attachment selection: A step in the prosthodontic treatment whereby a decision is made regarding the type of attachment to be used in the prosthesis based on implant angulation, interarch space, soft tissue (mucosal) height, and amount of retention needed.

attachment system: Design of a particular type of retentive mechanism employing compatible matrix and patrix corresponding components. Matrix refers to the receptacle component of the attachment system, and patrix refers to the portion that has a frictional fit and engages the matrix. Corresponding components are passive once engaged and offer resistance to displacement either through a direct mechanical mechanism or a frictional fit.

attenuation of radiation: The reduction in intensity of radiation as a result of scattering and absorption of radiation.

attrition: 1. The action of weakening and/or wearing down by rubbing or friction. 2. The mechanical deterioration and erosion of the occlusal surfaces of the teeth as a consequence of chewing or parafunction.

atypia: Not conforming to type; irregular.

atypical facial pain: A painful syndrome characterized by dull aching or throbbing, rather than paroxysms of pain, such as seen in trigeminal, glossopharyngeal, or postherpetic neuralgia, occurring in areas supplied by various nerve groups, including the fifth and ninth cranial nerves and the second and third cervical nerves. The distribution of atypical facial pain does not follow the established pathways of innervation of the major sensory nerves, however (i.e., trigeminal neuralgia). Attacks last from a few days to several months and often occur after dental care or sinus manipulation, but examination of the teeth, nose, sinuses, ears, and temporomandibular joints seldom reveals any abnormalities. A psychogenic or vascular etiology has been suggested.

augment: To make greater, more numerous, larger, or more intense.

augmentation: 1. The act of enlarging or increasing, as in size, extent, or quantity, beyond the existing size. See: Bone augmentation. 2. Grafting procedure designed to increase the volume of existing tissues, usually referring to bone for the purpose of adequate bony support around implants and/or improving tissue contours for esthetic purposes; also in alveolar ridge augmentation, bone grafts or alloplastic materials are used to increase the size of an atrophic alveolar ridge.

auricular prosthesis: Fixed/removable artificial replacement for all or part of a human ear.

auriculotemporal syndrome: A congenital or acquired condition (especially after surgery on the parotid gland) characterized by sweating and flushing in the periauricular and temporal areas when certain foods are eaten.

Also known as Frey's syndrome, Baillarger's syndrome, or Dupny's syndrome.

auscultation: The process of determining the condition of various parts of the body by listening to the sounds they emit.

autocrine: Transfer of chemical compounds as hormones and growth factors within the cell.

autogenous: Originating or derived from within the same subject; not derived from an external source; self-produced, autologous, endogenous.

autogenous bone graft: Bone graft, taken from an intraoral or extraoral site and placed in the same individual. Origin of the graft will determine whether it is cortical, corticocancellous, or cancellous in nature. Particulate grafts may be harvested with hand instruments or prepared by introducing chips into a bone mill. Block grafts can be harvested when a cortical component exists (i.e., symphysis, ramus buccal shelf, calvarium, or iliac crest), when volume is not sufficient, and/or if there is a need to retard resorption. Autogenous bone grafts are often mixed with allografts, alloplasts, or xenografts. Also called autograft or autotransplant.

autogenous graft: Tissue taken from the patient's own body and moved to a different site from its origin. Also called autograft or autotransplant. See: Autogenous bone graft, Bone graft, Soft tissue augmentation.

autoglaze: The creation of a glazed surface on a ceramic restoration by increasing the firing temperature to generate surface flow. Also called overglaze.

autograft: A tissue graft taken from a site that is different from the recipient site of the same individual receiving it. Also called autochthonous graft, autologous graft, autotransplant, and autoplast. See: Graft.

autoimmunity: An immune response to an organism's own tissues or components.

autologous: 1. Pertaining to self; defining products or components derived or transferred from one anatomic location to another within the recipient. 2. Autogenous.

autologous bone: See: Autogenous bone graft.

autologous graft: See: Autogenous graft.

autologous mixed lymphocyte reaction: A proliferative reaction of normal typical T lymphocytes when co-cultured with autologous HLADR-positive non-T lymphocytes.

autopolymer: A resin polymerized by a chemical reaction that occurs by adding an activator and a catalyst without adding heat.

autopolymerizing resin: Resin capable of polymerization via a chemical activator and catalyzing agent. Also called cold- or self-curing resin.

autoradiography: Photographic recording of radiation from radioactive material obtained by placing the surface of the radioactive material in proximity to a detector sensitive to the emitted spectrum, most commonly X-ray film or a charge coupled device.

available bone: Portion of an edentulous ridge that can be used for the placement of a dental implant.

avascular (nonvascular): Lacking in blood or lymphatic vessels. Avascular tissues may be normal, such as tooth enamel or some forms of cartilage, or may be a consequence of disease.

avascular necrosis: Cell death that occurs as a result of inadequate blood supply.

average axis facebow: A device that transfers the relationship of the maxilla and the mandibular axis of rotation to an articulator by recording standard anatomic landmarks for determining the transverse horizontal axis of the face.

average value articulator: An articulator that permits motion based on three mean mandibular measurements: an intercondylar distance of 10–11 cm, a condylar guidance of 33°, and an incisal guidance of 9–12°. Also known as a mean value articulator or Class III articulator.

avulsion: A forced and aggressive separation from the body; the action that results in a separation of a body part surgically or accidentally. See: Evulsion.

avulsion fracture: A separation of bone (or portion of bone) from its naturally occurring position by trauma or unintended force(s).

axial contour: The shape of a body in the dimension of its long axis. For teeth, it is the outline of the vertical portion of a tooth from the cementoenamel junction to its height of contour.

axial inclination: 1. The relationship of the long axis of a body to a designated plane. 2. In dentistry, the angle made by the long axis of a tooth, dental implant, or other object (i.e., implant guide pin) as it relates to a specified horizontal plane, such as the supporting bone or occlusal plane.

axial loading: Application of load, usually by the forces of occlusion, in the direction of the long axis of an implant body or tooth. Compare: Nonaxial loading.

axial reduction: Removal of tooth structure or its prosthetic equivalent (i.e., implant abutment) along its ideal long axis. The location and amount of reduction depend on the reason for altering or preparing. Compare: Incisal reduction, Occlusion reduction.

axial slice: A thin section from computed tomography scan data (usually 0.125–2.0 millimeters thick) transverse to the patient's length axis, ideally parallel to the plane of occlusion. See: Cross-sectional slice, Panoramic reconstitution.

axial surface: The exterior of a body that is oriented in its long axis.

axial wall: 1. The side of a body that is in its long axis. 2. In dentistry, the surface of a tooth preparation that is in its long axis.

axis: 1. A real or imaginary straight line passing through the center of a body, such as the mandible. 2. Long axis of a tooth – the central lengthwise line through the crown and the root. 3. A real or imaginary straight line around which a body may rotate.

axis of preparation: The prepared or intended path of insertion and removal for a dental restoration as it relates to its axial surface.

axis orbital plane: The horizontal imaginary line or plane determined by the transverse horizontal axis of the mandible as it correlates with the palpated lowermost point found at the inferior margin of either the left or right bony orbit (orbitale). This plane is used as a horizontal orientation point to position teeth and/or dental implants in the ideal horizontal position in relation to the temporomandibular joint and face.

axonotmesis: Nerve injury with loss of axonal continuity, but with maintenance of the myelin sheath. Sensory and/or motor functions are impaired. Recovery may occur after 1–3 months. It may be caused by a drill violating the mandibular canal, an anesthetic needle penetrating the nerve trunk, or excessive reflection. See: Neurapraxia, Neurotmesis.

azalide: New generation of macrolide derivatives with improved pharmacokinetic properties, tissue penetration, and activity against many gram-positive and gram-negative bacteria. See: Azithromycin.

azithromycin: An azalide antibiotic which inhibits bacterial protein synthesis, and is effective against a wide range of gram-positive, gram-negative, and anaerobic bacteria. It is used in the treatment of mild to moderate infections caused by susceptible organisms, and may be administered orally and intravenously. See: Azalide.

B

BAHA (abbrev.): Bone-anchored hearing aid.

B cell: White blood cell derived from bone marrow. As part of the immune system, B cells (or bursa-equivalent cells) may differentiate and become antibody-producing plasma cells. Also called B lymphocyte.

B lymphocyte: See: B cell.

bacteremia: The presence of bacteria in the bloodstream. The term is usually qualified as being transient, intermittent, or continuous in nature.

bacteria (plural), **bacterium** (singular): Members of a group of ubiquitous, single-celled microorganisms that have a prokaryotic (primitive) cell type. Many of these are etiologic in diseases that affect all life forms, including humans and other animals. See: *Aggregatibacter actinomycetemcomitans*, *Fusobacterium nucleatum*.

bacterial capsule: An extracellular coating usually composed of mucopolysaccharides produced by some bacteria. May increase an organism's virulence by interfering with the nonspecific immune system (phagocytosis) of the host.

bacterial collagenase: Any of various collagenases purified from a variety of microbes; they preferentially cleave collagen on the N-terminal side of glycine residues and occur in several classes of differing specificity. Bacterial collagenases are used in tissue disruption for cell harvesting.

bacterial leakage: Colonization and release of bacteria at the interface of an oral implant abutment and implant.

bacterial succession: A process of colonization by oral bacteria in a predictable, temporal pattern, with resident organisms altering the environment, allowing new organisms to become established or certain bacteria to achieve dominance.

bactericide: An agent capable of destroying bacteria. Also termed bacteriocide.

bacteriogenic: Caused by bacteria.

bacteriolytic: Characterized by or promoting the dissolution or destruction of bacteria.

bacteriostat: An agent that inhibits or retards the growth and multiplication of bacteria.

bacteriostatic: Inhibiting or retarding the growth of bacteria.

bacterium: See: Bacteria.

balanced articulation: Bilateral anterior and posterior occlusal contacts that occur simultaneously when the teeth are in centric and eccentric positions. This is determined not only by positions of the teeth but also by the influence of the temporomandibular joint.

balanced bite: See: Balanced articulation.

balanced occlusion: Existing or developed simultaneous harmonious occlusal contact of the teeth throughout the dental arch during mandibular centric and eccentric movements; especially important for removable complete dentures to achieve stability during function. See: Articulation.

balancing condyle: See: Nonworking side condyle.

balancing contact: See: Balancing occlusal contact.

Glossary of Dental Implantology, First Edition. Khalid Almas, Fawad Javed and Steph Smith.
© 2018 John Wiley & Sons, Inc. Published 2018 by John Wiley & Sons, Inc.

balancing interference: 1. Tooth contact not in harmony with balanced articulation on the side of the translating condyle as the mandible moves in lateral excursions. 2. Unwanted contact(s) of opposing occlusal surfaces on the nonworking side that are not in harmony with balanced articulation. See: Nonfunctional side.

balancing occlusal contact: See: Nonworking side occlusal contacts.

balancing occlusal surfaces: The occluding surfaces of dentures on the balancing side (antero-posteriorly or laterally) that are developed for the purpose of stabilizing dentures.

balancing side: The side from which the mandible moves (opposite the working side or primary chewing side) during lateral excursion. Also termed nonworking side.

ball abutment: See: Ball attachment.

ball attachment: Extracoronal type of attachment mechanism used to retain an overdenture, consisting of a spherical-shaped abutment and a metal housing. See: Metal housing.

ball attachment system: Specific design of a mechanical attachment in which the patrix fits into the matrix in a ball-and-socket type of relation. Each element is incorporated into either the natural tooth as part of a restoration or as an abutment on the implant with the reciprocal element incorporated into the prosthesis. The patrix, or ball, can be made of plastic or metal alloy of various diameters and with varied amounts of resistance.

bar: Round, half-round, or elliptically shaped metallic segment with greater length than width. A bar is commonly used to connect components of a prosthesis such as abutments, crowns, or parts of a removable partial denture. It also can be used to provide support, stability, and/or retention for a prosthesis. See: Dolder bar; Hader bar.

bar attachment system: Specific design of an attachment in which the patrix spans a specified width that the matrix matches. Each element is part of a prosthetic structure that spans two or more natural teeth and/or implants and is fixed intraorally with the matrix, which is incorporated within the prosthesis. Once the components are engaged by riders, clips, or micro plungers, there is resistance to displacement through either a mechanical mechanism or frictional fit.

bar clasp: A clasp retainer whose body extends from a major connector or denture base, passing adjacent to the soft tissues and approaching the tooth from a gingivooclusal direction bar clasp arm.

bar connector: A metal component of greater length than width that serves to connect the parts of a removable partial denture.

bar overdenture (implant): Removable partial or complete denture, which may be implant supported or implant tissue supported. Implants in this type of reconstruction are connected together with a bar incorporating attachment mechanisms for retention and/or support of the prosthesis. See: Clip bar overdenture.

bar splint: Connecting bar for adding rigidity and/or stability between teeth or implants. It is also used to fixate displaced or movable body parts as a result of trauma or surgery. See: Splinting.

barbiturate: A class of sedative-hypnotic drugs derived from barbituric acid, differing primarily in lipid solubility and hypnotic efficacy.

barium sulfate ($BaSO_4$): Finely ground radiopaque powder used as a marker in the construction of a radiographic template.

barrier membrane: A thin, flexible material used in guided bone regeneration (GBR) to locally augment deficient sites in implant patients. By creating a secluded space, the barrier prevents epithelial cells and fibroblasts from proliferating into the augmentation site, whereas the slower-growing angiogenic and osteogenic cells have exclusive access to the membrane-protected space. The first membranes were made of bioinert expanded polytetrafluoro-ethylene (e-PTFE), which is nonresorbable and therefore required removal with a second surgical procedure. Bioresorbable membranes, either of synthetic polymers or of animal-derived collagen, are often preferred in daily practice. Although their barrier function is limited in time, they do not require a second surgical procedure for membrane removal. Barrier membranes exclude undesirable cell types from entering the secluded area of the bony or periodontal defect during healing. Membrane configurations are designed for specific applications and vary in shape, size, and thickness. See: Guided bone regeneration (GBR); Guided tissue regeneration (GTR); Collagen membrane; Expanded polytetrafluoroethylene (e-PTFE) membrane.

barrier membrane exposure: See: Exposure.

basal bone: Supporting bone in the mandible that underlies and is continuous with the alveolar process and houses the major nerves and vessels. It also functions as a site of muscle attachment and is resistant to resorption. See: Bone.

base metal: Any metallic element that does not resist tarnish and corrosion. See: Noble metal.

base metal alloy: An alloy composed of metals that are not noble.

baseline data: 1. Measurements taken at the beginning of treatment with which subsequent measurements are compared. 2. In research, a known quantity or measurement with which subsequent data are compared.

baseplate: A rigid, comparatively thin layer of wax, shellac, or thermoplastic (heat, chemical, photo activated) polymer that conforms to the edentulous surface of a definitive cast. It is often intended to be a base that can have a wax occlusion rim or similar material attached for the purpose of recording a jaw position and/or setting prosthetic teeth in wax for try-in. See: Record base.

baseplate wax: A wax that has sufficient stiffness to be usable for making occlusion rims or waxing dentures or for performing other related procedures.

basic fibroblast growth factor (bFGF): See: Fibroblast growth factor (FGF).

basic multicellular unit (BMU): Functional unit consisting of cellular elements responsible for bone formation and resorption (i.e., remodeling).

basic structural unit (BSU): The unit of bone tissue formed by one basic multicellular unit (BMU). It is also referred to as an osteon.

basket endosteal dental implant: An endosteal dental implant with a body shaped like a perforated cylinder.

basophil: A granular leukocyte containing substances that contribute to inflammation, including leukotrienes and vascular amines such as histamine and serotonin; important in hypersensitivity reactions.

BCP (abbrev.): Biphasic calcium phosphate.

beam hardening artifact: An imaging artifact that appears as streaks and shadows adjacent to areas of high density such as dense bones, shoulders, dental restoration, and hips.

bed: The surgically prepared recipient site for a graft. See: Graft, Soft tissue.

Behçet's syndrome: A condition that is more common in men than women and is characterized by recurrent genital and oral ulcers plus ocular inflammation. The definitive cause is unknown.

bending moment: Rotary effect of a force potentially causing deformation through torque.

bending stress: Stress caused by a load that tends to bend an object. See: Compressive stress, Stress.

benign: Usually not threatening to health or life; not malignant.

benign mucous membrane pemphigoid: See: Pemphigoid.

benign paroxysmal positional vertigo (BPPV): Short, recurrent episodes of vertigo when carrying out certain lateralization and extension movements of the head. In implant dentistry, it may be a postoperative complication following surgery in the maxilla where osteotomes were used.

Bennett angle: The angle between the sagittal plane and the condylar path on the balancing side during lateral mandibular movements.

beta-lactam antibiotics: Antibiotics containing a beta-lactam ring; the penicillins, cephalosporins, monobactams (aztreonam), and carbapenems (imipenem-cilastatin).

beta-lactamase: A bacterial enzyme that accounts for the major resistance mechanism to beta-lactam antibiotics by opening the beta-lactam ring of penicillins and cephalosporins.

betamethasone: An oral, topical, and inhaled glucocorticoid with a long half-life. See: Glucocorticoid.

bevel: A slanting edge.

beveled flap: Section of soft tissue outlined by a surgical incision made at an acute angle to the gingival or mucosal tissue.

beveled incision: Technique by which incisions are made at an acute angle (less than 90°) to the gingival or mucosal surface, rather than perpendicularly.

bFGF (abbrev.): Basic fibroblast growth factor. See: Fibroblast growth factor (FGF).

BIC (abbrev.): Bone-to-implant contact.

bicortical implant anchorage: See: Bicortical stabilization.

bicortical stabilization: Practice of engaging both the superior and inferior cortices of bone at the time of implant placement. For an edentulous anterior mandible, the tip of the implant engages the inferior cortex while the neck of the implant engages the superior cortex to maximize initial stability of the implant. The engagement of a dental implant with the crestal cortical bone of the edentulous ridge and the cortical bone of the base of the mandible or the floor of the maxillary sinus or floor of the nasal cavity. It may also apply to the engagement of the facial and lingual cortices.

bidirectional crest distraction: Distraction approach designed to overcome the inherent difficulty in controlling the distraction vector in conventional, unidirectional devices. An additional inclination rod allows for buccal-oral (lingual) distraction in addition to vertical distraction.

bifurcation: The site where a division into two parts occurs, as where a tooth divides into two roots.

bilateral: Having or pertaining to two sides.

bilateral balanced articulation: The concurrent and synchronized anterior and posterior occlusal contact of teeth on both sides of the mouth in centric, lateral, and protrusive positions. Also known as balanced articulation.

bilateral distal extension removable partial denture: A removable dental prosthesis replacing the distal most tooth or teeth on each side of one arch of the mouth. See: Kennedy classification of removable partial dentures.

bilateral stabilization: See: Cross-arch stabilization.

billet: A length of metal/material that has a round or square cross-section. It is typically used to describe material disks used for milling.

bimeter: A device to measure biting force that has a central bearing plate of adjustable height.

bioabsorbable (syn): Absorbable. Property of a material to degrade or dissolve *in vivo*. Breakdown products are incorporated into normal physiologic and biochemical processes (e.g., bioabsorbable membranes or sutures).

bioabsorbable material: Solid polymeric material that can dissolve in body fluids without any change of the polymer or decrease in molecular mass.

bioacceptability: The quality of compatibility in a living environment in spite of adverse or unwanted side effects.

bioactive: Having an effect on, or eliciting a response from, living tissue. See: Bioinert.

bioactive fixation: Stabilization involving direct physical and/or chemical attachment mechanism(s) between biological tissues and a dental implant surface at the ultrastructural level.

bioactive glass: Ceramic material that stimulates or otherwise promotes biologic activity. It consists of silicophosphate chains that bond ionically to compounds such as CaO, CaF_2, Na_2O, ZnO, TiO_2, and NiO, among others. It may undergo ionic translocations *in vivo*, or exchange ions or molecular groups in an osseous recipient site, and thereby osseointegrate. Bioactive glass may be resorbable and is useful as a delivery system in bone engineering. See: Ceramic.

bioactivity: Effect of implant material that allows interaction and bond formation with living tissues. Implant bioactivity may depend upon material composition, topography, and chemical or physical surface variations.

bioadhesion: Result of a process whereby a chemical attachment between biologic and other materials is obtained.

bioceramics: Specially designed and fabricated ceramics for the repair or reconstruction of diseased, damaged, or missing parts of the body.

Bio-Col technique: Technique developed to preserve the ridge in the esthetic zone. A tooth is extracted via a low-trauma technique to maintain intact bony walls and surrounding gingival anatomy without flap reflection. The extraction socket is grafted up to the alveolar crest with an anorganic bovine bone substitute, covered with a collagen plug, and sutured in place with a horizontal mattress suture. A removable or fixed provisional restoration with an ovate pontic extending 3–4 mm subgingivally is placed, compressing the collagen plug and supporting the surrounding soft tissue. This technique has also been described in combination with immediate implant placement and with a buccal defect, whereby the defect is first lined with a collagen membrane.

biocompatibility: Condition whereby the body does not respond to a foreign substance (e.g., metal) but recognizes it immunologically as self. Biocompatible materials do not lead to acute or chronic inflammatory responses nor do they prevent proper differentiation of implant-surrounding tissues.

biocompatible: Capable of existing together; acceptable to the body. This term is used to describe blood, organs, or tissue that can be transplanted or transfused into a patient's body without being rejected. It describes a biodynamic process in which a material neither elicits an immune response nor is rejected by the host. Property of a material to elicit or perform without a negative host response (immune response or inflammation) in a specific application. In general, biocompatibility is measured on the basis of allergenicity, carcinogenicity, localized cytotoxicity, and systemic response.

biodegradable: Property of a material to degrade when placed in a biologic environment. See: Bioabsorbable.

bioengineering: Use of engineering in biomedical technology such as the movement analysis of body parts or prostheses. See: Tissue engineering.

biofeedback: A method of behavioral modification in which signals are relayed to the patient regarding the status of certain physiologic functions such as the heart rate and blood pressure.

biofilm: A multispecies community of microorganisms that adhere to each other and a surface, and are encased in an extracellular matrix. The extracellular matrix is a complex polymeric substance, and protects the microorganisms from environmental stresses. See: Plaque.

bioglass: See: Bioactive glass.

bioinert: Describes a biomaterial that does not elicit a biologic response or is unaffected by the adjacent biologic environment.

biointegration: The bonding of living tissue to the surface of a biomaterial or implant, independent of any mechanical interlocking mechanism. It is often used to describe the bond to hydroxyapatite-coated dental implants. See: Osseous integration.

biologic width: 1. The combined apicocoronal height of connective tissue and epithelial attachment. It exists around teeth as well as around dental implants once exposed to the oral cavity. 2. Structure of the attachment apparatus containing connective tissue attachment, junctional epithelium, and gingival sulcus. **Normal b. w.**: measures 1 mm for each structure, including the connective tissue attachment, junctional epithelium, and gingival sulcus.

biomaterial: Any substance other than a drug that can be used for any period of time as part of a system that treats, augments, or replaces any tissue, organ, or function of the body.

biomechanical load model: Simulation or model of load pattern in and adjacent to a structure. See: Biomechanics.

biomechanical test: A test that measures the physical properties of any biomechanical device, device–tissue interface (e.g., bone–implant), or the properties of tissues themselves.

biomechanics: 1. The study of mechanics as it relates to a living structure, specifically the forces exerted by muscles and gravity on skeletal structures. 2. The analysis of biology from a functional aspect. 3. Engineering principles applied to living organisms. See: Dental biomechanics.

biometry: Statistical analysis of biological data.

biomimetic: Able to replicate or imitate a body structure (anatomy) and/or function (physiology). See: Tissue engineering.

biomineralization: Formation or accumulation of minerals into biologic tissues such as bone and teeth. The process of biologic mineralization is not completely understood. Interstitial fluids are supersaturated with mineral hydroxyapatite, and calcium binding proteins such as osteocalcin are deposited and may play a role in the formation of crystal nuclei.

BIONJ (abbrev.): Bisphosphonate-induced osteonecrosis of the jaw. See: Bisphosphonate-related osteonecrosis of the jaw.

Bio-Oss: See: Bovine-derived anorganic bone matrix.

biopsy: The removal and examination, usually microscopic, of tissue for the purpose of establishing a histopathological diagnosis. **aspiration b.**: The aspiration of fluid through a needle for the purpose of establishing a diagnosis. **Excisional b.**: The removal of an entire lesion, including a significant margin of contiguous, normal-appearing tissue for microscopic examination and diagnosis. **Incisional b.**: The removal of a selected portion of a lesion and, if possible, adjacent normal-appearing tissue for microscopic examination and diagnosis.

bioresorbable: The capacity to become lyzed or assimilated *in vivo*.

bioresorbable material: Solid polymeric material that shows bulk degradation and further resorbs *in vivo*, resulting in total elimination of the initial foreign material. Compare: Resorbable.

biostatistics: The science of the application of statistical methods to biologic facts, as the mathematical analysis of biologic data. See: Biometry.

bio-stimulating laser: See: Low-level laser therapy.

biotype: The thickness or dimension of the soft and hard tissue surrounding natural teeth or dental implants.

biphasic calcium phosphate (BCP): Alloplastic bone substitute consisting of 60% hydroxyapatite and 40% beta-tricalcium phosphate used in intraoral grafting procedures. The granules are 90% porous and with interconnected pores of 100–500 microns. See: Calcium phosphate, Tricalcium phosphate.

bisphosphonate (BP): (syn): Diphosphonate. Group of drugs used to manage osteoporosis and Paget's disease, or to treat hypercalcemia of malignancy or metastatic bone lesions. Its mechanism of action involves the suppression of osteoclasts, thereby reducing bone resorption. Two main groups exist: nitrogen containing and nonnitrogen containing, with subgroups of either oral or intravenous administration. See: Bisphosphonate-related osteonecrosis of the jaw (BRONJ).

bisphosphonate-associated osteonecrosis (BON): See: Bisphosphonate-related osteonecrosis of the jaw (BRONJ).

bisphosphonate-induced osteonecrosis of the jaw (BIONJ): See: Bisphosphonate-related osteonecrosis of the jaw.

bisphosphonate-related osteonecrosis of the jaw (BRONJ): A complication characterized by exposed necrotic bone in the maxillofacial region that does not heal within 8 weeks after diagnosis and proper care, in a patient under current or previous bisphosphonate treatment and who has not received radiation in the head and neck area. Risk factors include route of administration (intravenous versus oral), duration of therapy, and type of bisphosphonate (nitrogen containing or not). See: Bisphosphonate.

biteplane (biteplate): A tooth-and-tissue-borne appliance usually constructed of plastic and wire and worn in the palate; used as a diagnostic or therapeutic adjunct.

bite splint: See: Occlusal guard.

biting force: Force generated by contraction of elevator muscles of mandible acting against the maxilla.

black space: See: Black triangle.

black triangle: (syn): Black space. 1. Condition when a void is present in the interproximal space apical to the contact point. 2. Missing papilla between teeth when the interproximal bone has been reduced in height. The coronal-apical distance between the bone crest level and the contact point of adjacent teeth will determine if a papilla can be consistently maintained. A similar relationship has been shown for single-tooth implants.

blade: Flat instrument with one or more sharp edges used for cutting.

blade endosteal dental implant: A dental implant placed in bone. It has a wedge-shaped body that is narrow in a buccal-lingual direction with openings or vents in its body through which tissue may grow. An abutment portion transverses the mucogin-gival tissues that offer support or retention of a dental prosthesis. It may or may not be osseointegrated.

blade implant: Design-specific type of implant categorized as an endosteal implant. Blade implants can vary in width and length and are intended to be placed within bone as a one-piece implant. Both the implant that is the endosteal portion and the transmucosal component that serves as an abutment intraorally are included. See: Blade endosteal dental implant and Implant, oral.

blanching: To make or become white or pale, usually in reference to periimplant or periodontal soft tissues (e.g., during pros-thetic try-in/insertion).

blasted implant surface: Treatment of a surface by grit blasting to increase its surface area by subtraction. See: Subtractive surface treatment.

bleeding: Condition involving the loss of blood internally (when blood leaks from blood vessels inside the body); externally through a natural opening (such as the oral cavity); or externally through a break in the skin.

bleeding on probing: A clinical examination parameter of the natural tooth or implant gingiva or soft tissue sulcus that is used to evaluate the health of that tissue. Lack of bleeding on probing may indicate health but bleeding may or may not indicate diseased tissue. A probing force of 0.25 N is generally accepted as the appropriate probing force.

block bone graft: Includes blocks harvested either from the mandibular symphysis or ramus buccal shelf that are used for localized ridge augmentation procedures. See: Alveolar ridge augmentation, Bone graft.

block graft: Graft consisting of a monocortical piece of autogenous bone (e.g., chin or ramus), or a piece of bone replacement graft, usually stabilized in the recipient site with screws.

block out: 1. Removal of unwanted undercuts on a cast. 2. The activity of applying wax or another similar provisional substance to portions of a cast that have unnecessary or unwanted undercuts. Desired undercuts that are essential for fabricating the prosthesis are left as such.

blood cell: Element found in peripheral blood. In humans, the normal mature form is a nonnucleated, yellowish, biconcave disk, adapted by virtue of its configuration and its hemoglobin content to the transport of oxygen. See: Erythrocyte.

blood clot: Semi-solidified mass in the bloodstream formed of an aggregation of blood factors, primarily platelets and fibrin, with entrapment of cellular elements. Also called coagulum.

blood platelet: See: Platelet.

BMD (abbrev.): Bone mineral density.

BMP (abbrev.): Bone morphogenetic protein.

BMPR (abbrev.): Bone morphogenetic protein receptors.

BMU (abbrev.): Basic multicellular unit.

Boley gauge: A caliper-type sliding gauge used for measuring thickness and linear dimension.

bolus: A rounded mass of food or pharmaceutical preparation ready to be swallowed.

BON (abbrev.): Bisphosphonate-associated osteonecrosis.

bond: 1. The linkage between two atoms or radicals of a chemical compound. 2. The force that holds two or more units of matter together. See: Secondary bonds, Van der Wall's bond.

bond strength: The force required to break a bonded assembly with failure occurring in or near the adhesive/adherens interface.

bonding: 1. Joining together securely with an adhesive substance such as cement or glue. 2. The procedure of using an adhesive, cementing material, or fusible ingredient to combine, unite, or strengthen. 3. An adhesive technique in dentistry involving conditioning of enamel and/or dentin so as to create tags in the tooth structure for mechanical retention of restorative material.

bonding agent: A material used to promote adhesion or cohesion between two different substances, or between a material and natural tooth structures.

bone: The mineralized connective tissue that constitutes the majority of the skeleton. It consists of an inorganic component (67%) (minerals such as calcium phosphate) and an organic component (33%) (collagenous matrix and cells). **Alveolar b.**: Bony portion of the mandible or maxilla in which the roots of the teeth are held by periodontal ligament fibers. Alveolar bone is formed during tooth development and eruption. **Alveolar b. proper**: Compact bone that composes the alveolus (tooth socket). Also known as the lamina dura or cribriform plate, the fibers of the periodontal ligament insert into it. **Basal b.**: Bone of the mandible or maxilla, excluding the alveolar bone. **Bundle b.**: Type of alveolar bone, so called because of the continuation into it of the principal (Sharpey's) fibers of the periodontal ligament. **Buttressing b.**: Excessive bone formation occurring on the marginal alveolar bone which is theorized to occur as a result of traumatogenic occlusion. **Cancellous b.**: syn. Medullary bone, Spongy bone, Trabecular bone. Bone in which the trabeculae form a three-dimensional latticework with the interstices filled with bone marrow. **Compact b.**: Bone substance that is dense and hard. **Cortical b.**: syn. Compact bone. The noncancellous hard and dense portion of bone consisting largely of concentric lamellar osteons and interstitial lamellae. **Lamellar b.**: Mature bone, organized in layers (lamellae) that may be concentrically arranged (compact bone) or parallel (cancellous bone). **Woven b.**: (syn): Nonlamellar bone, Primary bone, Primitive bone, Reactive bone. Immature bone encountered where bone is actively healing or being regenerated.

bone-anchored hearing aid (BAHA): Electronic device affixed to the temporal bone in the periauricular area with skin-penetrating implant abutments for the amplification of sound in hearing-impaired patients.

bone atrophy: A decrease in bone mass exhibited as resorption that is represented internally by a decrease in density.

bone augmentation: Placement of an autogenous graft and/or a bone replacement graft, or any procedure that corrects a hard tissue deficiency.

bone biopsy: Bone sample harvested from an area of interest for analysis.

bone cell: Bone cells include osteoblasts, which are responsible for bone formation, and osteoclasts, which are responsible for bone resorption.

bone collector: See: Bone scraper, Bone trap.

bone condenser: See: Osteotome.

bone condensing: See: Osteotome technique.

bone conduction: The transmission of sound from the skull bones to the inner ear. Also known as cranial conduction, osteotympanic conduction, and tissue conduction. See: Osteoconduction.

bone core: See: Bone biopsy.

bone curettage: Removal of soft tissue either from a bony surface by scraping with a curette in preparation for implant placement and/or alveolar ridge augmentation, or from a bony cavity following the removal of pathology.

bone defect: See: Alveolar defect, Ridge defect.

bone "density": 1. **Clinical**: Tactile assessment of bone quality reflecting the percentage of calcified bone to marrow, determined during osteotomy preparation. Usually classified from D1 (dense) to D4 (porous). 2. **Histological**: The "density" is calculated from the percentage of all bone tissue that is constituted by mineralized bone. 3. **Radiographic**: An estimate of the total amount of bone tissue (as bone mineral) in the path of one or more X-ray beams, as measured by Hounsfield units. When in quotes, "density" is as defined in absorptiometry, and does not mean density as used in physics. Other classifications exist. **bone derivative**: A substance extracted from bone, such as bone morphogenetic proteins.

bone expander: See: Osteotome.

bone expansion: Manipulation of a bony ridge with flat and rounded osteotomes for recontouring the cortical ridge to gain more bone width than originally present, usually to accommodate placement of a dental implant. See: Ridge expansion.

bone factor: Relative response of alveolar bone to positive or negative stimulations; the ratio of osteogenesis to osteolysis.

bone fibers: See: Sharpey's connective tissue fibers.

bone fill: Clinical restoration of bone tissue in a treated osseous defect. It addresses neither the presence nor absence of histologic evidence of new connective tissue attachment nor formation of a new periodontal ligament in the case of tooth-supporting bone. Measurement can be accomplished radiographically, clinically (by reentry), or histologically.

bone fracture: Break in bone, usually the result of trauma. It can also be caused by an acquired disease of bone or by abnormal formation associated with bone disease. Fractures are further classified by their character and location: greenstick, spiral, comminuted, transverse, compound, and compression.

bone fusing: See: Osseous integration.

bone graft: Bone taken from a donor site of the patient (autogenous) or from an outside source (allograft, alloplastic, or xenograft). A bone graft is used in the alveolar ridge to augment a bone deficiency. It can be used with simultaneous or subsequent implant placement. Source of an autogenous bone graft may be intraoral or extraoral in origin. Intraoral sources include adjacent cortical bone, anterior nasal spine, retromolar area, maxillary tuberosity, ramus, buccal shelf, and the mandibular symphysis. Extraoral sources of bone grafts include cranium, iliac crest, and tibia. Depending on the source, the graft is either more cortical or more cancellous in nature. See: Allogeneic bone graft, Alloplastic graft, Alveolar ridge augmentation, Autogenous bone graft, Onlay graft, Xenograft.

bone grafting: A surgical procedure performed to establish additional bone volume, using autogenous bone and/or a bone replacement graft, prior to or simultaneously with dental implant placement.

bone harvest: Acquisition of bone from a patient for an autogenous graft, from deceased individuals for an allogeneic graft, or from animals for a xenograft.

bone healing: Cellular events, recapitulating embryogenesis. After initiation of woven bone formation, deposition of parallel-fibered bone ensues. These two primary types of bone repair the defect within weeks; thereafter, the formation of perivascularly arranged lamellar bone takes place with simultaneous resorption of the two primary bone types. This substitution, which gives strength to the bone, may take months to years, depending upon the size of defect. Finally, a structural rearrangement of trabeculae in response to function (Wolff law) takes place. Healing of fractures of long bones may often be characterized by a callus formation in the initial stages, where woven bone is mixed with cartilage, resulting in a clinically as well as radiologically visible thickening of the fracture site. This callus will disappear along with the osseous maturation.

bone–implant contact (BIC): Direct contact of bone with the surface of an endosseous implant as seen microscopically. The ratio of bone contact to implant surface (percent) is used to evaluate implant surface topographies and materials.

bone–implant interface: Line of demarcation between the nonliving surface of an endosseous implant and the living bone it contacts. Numerous factors may influence the degree to which bone heals in contact with the implant surface, including surface texture, surface contamination, time since placement, and extent of functional loading, among others. See: Implant interface. **Immediate loading considerations for b.–i. i.**: See: Primary stability; Secondary stability. **Implant design and b.–i. i.**: Architecture of the implant stack or its overall design, including thread design and pitch. It affects the ability of the implant to be placed into its osteotomy with primary stability and is deemed necessary for osseointegration to occur. **Micromotion and b.–i. i.**: Micromotion during initial osseointegration may precipitate failure of osseointegration to occur. See: Micromotion.

bone induction: Interaction among pluripotential cells and bone morphogenetic proteins (BMPs) that converts these cells to osteoblasts. See: Osteoinduction.

bone loss: Physiologic loss of bone mass. The peak of mineral density is reached between 30 and 40 years of age; women lose about 35% of cortical bone and 50% of trabecular bone, whereas men lose about two-thirds of these amounts. See: Osteoporosis.

bone loss (implant): Physiologic or pathologic bone resorption around a dental implant. See: Crestal bone loss, Early crestal bone loss, Implant periapical lesion, Periimplantitis.

bone marrow: Nonmineralized tissue found within bone containing hematopoietic and/or fatty tissues.

bone mass: Amount of bone, often estimated by absorptiometry, viewed as a volume minus the marrow cavity. Optimal balance in the composition of the bone is reached between 30 and 40 years of age.

In this age period, the ratio of cortical and trabecular bone to bone marrow assures that maximum strength is reached by a minimum of bone mass.

bone matrix: The intercellular substance of bone consisting of collagenous fibers embedded in an amorphous ground substance and inorganic salts. Contains collagen type I (90%) and noncollagenous protein (about 10%): osteonectin, osteopontin, bone sialoprotein, and growth factors (cytokines) such as insulin-like growth factors (IGF1 and IGF2), transforming growth factor beta 1 (TGF-β1), platelet-derived growth factor (PDGF), acidic and basic fibroblast growth factors (aFGF and bFGF), and bone morphogenetic proteins (BMPs).

bone mill: Device used to mechanically transform harvested autogenous bone into a suitable particle size for grafting procedures.

bone milling: A process used to particulate harvested bone into progressively smaller particles.

bone mineral: Mineral in bone composed of calcium carbonate (10%), calcium and magnesium fluoride (5%), and calcium phosphates (85%), present primarily as hydroxyapatite.

bone mineral density (BMD): Density of bone expressed in cm^2, measured by dual-energy X-ray absorptiometry (DEXA). Used as a measure of bone health and in the diagnosis of osteoporosis.

bone modeling: Processes producing functionally purposeful skeletal organs aimed at characteristic adult shape and form; includes longitudinal, transversal, and appositional growth.

bone morphogenetic protein (BMP): Special group of the transforming growth factor beta (TGF-β) superfamily of growth factors with the unique property of stimulating mesenchymal stem cells to differentiate toward a chondro- and osteoblastic lineage. BMP-2, BMP-3, and BMP-7 have proven to be powerful stimulators of bone healing. Several BMPs such as BMP-2, BMP-4, and BMP-7 are known to induce the expression of core-binding factor alpha 1 (CBFα1). See: Isoforms. **Osteoinductive**

properties of b. m. p.: The BMP family of proteins, most notably BMP-2, BMP-4, and BMP-7, are known to promote *de novo* bone formation through the process of osteoinduction. Bone may be formed with a cartilage intermediate stage, as in the situation of endochondral bone formation, or directly, as in intramembranous bone formation.

bone morphogenetic protein 2 (BMP-2): Polypeptide that belongs to the transforming growth factor beta (TGF-β) superfamily of proteins. Like other BMPs, it plays an important role in the development of bone and cartilage. It is involved in the Hedgehog pathway, TGF-β signaling pathway, and cytokine–cytokine receptor interaction, as well as cardiac cell differentiation and epithelial to mesenchymal transition.

bone morphogenetic protein 4 (BMP-4): Polypeptide belonging to the transforming growth factor beta (TGF-β) superfamily of proteins. Like other BMPs, it is involved in bone and cartilage development, specifically tooth and limb development and fracture repair, and has been shown to be involved in muscle development and bone mineralization.

bone morphogenetic protein 5 (BMP-5): Polypeptide member of the transforming growth factor beta (TGF-β) superfamily of proteins. BMP-5 may play a role in certain cancers. Like other BMPs, BMP-5 is inhibited by molecules chordin and noggin. It is expressed in the trabecular meshwork, lung, liver, and optic nerve, and may be involved in the development and normal function of these organs.

bone morphogenetic protein 7 (BMP-7): Member of the transforming growth factor beta (TGF-β) superfamily of proteins. Similar to other members of the BMP family of proteins, it plays a key role in the transformation of mesenchymal cells into bone and cartilage. It is inhibited by noggin. BMP-7 may be involved in bone homeostasis and is expressed in the brain, kidneys, and bladder. It has been shown to induce SMAD-1 as well as multiple biomarkers of osteoblast differentiation. Also called Osteogenic protein 1.

bone morphogenetic protein receptors (BMPR): Transmembrane receptors that are present in a wide variety of cells and mediate BMP signals. They comprise serine or threonine kinase receptors composed of subtypes I and II.

bone necrosis: See: Osteonecrosis.

bone-plate device with external activation screws: See: Alveolar distraction osteogenesis.

bone preparation: Act of readying the bony site for implant, transplant, or graft placement. To achieve implant osseointegration, a low-trauma preparation of the implant bed is necessary. Bone preparation with several drills of increasing diameter is performed using copious saline solution to provide cooling.

bone quality: A qualitative assessment of bone based on its density.

bone reduction guide: A stereolithographic guide used to assist in accurate reduction of excess bone in the mandible or maxilla.

bone regeneration: Renewal or repair of lost bone tissue. Also: Cellular events during wound healing; recapitulation of cellular events of embryogenesis. The quantitative extent is defect dependent and influenced by cellular race.

bone regeneration strategies: Use of polypeptide growth factors as mediators to promote osteoblast migration, mitogenesis, or matrix synthesis leading to bone regeneration. See: Growth factor.

bone remodeling: Basic physiologic remodeling of bone takes place in a biologically coupled system of activation, resorption, and formation (ARF). Histomorphologically, the process starts in cortical bone as a cutting cone, consisting of a group of osteoclasts, digs a tunnel with a breakdown of 20 μm per day with a simultaneous increase in diameter of the tunnel in magnitude of 5 μm per day until a width of approximately 100 μm in radius is reached.

bone remodeling rate (BRR): The turnover or replacement of packets of bone tissue called basic multicellular units, or BMUs, in all or part of a bone structure without a change in shape.

bone remodeling unit (BRU): A group of osteoblasts and osteoclasts involved in bone remodeling. See: Remodeling (bone).

bone replacement graft: Any material other than autogenous bone, which is used as a hard tissue graft, in an attempt to stimulate new bone formation in an area where bone formerly existed.

bone resorption: Loss of bone due to osteoclastic activity. See: Resorption.

bone scaffold: Process of bone formation that occurs through the utilization of a scaffolding matrix that may deliver cells, genes, or proteins. The scaffold may be osteoinductive or osteoconductive and serves to maintain the architecture of the anatomic defect.

bone scraper: Device used to harvest bone particles through surface shavings for grafting purposes.

bone sounding: Simple preoperative procedure performed under local anesthesia using a fine needle with a rubber stopper. The needle is used to penetrate soft tissues to assess the form and volume of the existing alveolar ridge.

bone spreader: See: Osteotome.

bone stimulation: Initiation of bone formation around endosseous implants by pulsed electromagnetic fields. Must be performed within very early stages of healing, i.e., during the first and second weeks; after 2 weeks, no effect can be measured. This principle has only been used in animal studies.

bone strength: Resistance of bone fracture. Bone strength depends upon bone structure. The denser the trabecular pattern, the stronger is the bone. This compressive strength of the vertebral bodies decrease with age. See: Osteoporosis.

bone structural unit (BSU): Represents the end result of a remodeling cycle of mature bone. In cortical bone, it constitutes a Haversian system after a cortical remodeling unit has taken place. In cancellous bone, it is a wall or packet. See: Bone remodeling unit (BRU), Basic multicellular unit (BMU).

bone substitute: Nonviable biomaterial for reconstruction of bone, producing only a scaffold for formation of new bone. Supports the inherent potential for bone regeneration. It may be resorbable or remain in an unchanged version at the site of implantation. It also may assist in preservation of contour of an osseous reconstruction. See: Osteoconduction.

bone tap: See: Tap.

bone trap: Device connected to the surgical suction to collect fine bone slurry within the surgical field during the drilling of bone or harvest of a bone block for alveolar ridge augmentation or maxillary sinus floor elevation. Collected bone can be added to the particulate graft.

bone trephine: Hollow, cylindrical cutting bur of various diameters used to harvest cylindrical bone blocks.

bone turnover: See: Turnover (bone).

bony ankylosis: The bony union of the constituents of a joint that results in complete immobility of the joint.

bony defect: Alteration in the morphologic features of bone.

border movement: When observed in a designated plane, it is the mandibular movements at the boundaries permitted by anatomic structures. The movements are reproducible and unique for each individual. All mandibular movements are determined by the parameters of the border movements.

border seal: The physical contact established by the alveolar mucosa to drape the molded borders of an oral removable prosthesis in an attempt to create negative pressure that aids in the retention of the prosthesis and the prevention of the ingress of fluids, air, and food into the intaglio surface.

border tissue movements: The action of the alveolar mucosa aided by muscles and tissues proximal to the borders of the denture. Usually recorded during border molding to fashion the denture edges.

bovine-derived anorganic bone matrix: Particular anorganic bovine bone substitute with a calcium-deficient carbonate hydroxyapatite having a crystal size of approximately 10 nm. All proteins are removed from the bovine xenograft via various chemical and physical processes.

Its porous structure, like normal bone, is osteoconductive but resistant to resorption, although osteoclasts are identified in lacunae on the surfaces. The surface area is very large, and the modulus of elasticity is similar to that of normal bone.

bovine hydroxyapatite material: See: Bovine-derived anorganic bone matrix.

BP (abbrev.): Bisphosphonate.

BPPV (abbrev.): Benign paroxysmal positional vertigo.

bridge: Slang. See: Fixed dental prosthesis.

BRONJ (abbrev.): Bisphosphonate-related osteonecrosis of the jaw.

BRR (abbrev.): Bone remodeling rate.

BRU (abbrev.): Bone remodeling unit.

Brunski and Hurley model: Set of equations that allows the user to predict the forces and moments acting on each implant in a group of implants that support a loaded prosthesis.

bruxism: 1. The parafunctional grinding, clenching, or clamping of teeth. 2. A habit that consists of the involuntary recurrent or spasmodic nonfunctional grinding, clenching, or clamping of teeth in other than desired functional movements of the mandible (chewing), which results in occlusal damage. Also known as tooth grinding, occlusal neurosis.

bruxomania: The grinding or clenching of teeth occurring as a neurotic habit while awake.

BSE (abbrev.): Backscattered electron. See: Backscattered electron (BSE) imaging.

BSU (abbrev.): Bone structural unit. See: Osteon.

buccal: Pertaining to or adjacent to the cheek.

buccal flange: The portion of the denture that extends from the cervical margins of the denture teeth to the border seal areas.

buccal index: An impression record of the facial aspect of teeth relative to a cast.

buccal mucosal incision: Incision made in buccal nonkeratinized mucosa; not routinely used in implant surgery.

buccal plate: (syn): Labial plate. Bony wall at the buccal aspect of an alveolus consisting of alveolar bone proper, cortical bone, with or without intervening cancellous bone.

buccal vestibule: Portion of the oral cavity that is bounded on one side by the teeth, gingiva, and alveolar ridge (in the edentulous mouth, the residual ridge) and on the lateral side by the cheek posterior to the buccal frenula.

buccolingual relationship: A reference to the position as it relates to the cheek and tongue in the coronal plane.

buccoversion: The divergence of a tooth from its customary alignment in the dental arch to a direction toward the cheek or lips.

BULL (abbrev.): Buccal of the Upper, Lingual of the Lower (cusps); applies to Clyde H. Schuyler's rules for occlusal adjustment of a normally related dentition in which those cusps contacting in maximum intercuspation (mandibular buccal and maxillary lingual) are favored by adjustment of those cusps that are not in occlusal contact in maximum intercuspation (maxillary buccal and mandibular lingual); also called the Bull rule.

bulla: A vesicle or blister >5 mm in diameter.

bundle bone: Bone of ectomesenchymal origin that lines the tooth alveolus and also forms the cribriform plate. It is characterized by perpendicular striations formed by the insertion of Sharpey's fibers and blood vessels derived from the periodontal ligament. This tooth-related bone structure plays an important role during initial ridge alterations following extraction. Radiographically, it is called the lamina dura.

burnish: To make shiny or lustrous by rubbing; also to facilitate marginal adaptation of restorations by rubbing the margin with an instrument.

burnishibility: The ability or ease with which a material can be burnished.

butt: To bring any two flat-ended surfaces into contact without overlapping, as in a butt joint.

button implant: See: Mucosal insert.

buttressing bone: Marginal linear aspect of bone, which may be formed in response to heavy occlusal forces.

C

Ca: Acronym for carcinoma or cancer.

CAD (abbrev.): Computer-aided design.

CAD/CAM: Acronym for computer-aided design/computer-assisted machining or computer- aided design/computer-aided manufacturing. See: Computer-aided design/ Computer- assisted manufacture (CAD/ CAM).

CAD/CAM (dentistry): Using computer technologies to design and produce different types of dental restorations, including crowns, veneers, inlays and onlays, fixed prostheses, dental implant restorations, and orthodontic appliances. See: Computer-aided design and drafting and computer-aided manufacturing.

CAD/CAM abutment: Prosthetic implant component fabricated through the use of computer- aided design and/or computer-assisted manufacture (CAD/CAM).

CADD (abbrev.): Computer-aided design and drafting.

calcified algae: A unique subset of marine seaweeds that incorporate calcium carbonate, essentially, limestone, into their thalli.

calcium carbonate ($CaCO_3$): See: Coralline.

calcium hydroxide: An odorless white powder that is very slightly soluble in water and insoluble in alcohol. Aqueous and nonaqueous suspensions of calcium hydroxide are often employed as cavity liners to protect the dental pulp from the irritant action of restorative materials; also used in pulp capping, pulpotomy, and apexification procedures.

calcium phosphate: 1. Mineral needed for the mineralization of the new bone in a graft site. Its source is usually from the surrounding bone and may be also introduced through the blood supply. 2. Class of ceramics with varying calcium-to-phosphorus ratios, which can form a direct bond with bone. It can also be used as a bone substitute.

calcium sulfate: Used in bone regeneration as an alloplastic graft, a graft binder, or a graft extender, and as a barrier. This biocompatible material ($CaSO_4$) resorbs following implantation. It has been shown that tissue will often migrate over calcium sulfate if primary closure cannot be obtained. Calcium sulfate has been proposed as a delivery vehicle for growth factors and antibiotics. See: Medical-grade calcium sulfate (MGCS).

calcium sulfate plaster: A pasty composition of $CaSO_4$ and water used as a medicated or protective dressing that hardens upon drying.

calculus: In dentistry, a chalky or dark deposit attached to tooth structure, essentially made of mineralized microbial plaque. Found on tooth structure in a supragingival and/or subgingival location.

Caldwell–Luc: Surgical procedure named after American physician George Caldwell and French laryngologist Henry Luc. Its original indication was for the relief of chronic sinusitis by improving drainage of the maxillary sinus through an incision into the canine fossa.

Caldwell-Luc approach: Surgical approach using a window into the buccal bone wall of the maxillary sinus. The goal is sinus floor elevation to allow simultaneous or subsequent

Glossary of Dental Implantology, First Edition. Khalid Almas, Fawad Javed and Steph Smith.
© 2018 John Wiley & Sons, Inc. Published 2018 by John Wiley & Sons, Inc.

implant placement in sites with insufficient bone height.

calibration: A comparison between measurements; one of known magnitude or correctness made or set with one device and another measurement made as similar as possible with a second device. The device with the known or assigned correctness is called the standard. The second device is the unit under test, test instrument, or any of several other names for the device being calibrated. Successful calibration has to be consistent and systematic. At the same time, the complexity of some instruments requires that only key functions be identified and calibrated. Under those conditions, a degree of randomness is needed to find unexpected deficiencies.

callus: The tissue that forms between and around fractured bone segments to maintain structural integrity and facilitate bone regeneration.

calvaria: The dome-like superior portion of the cranium, derived from the membranous neurocranium, and consisting of the frontal and parietal bones and the squamous parts of the occipital and temporal bones. Bone may be harvested from this site for grafting purposes.

calvarial graft: Autogenous bone graft harvested from the dome-like superior portion of the cranium, most frequently from the parietal region, generally on the right side (nondominant hemisphere) behind the coronal suture, and approximately 3 cm lateral to the sagittal suture.

CAM (abbrev.): Computer-aided manufacturing.

CAM abutment: Abutment which is designed by casting a waxed castable abutment, which is subsequently scanned, digitized, and fabricated through computer-aided manufacturing.

Campylobacter rectus: Previously named *Wolinella recta*. Surface translocating gram-negative, motile, facultative bacteria that are frequently observed as helical, curved, or straight bacterial cells. This bacterium is found in patients with periodontitis. The bacteria display flagella located at one pole of their cell body that results in a motility that is described as rapid and darting.

canaliculus: Minute canal extending to the lacunae of bone. See: Osteocyte.

cancellous bone: The lattice-like, reticular, or spongy or part of bone; the tissue found in the medulla of the bone; it has a variable trabecular pattern and is made of interstitial tissue that may be hematopoietic. Also used to describe a graft derived from cancellous bone, which is a spongy type of bone containing a trabecular structure with red bone marrow and most of the bone vasculature. See: Bone, Trabecular bone.

cancellous bone graft: Graft consisting of medullary bone.

cancer: See: Neoplasm.

cancer reconstruction: Tumor resection of the jaws often leads to discontinuity defects that need extensive bone reconstruction and restoration with implant-supported prostheses.

***Candida* ssp**: A yeast-like fungus often found in association with oral diseases such as "thrush" (oral candidiasis). Usually stains gram positive, is aerobic, and is significantly larger than bacteria. Most frequently encountered species is *C. albicans.*

Candida albicans: The utmost pathogenic species of *Candida*, which under some circumstances may cause infections; however, typically it is an innocuous inhabitant of mucous membranes.

candidiasis (thrush): An infection caused by the fungus genus *Candida*. It is associated with multiple influencing factors that include (1) the use of broad-spectrum antibiotics, (2) diabetes mellitus, (3) xerostomia, (4) suppression of the immune system, and (5) pregnancy. Clinically, it appears as soft, white, curd-like plaques that can be wiped off, leaving an erythematous area.

canine eminence: The labial prominence on the maxillary alveolar process corresponding to the position of the root of the canine tooth.

canine guidance: See: Canine protected articulation.

canine protected articulation: A form of mutually protected articulation in which the vertical and horizontal overlap of the canine teeth disengage the posterior teeth in the excursive movements of the mandible. Compare: Anterior protected articulation.

canine protected occlusion: Regarding implant dentistry, a tooth arrangement that protects implant-supported prosthetic crowns from off-axial loads or lateral forces that may be detrimental or cause an overload of the supporting bone. Generally, the mandibular canine cusp articulates or slides against the maxillary canine lingual surface to cause a separation of the posterior teeth so off-axial load is avoided.

canine protection: A form of articulation in which the overlap of the canine teeth disengages the posterior teeth in excursive movements. See: Guidance, Canine, Canine protected articulation.

cantilever: A projecting beam or member supported on one end only.

cantilever fixed dental prosthesis: A fixed dental prosthesis in which the pontic is cantilevered, i.e., is retained and supported only on one end by one or more abutments.

cap attachment: See: Metal housing.

cap splint: A plastic or metallic device that is cemented on to the clinical crowns; used to treat upper or lower jaw fractures.

capillary attraction: An increase or decrease in the height of a liquid as it contacts the retaining walls of a container.

Capnocytophaga **ssp**: Gram-negative, capnophilic (carbon dioxide loving), fusiform bacilli found as normal oral flora in humans. May be associated with systemic disease, usually in leukemic and/or granulocytopenic patients.

capnophilic: Refers to a type of organism that grows optimally under conditions of increased (above atmospheric levels) partial pressure of carbon dioxide, e.g., *Capnocytophaga* ssp.

capsular fibrosis: As related to the temporomandibular joint, a contracture of the capsular ligament due to a fibrotic change.

capsular ligament: Referencing the temporomandibular joint, a thin, loose, envelope-like fibrous band of tissue that connects the head of the mandible's condyle with the glenoid fossa. It is attached superiorly to the circumference of the glenoid fossa, anteriorly to the articular tubercle, and inferiorly to the condyle of the mandible.

carat: A standard of gold fineness. The percentage of gold in an alloy, stated in parts per 24. Pure gold is designated 24 carat.

carbide bur: A rotary cutting instrument made from tungsten carbide.

carbon fiber: Filaments made by high-temperature carbonizing of acrylic fiber. Used in the production of high-strength composites.

cardiopulmonary resuscitation (CPR): An emergency procedure involving manual compression of the chest overlying the heart and forcing air into the lungs, maintaining circulation when circumstances render the heart unable to pump blood.

cartilage: A derivative of connective tissue arising from the mesenchyme. Typical hyaline cartilage is a flexible, rather elastic material with a semi-transparent glass-like appearance. Its ground substance is a complex protein through which is distributed a large network of connective tissue fibers.

case–control study: Study design used to identify factors that may contribute to a medical condition by comparing a group of patients who have that condition (experimental group) with a group of patients who do not (control group).

case history: The data collected about an individual, family, environmental factors (including medical/dental history) and any other information that may be useful in analyzing and diagnosing conditions, or for instructional purposes; best termed the patient history.

case report: A type of documentation in which diagnosis, treatment, and outcome of a patient are described.

case sequencing: The order of treatment for a patient undergoing dental implant therapy, including time of treatment as it relates to healing and prosthodontic restoration.

case series: Analysis of a series of patients with a certain diagnosis and treatment of interest. There is no control group involved.

cast: 1. Three-dimensional image of an actual body part reproduced in a castable material. See: Diagnostic cast, Master (definitive) cast, Preliminary cast. 2. A positive reproduction of a shape created by pouring a material that hardens into a mold, matrix, or impression of the needed shape.

cast clasp: A removable dental prosthesis clasp fabricated by the lost-wax casting process.

cast connector: A cast metal union between the retainer(s) and pontic(s) in a fixed dental prosthesis.

cast metal core: The base restoration (core) indirectly made by using a lost-wax casting technique for the purpose of supporting a fixed dental prosthesis.

cast post-and-core: A one-piece foundation restoration for an endodontically treated tooth that comprises a post within the root canal and a core replacing missing coronal structure to form the tooth preparation.

cast relator: An instrument that orients opposing dental models in an arbitrary manner without correlation to anatomic landmarks.

cast, study or diagnostic: A positive reproduction of the teeth and associated structures formed by pouring dental stone or dental plaster into a matrix or impression. It is made for the purpose of evaluating dental structures and occlusal analysis.

castable: A material that can be cast. The material can be in a liquid state due to heating or mixing a powder and a liquid; once poured or injected into a mold, it solidifies.

castable abutment: (syn): UCLA abutment. A prefabricated component, with or without a prefabricated cylinder, used to make a custom abutment for a cement-retained or screw- retained prosthesis, by waxing its plastic burnout pattern and subsequently casting the abutment through a lost-wax technique. See: Prefabricated cylinder.

castable ceramic: Regarding dentistry, a glass-ceramic material that can be cast using the lost-wax method.

casting: A reproduction of an object formed by pouring or injecting a fluid into a mold that then becomes a solid.

casting ring: A metal cylinder in which a refractory pattern is made and used in the casting process for a dental prosthesis.

casting wax: A wax composite with acceptable characteristics that can be used for making wax patterns that are placed in an investing material. Then, once the investment has set, heat is applied and the wax is "lost" from the investment. The investment is then subject to the casting process where a liquid is poured into the investment to replace the lost wax. The liquid solidifies and the investment material is then removed, leaving a cast object that is a duplicate of the wax pattern.

CAT (abbrev.): Computed axial tomography. See: Computed tomography (CT) scan.

CAT scan (abbrev.): Computed axial tomography scan.

catalyst: Substance that accelerates a chemical reaction without affecting the properties of the materials involved.

cathode: The negative pole in electrolysis.

cautery: Applying a caustic substance, electric current, hot instrument, or other agent to burn or destroy tissue and control bleeding during surgery. From the Greek term *kauterion*, meaning branding iron.

cavernous resorption: See: Resorption.

cavity varnish: An organic solvent (chloroform or ether) that contains a mixture of copal resin or other synthetic resins and is used to protect a tooth from the constituents of the restorative material(s).

CBA (abbrev.): Cost-benefit analysis.

CBCT (abbrev.): Cone beam computed tomography.

CBFα1 (abbrev.): Core-binding factor alpha 1.

CCD (abbrev.): Charge-coupled device.

CD (abbrev.): Complete denture.

CDA (abbrev.): Certified dental assistant.

CD antigens: Cell surface molecules that are distinguishable with specific monoclonal antibodies and may be used to differentiate cell populations. Examples of clusters of differentiation (CD) antigens include CD4, CD8, and CD40.

CDL (abbrev.): Certified dental laboratory.

CDMP1 (abbrev.): Cartilage-derived morphogenetic protein-1.

cDNA: A fragment of DNA complementary to a specific RNA sequence, synthesized from it *in vitro* by reverse transcription. cDNA probes can be used for the identification of pathogenic bacteria in dental plaque samples.

CDT (abbrev.): Certified dental technician.

CEA (abbrev.): Cost-effectiveness analysis.

cell: Microscopic mass of protoplasm enveloped by a semi-permeable membrane. Smallest structural unit of living matter able to function independently. See: Erythrocyte, B cell, Blood.

cell-occlusive membrane: See: Barrier membrane.

cellular process: All of the functions that cells perform to survive, including molecular transport, protein synthesis, DNA replication, reproduction, respiration, cellular metabolism, and signaling.

cellulitis: A widespread inflammation, usually related to an inflammatory condition contained within loose subcutaneous tissue. Often associated with a bacterial infection and is frequently a precursor to abscess formation.

cement: 1. To unite or make firm by or as if by cement; to lute. 2. Substance used to bind surfaces or objects together. Commonly stored as separate powder and liquid components that, when mixed together, become a luting agent upon hardening. To cement is to join surfaces by means of an appropriate medium. **Permanent c.**: Binding or luting agent intended for long-term use, e.g., zinc phosphate cement, which is composed of powder (zinc and magnesium oxides) and liquid (phosphoric acid, water, buffer agents). Other types include resin and glass-ionomer cements. **Temporary c.**: Binding or luting agent intended for short-term use, e.g., zinc oxide (powder) eugenol (liquid) mixture.

cemental lamella: One of the layers of cementum.

cementation: 1. The process of attaching parts by means of cement. 2. Attaching a restoration to natural teeth by means of a cement (GPT-4).

cementodentinal junction: The area of union of the dentin and cementum.

cementoenamel junction: The meeting point on any tooth between the root cementum and the crown enamel. See: Junction.

cementogenesis: The creation or development of cementum.

cementoid: The uncalcified surface layer of cementum including incorporated connective tissue fibers.

cement-retained: The use of dental cement for the retention of a prosthesis to an abutment, or transmucosal portion of a one-piece dental implant. See: Attachment-retained, Screw-retained.

cementum: The thin, calcified tissue of ectomesenchymal origin covering the roots of teeth in which embedded collagen fibers attach the teeth to the alveolus.

cementum fracture: The tearing or splintering of the cementum from the tooth's root surface. Superficial disruptions of a tooth root that result in the displacement of cementum fragments.

center of ridge: The midline of the residual ridge in a buccolingual dimension, as viewed from the occlusal aspect.

central bearing: A device that applies a single point force that is applied as centrally as possible at the center of support between the maxillary and mandibular jaws. It distributes the closing forces evenly throughout the supporting structures when recording maxillomandibular jaw relationships. It is also used to detect errors in occlusion.

central bearing point: The precise location of contact for a central bearing device.

central bearing tracing: The recorded path of motion on the horizontal plate of the central bearing tracing device.

central bearing tracing device: A device that is used to balance occlusal forces when measuring maxillomandibular jaw relationships or to map the full envelope of mandibular movement. It consists of a plate attached to a dental arch and a tracking device that records movement.

centric: 1. Located in or at a center. 2. Oriented around or directed toward a center.

centric occlusion: The maximum balanced intercuspation of maxillary and mandibular teeth; may or may not coincide with centric relation. Positional relationship of occluding tooth surfaces when the mandible is in centric relation. The coincidence of centric occlusion and centric relation is desirable when creating an occlusion, but the maximal intercuspal relationship may not always exist. See: Maxillomandibular relationship.

centric position: The position of the mandible in either centric occlusion or centric relation.

centric prematurity: An occlusal contact or interference that occurs before a balanced and stable jaw-to-jaw relationship is reached in centric occlusion or centric relation.

centric range: The physical distance that exists between centric relation and maximum intercuspation as viewed in the horizontal and sagittal planes.

centric relation: 1. The maxillomandibular relationship in which the condyles articulate with the thinnest avascular portion of their respective disks with the complex in the anterior-superior position against the shapes of the articular eminences. This position is independent of tooth contact. This position is clinically discernible when the mandible is directed superior and anteriorly. It is restricted to a purely rotary movement about the transverse horizontal axis (GPT-5). 2. The most retruded physiologic relation of the mandible to the maxillae to and from which the individual can make lateral movements. It is a condition that can exist at various degrees of jaw separation. It occurs around the terminal hinge axis (GPT-3). 3. The most retruded relation of the mandible to the maxillae when the condyles are in the most posterior unstrained position in the glenoid fossae from which lateral movement can be made at any given degree of jaw separation (GPT-1). 4. The most posterior relation of the lower to the upper jaw from which lateral movements can be made at a given vertical dimension (Boucher). 5. A maxilla to mandible relationship in which the condyles and disks are thought to be in the midmost, uppermost position. The position has been difficult to define anatomically but is determined clinically by assessing when the jaw can hinge on a fixed terminal axis (up to 25 mm). It is a clinically determined relationship of the mandible to the maxilla when the condyle disk assemblies are positioned in their most superior position in the mandibular fossae and against the distal slope of the articular eminence (Ash). 6. The relation of the mandible to the maxillae when the condyles are in the uppermost and rearmost position in the glenoid fossae. It may not be possible to record this position in the presence of dysfunction of the masticatory system. 7. A clinically determined position of the mandible placing both condyles into their anterior uppermost position. This can be determined in patients without pain or derangement in the TMJ (Ramsfjord).

centric relation record: A registration of the relationship between the maxilla and mandible when the mandibular condyles are in centric relation. The record may be taken intraorally or extraorally.

centric slide: The physical movement of the mandible as it transits from centric occlusion to maximum intercuspation.

centric stop: Occlusal contacts of opposing teeth that maintain the occlusal vertical dimension between the maxillary and mandibular arches.

cephalogram: See: Cephalometric radiograph.

cephalometric radiograph: A standardized radiograph of the head used for making cranial measurements.

cephalometric tracing: A line diagram that is a copy of the structural landmarks of the orthodontically relevant craniofacial markers and facial bones. It is made by drawing on a thin paper sheet placed on a cephalometric radiograph through which light is projected.

cephalometry: 1. The science of measuring the dimensions of the head. 2. In dentistry, it is the determination of the permutations of angles, lines, and planes derived from tracings of landmarks on frontal and lateral radiographic head films. The measurements are used to assess growth, development, and treatment responses of the craniofacial bones as it relates to diagnosis, in-treatment evaluations, or completed orthodontic treatment.

cephalosporins: Broad-spectrum beta-lactam antibiotics chemically related to and having the same mechanism of action as the penicillins, disrupting the synthesis of the peptidoglycan layer of bacterial cell walls.

cephalostat: A device used to precisely and predictably position the head so as to create spatially oriented and reproducible radiographs or photographs.

ceram: A fine-grained glass-ceramic material that is derived from applying heat to a specific form of glass.

ceramic: 1. A broad class of materials made from a variety of nonmetallic compounds with a metallic component, which are fired at high temperatures to achieve their physical characteristics of high hardness, brittleness, low thermal and electrical conductivity, and high corrosion resistance. They are generally oxides but can also be composed of calcium phosphates, alumina, zirconia, nitrides, borides, carbides, silicides, and sulfides, alone or in combination with glass or metals (cermets). In dentistry, the term is used liberally to include all materials that mimic the optical qualities of natural tooth structure or gingivae and have the characteristics of this class. They are also sometimes used as synthetic osseous grafting materials and biocompatible surface coatings. 2. Of or relating to the application of ceramics. See: Alloplast, Bioactive glass.

ceramic abutment: Prosthetic implant component composed of a ceramic biomaterial that is considered an esthetic material as compared to unesthetic metal. The ceramic material used in fabrication of a prosthetic implant component varies, as does the fabrication method of various manufacturers, which can include use of CAD/CAM technology.

ceramic crown: 1. A fixed dental prosthesis, fabricated entirely with ceramic materials. It is cemented, bonded, or screwed to an underlying implant fixture, abutment, or framework. 2, A fixed dental prosthesis that is fabricated entirely with ceramic materials and cemented or bonded to an underlying natural tooth. See: Ceramic restoration, Crown.

ceramic flux: A glass modifier that disrupts the oxygen–silica bonds and in doing so increases fluidity. The bonds are disrupted by the addition of metallic ions, such as calcium carbonate, potassium carbonate, or sodium carbonate.

ceramic onlay: An indirect, intracoronal restoration involving coverage of one or more cusps fabricated entirely with ceramic materials and generally bonded to natural tooth.

ceramic restoration: Artificial substitute for tooth structure and anatomy fabricated entirely of ceramic material that covers and restores the remaining coronal portion of the tooth.

ceramics: 1. Relating to the science of manufacturing and use of ceramic, particularly bioceramic compounds. 2. The art of fabricating dental restorations using ceramic alone or in combination with other materials.

ceramist (ceramicist): A laboratory technician who specializes in the art and science of dental ceramics.

cermet: 1. Any mixture of ceramic and metal particles used as a restorative material. 2. A ceramo-metal compound, often used as a friction-reducing coating (i.e., titanium nitride).

Certified dental laboratory: In the United States, a dental laboratory that has met established specific standards for personnel skills, laboratory facilities, and infection control and is certified by the National Board for Certification of Dental Laboratories.

Certified dental technician: In the United States, a dental technician who has met established specific standards and is certified by the National Board for Certification of Dental Laboratories.

cervical: 1. In anatomy, pertaining to the cervix or neck. 2. In dentistry, pertaining to the region at or near the cementoenamel junction.

cervix: A narrow or constricted portion; in dentistry, it refers to the constricted region where the crown meets the root of a tooth. See: Implant neck.

chamber, pulp: The segment of the pulp cavity located inside the anatomic crown portion of the tooth.

chamfer: 1. A tooth preparation line design in which the gingival aspect and external axial surface meet at an angle >90° but <180°. 2. A small channel or trench.

chamfer angle: 1. The angle formed by the surface plane of the prepared chamfer and the vertical component of the unprepared tooth. 2. The angle formed by the surface plane of the restorative finish line of an implant abutment and its long axis.

characterization: To change by applying distinct markings, indentations, coloration, and similar unique methods of demarcation on a tooth or dental prosthesis to improve the natural appearance.

characterize: To define in a unique, distinguishing manner.

characterized denture base: A denture base with coloring that mimics the color, hues, and shades of naturally occurring oral tissues.

charge-coupled device (CCD): A device for the movement of electrical charge, usually from within the device to an area where the charge can be manipulated (e.g., conversion into a digital value). This is achieved by "shifting" the signals between stages within the device one at a time. Charge-coupled devices are widely used for digital imaging.

cheilitis: Inflammation occurring in the lip.

cheilitis, angular: Inflammation affecting the corner angles or commissures of the mouth.

cheiloplasty: Plastic surgery performed on the lip.

cheilosis: A disorder of the lips and angles of the mouth characterized by fissures; often associated with a riboflavin deficiency.

chemoattractant: A chemical or biological mediator that causes movement of cells along a concentration gradient to the area with the highest concentration of the chemical.

chemotaxis: The migration of cells along a concentration gradient of an attractant.

chemotherapy: The treatment or control of a disease by chemical agents.

chewing: See: Mastication.

chewing cycle: See: Mandibular movement.

chin graft: A bone graft harvested from the facial aspect of the mandibular symphyseal area, between the mental foramina, apical to the roots of the teeth, and usually above the lower border of the mandible.

chisel: An instrument with a beveled cutting edge used for cutting or cleaving hard tissue.

Chi-square test: A statistical method used to determine whether observed frequencies are significantly different from expected frequencies and whether there is a statistically significant difference.

chlorhexidine gluconate: A bis-biguanide antimicrobial, used as an oral rinse or local antiseptic. Its mechanism of action involves the lysis of bacterial membranes.

chondrocyte: Mature cartilage-forming cell embedded in cartilage. Highly specialized connective tissue designed to withstand high compressive forces. Cartilage is nourished via diffusion. In endochondral ossification, the chondrocytes undergo apoptosis associated with vascularization, bone formation, and resorption of cartilage.

chondroitin sulfate: Plays a major role in maintaining the high osmotic tension essential to the elasticity of hyalin cartilage. Hyalin cartilage is composed of collagen type II that forms a meshwork, enclosing giant macromolecular aggregates of proteoglycans.

Chondroitin sulfate is a main part of this ground substance.

chroma: 1. The purity of a color, or its departure from white or gray. 2. The intensity of a distinctive hue; saturation of a hue. See: Saturation.

chromosome: One of the nuclear bodies that carries hereditary factors in cells. There are 46 in humans.

chronic: Continuing over a long period of time. Used to describe a disease state of long duration.

chronic abscess: Abscess of comparatively slow development with minimal evidence of inflammation. Symptoms include intermittent discharge of purulent matter and long- standing collection of purulent exudate. May follow an acute abscess. Compare: Residual abscess.

chronic closed lock: A clinical situation where the temporomandibular joint has restricted motion over a long period of time. An anterior dislocation of the intraarticular disk causes this clinical situation. Chronic pain is typically observed.

chronic infection: Ongoing and often slowly progressing infection. Usually develops from a acute infection and can last for days to months to a lifetime.

chronic pain: Pain marked by an extended duration or frequent recurrence.

chronic periodontitis: See: Periodontitis.

CHS (abbrev.): Crown height space.

cicatrix: Observed fibrous connective tissue that results from wound healing. See: Scar.

cingulum: 1. An anatomical band or encircling ridge. 2. The lingual lobe of many anterior teeth; a convex protuberance at the lingual cervical one third of the anatomic crown.

circulation, blood: General term for blood supply and flow through blood vessels, organs, and tissues.

circumferential clasp: A retainer that encircles a tooth by more than 180°, including opposite angles, and which generally contacts the tooth throughout the extent of the clasp, with at least one terminal located in an undercut area.

circumferential subperiosteal implant: See: Subperiosteal implant.

circumvallate papilla: See: Papilla.

citric acid: A tricarboxylic acid that is useful as a near-saturated solution (pH = 1.4) to detoxify (cleanse) root surfaces that are contaminated and expose intrinsic collagen fibers in the hope of achieving new tissue attachment.

clamp, abutment: See: Abutment clamp.

clamping force: The result of the elastic deformation of a screw after application of torque drawing two components together. See: Preload.

clarithromycin: A semi-synthetic macrolide antibiotic used in the treatment of orofacial infections caused by gram-positive cocci and susceptible anaerobes. Its mechanism of action involves the prevention of bacteria from growing by interfering with protein synthesis. Alternative drug used for antibiotic prophylaxis.

clasp: The component of the clasp assembly that engages a portion of the tooth surface and either enters an undercut for retention or remains entirely above the height of contour to act as a reciprocating element. Generally, it is used to stabilize and retain a removable dental prosthesis.

- **Class I articulator**: See: Articulator.
- **Class I malocclusion**: See: Angle's classification of malocclusion.
- **Class I removable partial denture**: See: Kennedy classification of removable partial dentures.
- **Class II articulator**: See: Articulator.
- **Class II malocclusion**: See: Angle's classification of malocclusion.
- **Class II removable partial denture**: See: Kennedy classification of removable partial dentures.
- **Class II, Division I malocclusion**: See: Angle's classification of malocclusion.
- **Class II, Division II malocclusion**: See: Angle's classification of malocclusion.
- **Class III articulator**: See: Articulator.
- **Class III malocclusion**: See: Angle's classification of malocclusion.
- **Class III removable partial denture**: See: Kennedy classification of removable partial dentures.

- **Class IV articulator**: See: Articulator.
- **Class IV removable partial denture**: See Kennedy classification of removable partial dentures.

clavulanic acid: A beta-lactamase inhibitor sometimes combined with penicillin group antibiotics to overcome certain types of antibiotic resistance. See: Amoxicillin.

clean technique: Surgical procedure that takes place in a clinic setting. All instruments, implants, grafts, and irrigation solution used are sterile. Surgeons wear sterile gloves, but hospital operating room-level sterility is not achieved. The surgeons and assistants wear nonsterile attire and the patient is not necessarily covered by sterile drapes. See: Sterile technique.

clearance: 1. A physical state in which physical masses may pass each other without interference. 2. The gap between two bodies. 3. A measure of the body's ability to eliminate a drug.

cleft, gingival: A vertical opening, slit, or fissure in the gingiva.

cleft lip and/or palate: Most common craniofacial anomaly, occurring 1 in 600–700 live births, characterized by failure of fusion between embryologic processes during facial morphogenesis. Failure of fusion between the medial and lateral nasal and the maxillary processes results in a cleft of the lip and/or alveolar process, whereas failure of fusion between the lateral palatine processes results in a cleft of the palate. The cleft may be complete or incomplete, and it can occur unilaterally or bilaterally. Cleft lip may occur without clefting of the alveolar process or palate, and cleft palate can also occur as an isolated phenomenon.

clicking: A series of clicks, such as the snapping, cracking, or noise evident on excursions of the mandible; a distinct snapping sound or sensation, usually audible (or by stethoscope) or on palpation, which emanates from the temporomandibular joint(s) during jaw movement. It may or may not be associated with internal derangements of the temporomandibular joint.

clindamycin: Lincosamide antibiotic used in the treatment of orofacial infections caused by anaerobic bacteria. It is also active against aerobic bacteria, such as streptococci and staphylococci. Alternative drug used for antibiotic prophylaxis. Pseudomembranous colitis has been reported as a common side effect (0.01–10%) of patients taking this medication.

clinical: 1. Of or related to or conducted in or as if within a clinic. 2. Analytical or detached – clinically.

clinical attachment level: Distance from the cementoenamel junction or implant collar to the tip of a periodontal probe during soft tissue diagnostic probing. Health of the attachment apparatus can affect the measurement.

clinical crown: The portion of a tooth that projects above the free gingival margin.

clinical implant performance scale: Quantitative scale to compare different implant systems in different indications, including the complications that occur and treatment procedures necessary in the aftercare period.

clinical record: Information comprising a patient's medical and dental history, clinical findings, diagnosis, prognosis, plan of therapy, and progress of treatment.

clinometer: A device (also called an inclinometer) for measuring angles of elevation, slope, tilt, inclination, or depression. The device is used to measure range of motion in joints and for measuring angles in the body, particularly in the pelvis, back, and neck.

clinometric: Of, relating to, or ascertained by a clinometer.

clinometry: The art or operation of measuring the inclination of strata.

clip: A retentive element within an overdenture used for its fixation to a bar. See: Bar overdenture.

clip bar overdenture: Overdenture prosthesis receiving partial retention from a bar clip. It is embedded in the impression surface of the restoration.

clone: Refers to the progeny of a somatic cell all having identical genotype.

closed architecture: Software or hardware restricted to a specific company's digital equipment or digital workflow.

closed curettage: Elimination of tissue or biological debris contiguous to a tooth via entry into the gingival crevice without flap reflection. See: Curettage.

closed lock: An internal (Type II) imbalance of the temporomandibular joint in which the condyle is blocked from sliding under the anteriorly and medially displaced articular disk.

closed reduction of a fracture: Repositioning of bone fragments through manipulation only, that is, without surgical intervention.

closed-tray impression: (syn): Indirect impression. Impression technique that uses an impression coping with positioning features, around which a rigid elastic impression material is injected. After removal of the impression, the coping is unthreaded from the mouth, connected to a laboratory analog and repositioned into the impression prior to pouring. See: Open-tray impression.

closest speaking space: The interdental clearance provided by the maxillary and mandibular incisor teeth during speaking jaw motion while pronouncing fricatives and sibilants.

closure force: Force generated by muscles of mastication. See: Biting force.

closure screw: Surgical component inserted into the head of the implant or the occlusal surface of an implant. It is intended to obturate the access opening of the implant so as to prevent debris from flowing into or plugging the access. See: Cover screw.

clot: See: Blood clot.

cloud computing: The practice of using a network of remote servers hosted online to store, manage, and process data, rather than a local server or a personal computer.

cloud sourcing: Process by which specialized cloud products and services and their deployment and maintenance are outsourced to and provided by one or more cloud service providers.

cloud storage: A model of data storage in which the digital data is stored in logical pools, and the physical storage spans multiple servers (and often locations). The physical environment is typically owned and managed by a hosting company. Cloud storage providers are responsible for keeping the data available, accessible, and secure. They also ensure that the physical environment is protected and running. People and organizations buy or lease storage capacity from the providers to store user, organization, and other critical data.

cluster (implant) failure: The occurrence of multiple dental implant failures in one or a minute group of patients derived from a large pool of subjects.

clutch coll: A device affixed to the maxillary and mandibular arches to support components that record mandibular movement.

CMV (abbrev.): Cytomegalovirus. A DNA virus, genetically distinct from other herpesviruses, that grows more readily in fibroblasts than in epithelial and lymphoid cells; causes cytomegalic inclusion disease and mononucleosis, and is secreted in renal transplant patients.

CNC (abbrev.): Computer numerical control machining.

co-adapted: In dentistry, the proper realignment of displaced parts back to their original position, as in the fractured incisal edge of a central incisor that may be co-adapted and bonded back to its original position.

coagulation: The process of changing liquid to solid, especially of blood; clotting.

coagulum: A clot or a coagulated mass.

coagulum, osseous: See: Osseous coagulum.

coaptation: Proper alignment of the displaced edges of a wound or the ends of a fractured bone.

coating: 1. Abutment: Surface treatment for an abutment to alter its optical transmission characteristics. 2. A substance applied to all or a portion of the dental implant. See: Additive surface treatment, Textured surface.

coccobacillus: A descriptive term of bacterial cell morphology referring to a structure intermediate in shape between a true coccus and a bacillus (rod).

cohesion: 1. The act or state of sticking together tightly. 2. The force whereby molecules of matter adhere to one another; the attraction of aggregation. 3. Molecular attraction by which the particles of a body are united throughout their mass.

cohort study: Study in which subjects who presently have a certain condition and/or receive a particular treatment are followed over time and compared with another group who are not affected by the condition under investigation.

col: Taken from a geography term meaning the pass or depression between two mountains; in dentistry, it refers to the gingival depression between the teeth that connects the facial and lingual papillae. It follows the shape of the interproximal contact in healthy gingiva.

cold-curing resin: See: Autopolymerizing resin.

collagen: A molecule characterized by a triple helical structure and a high content of glycine, proline, and hydroxyproline. It is the major constituent of connective tissue fibers, the organic matrix of bone, dentin, cementum, and basal laminas. Collagen is synthesized by fibroblasts, chondroblasts, osteoblasts, and odontoblasts. Several types are found in the human body. Type 1 collagen is one of the first products synthesized by the body when bone formation occurs.

collagenase: A metalloproteinase that catalyzes the breakdown of collagen, a key component of the extracellular matrix. It is also responsible for the cleavage of procollagen, which is secreted by the cell during the normal process of collagen production.

collagen fiber: See: Fiber.

collagen fleece: Collagen fleece is made from the natural collagen of porcine dermis. The 3D structure of the collagen is preserved by gentle processing and, through the aggregation of thrombocytes, promotes the formation and stabilizing of blood clots during the initial wound healing phase. Collagen fleece is used, for example, to treat soft tissue extraction points and minor bone defects. In addition to its outstanding adhesive properties, the fleece retains its shape and structure when wet. When hydrated, it forms a smooth gel which can be easily draped. It is also used as a natural local hemostyptic, which is volume stable and fully resorbed after 2–4 weeks.

collagen membrane: Resorbable barrier membrane made of heterogenic collagen, developed for guided tissue regeneration (GTR) or guided bone regeneration (GBR) techniques. The resorption time of collagen membranes can be controlled using methods of collagen cross-linking. See: Barrier membrane.

collar: See: Implant collar.

collateral ligaments: In the jaw, this refers to paired ligaments that limit motion of the lower jaw within the confines of physiologic motion. Ligaments connect bone to bone and do not stretch, so when working collaterally they limit joint movement. One example of collateral ligaments is in the temporomandibular joint, where they assist in the hinging motion of the joint and prevent the head of the condyle from popping out of the joint.

colonization: Formation and establishment of population groups of the same type of microorganism, such as in the periodontal pocket.

color: 1. To apply colors. 2. To produce color or color effects. 3. To apply or combine colors to produce an effect.

color matching: Art and science of combining the attributes of color and color mixtures to include the properties of hue, value, saturation, opacity, translucency, and pigment loading.

color rendering index: A number from 1 to 100 given to a light source to indicate its relative equivalence to pure white light which has a color rendering index (CRI) of 100. The closer the number is to 100, the more it resembles pure white light.

color scale: An orderly arrangement of colors showing graduated change in some attribute or attributes of color as a value scale.

combination clasp: A clasp for a removable dental prosthesis that has a circumferential retainer comprising a wrought wire retentive clasp and a cast reciprocal (stabilizing) arm.

combination syndrome: The clinical changes observed when an edentulous maxillary arch is opposed by a mandible with retained anterior teeth that may or may not be extruded and missing posterior teeth. Over time, there is a loss of bone in the premaxilla and in the edentulous posterior mandible, overgrowth of the maxillary tuberosities, and hyperplasia of the hard palate mucosa. Also referred to as anterior hyperfunction syndrome, or Kelly syndrome.

comfort cap: Element designed to fit over a component such as the transmucosal abutment. Intended to cover the component to protect the intraoral tissues from a detectable edge and/or prevent damage to the exposed surfaces of the component. See: Healing abutment.

commercially pure titanium (CP-Ti): Biocompatible metal commonly used for dental implants. It is an alloy of approximately 99 wt.% titanium and small amounts (from 0.18 to 0.40 wt.%) of oxygen with trace amounts (less than 0.25 wt.%) of iron, carbon, hydrogen, and nitrogen. Commercially pure titanium is classified in multiple grades. The amount of oxygen determines the grade of the alloy. See: Titanium, Titanium alloy.

comminute: The reduction of food into small parts, comminution.

comminuted fracture: A complex bone fracture characterized by breaks in several places in the same area, crushed and/or splintered.

commissural: (adj): See: Commissure.

commissure: A meeting point or junction between two anatomic structures, such as the corners of the mouth.

commissure splint: A device placed between the lips that helps increase the separation between them. Such a device is often used when surgical, electrical, or chemical damage of the lips has caused contracture or restriction of the lips. Also known as a lip splint.

compact bone: Concentrically arranged dense bone solidly filled with inorganic salts and organic ground substance with the presence of small spaces called lacunae filled with osteocytes (bone cells). See: Bone, compact, cortical.

compatible: Refers to the interchangeability of prosthetic components of one implant system to another. See: Biocompatible.

compensating curve: The curve created by the alignment of the occlusal and incisal surfaces of artificial teeth that compensates for the condylar path when the mandible moves from centric to eccentric positions and provides for a balanced occlusion. The compensating curve corresponds to the curve of Spee in a natural dentition. See: Curve of Spee.

complaint: A symptom, malady, ailment, disorder, or disease reported by a patient.

complement: A group of serum proteins involved in the control of inflammation, the activation of phagocytes, and the lytic attack on cell membranes. The system can be activated by interaction with antigen-antibody complexes or by bacterial substances.

complementary colors: 1. Two different colors that form a neutral color when mixed together in correct proportions; complementary colored light creates white light upon mixture in an additive process, and mixtures are determined by the laws of additive color. If complementary, colorants mixed together form gray or black, and mixtures are determined by the laws of subtractive colorant mixtures. 2. Colors directly opposite on the color wheel. Complementary colorants form gray or black when mixed. Also follows the laws of subtractive color.

complete arch subperiosteal implant: A device placed under the periosteum on the residual ridge to provide abutments for supporting a removable or fixed dental prosthesis in a fully edentulous arch. Usage of such implants should be described by means of the relationship to their bases of support, the alveolar bone. As such, at placement, the implant is described as an eposteal dental implant. See: Eposteal dental implant.

complete cleft palate: A cleft or opening that extends through the anterior portion of the alveolar ridge as well as the primary and secondary palates.

complete crown: A restoration, frequently made of cast metal or a ceramic material, that covers all five surfaces of a tooth: mesial, distal, occlusal, facial, lingual.

complete denture: Prosthesis, usually removable, used to replace all of the dentition and related structures of the maxillary or mandibular arch.

complete denture prosthetics: 1. The replacement of the natural teeth in at least one arch using man-made materials. 2. The art and science of restoring the appearance and function of an edentulous mouth.

complete denture prosthodontics: The art and science related to knowledge and skills about restoring an edentulous arch with a dental prosthetic device.

complete facial moulage: A process consisting of an impression that records the soft tissue contours of the face.

complete subperiosteal implant: See: Subperiosteal implant.

compliance: Action in accordance with recommendation(s).

complicated fracture: A break or disruption in an osseous structure that then causes an injury to adjacent structures like organs, nerves, or blood vessels.

complication: Unexpected deviation from the normal treatment outcome. It is generally classified as either technical or biological, e.g., surgical complication, hemorrhage, damage to the inferior alveolar nerve, infection, delayed wound healing, or lack of osseointegration. See: Esthetic complication.

compomer: A polyacid-modified composite resin containing an acid-modified dimethacrylate resin, glass ionomer fillers, and a photo initiator.

component, implant: See: Implant component.

components of occlusion: The structures related to how the teeth interact, which includes the temporomandibular joints, muscles that are related, the teeth, jaws, and other supporting or related soft and hard tissues.

composite bone: Transitional state between woven and lamellar bone, in which a woven bone lattice filled with lamellar bone can be seen histologically.

composite graft: Graft composed of multiple graft types (e.g., autogenous-synthetic graft or autogenous-xenograft), which may be mixed or layered within the defect.

composite resin: A highly cross-linked polymeric material reinforced by a dispersion of amorphous silica, glass, crystalline, or organic resin filler particles and/or short fibers bonded to the matrix by a coupling agent.

compound joint: A joint in the body that involves three or more bones.

compressive stress: Stress caused by a load (two forces applied toward one another in the same straight line) that tends to compress or shorten an object. See: Bending stress, Stress.

compromised osteogenesis: Any interference with osteogenesis. Lack of primary stability during the placement of implants in the osteotomy site may lead to fibrous integration of the implant, instead of osseointegration.

computed axial tomography (CAT): Imaging technique that uses a combination of X-rays and computer technology to generate a three-dimensional, panoramic, or cross-sectional image of a bodily structure. Data acquisition is through a series of scans along a single axis of a bodily structure, in implant dentistry parallel to the occlusal plane. It can be used for the treatment planning of dental implants with software-based planning.

computed tomography (CT): A radiologic two-dimensional representation of a three-dimensional depiction of a patient's anatomic structures. The images formed depict anatomic osseous structures that can be measured and examined for dental implant placement. A computer is used to arrange the collected radiographic images into a single view. See also: Cone beam computed tomography.

computer-aided design (CAD): The use of computer programs to create two- or three- dimensional (2D or 3D) graphical representations of physical objects. CAD software may be specialized for specific applications.

computer-aided design and drafting (CADD): The use of computer technology for the process of design and design documentation. Computer-aided drafting describes the process of drafting with a computer. CADD software provides the user with input tools for the purpose of streamlining design processes, drafting, documentation, and manufacturing processes.

computer-aided design/computer-aided manufacturing (CAD/CAM): Process for direct preparation of an object from computer-acquired or computer-generated data.

computer-aided design/computer-assisted manufacture (CAD/CAM): Computer technology used to design and manufacture various components.

computer-aided manufacturing (CAM): The use of computer software to control machine tools and related machinery in the manufacturing of work pieces. Its primary purpose is to create a faster production process and components and tooling with more precise dimensions and material consistency. In some cases, it uses only the required amount of raw material (thus minimizing waste), while simultaneously reducing energy consumption.

computer-aided navigation: Computer system for intraoperative navigation, which provides the surgeon with current positions of the instruments and operation site on a three-dimensional reconstructed image of the patient that is displayed on a monitor in the operating room. The system aims to transfer preoperative planning on radiographs or computed tomography scans on the patient, in real-time, and independent of the position of the patient's head.

computer-assisted manufacture surgical guidance: Computed tomography imaging augmented by implant placement planning to fabricate a surgical template for osteotomy localization during surgery.

computer-assisted surgical guide: See: Stereolithographic guide.

computer numerical control machining (CNC): Numeric set of instructions generated from CAM software that governs the machine movements of a milling apparatus or 3D printer in order to fabricate an object.

computer simulation (computer model or computational model): A computer program, or network of computers, that attempts to simulate an abstract model of a particular system.

concrescence: When the roots of adjacent teeth are joined via cementum deposits.

concretion: A predominantly inorganic mass in a cavity or in the tissue of an organism.

condensation: The process of using force to ensure continuity of the matrix phase and removal of excess mercury when compacting dental amalgam.

condensing osteitis: See: Osteitis, condensing.

conditioned reflex: A learned response to a stimulus.

condylar agenesis: A congenital anomaly depicted by the absence of the condyle.

condylar articulator: A device that replicates the position and movement of the jaws whereby the artificial condyle is represented by a metallic ball that interacts with a plane to represent the articulating surface of the temporomandibular joint. These articulators can be arcon instruments, where the metallic condyle is positioned in a similar manner to a naturally occurring condyle and moves against the artificial articulating surface, or nonarcon instruments, where the metallic plane moves against the metallic ball, unlike that which occurs in a human temporomandibular joint.

condylar axis: A theoretical line traversing through the center of the mandibular condyles and around which the mandible rotates.

condylar dislocation: A dislocation of the mandibular condyle, typically forward of the articular eminence; it is not self-correcting or self-reducing.

condylar displacement: When the condyle is not in its natural position.

condylar guidance: 1. The segment of an articulator that is located in the superior posterior region of the nonmobile member that is designed to control the movement of the movable member. 2. The pathway that the condyles traverse during translatory movements; the inclination of the path can be measured in degrees relative to the Frankfort plane.

condylar subluxation: A self-reducing incomplete or partial disarticulation of the condyle from its glenoid fossa.

condyle: A rounded articular prominence found on the end of a bone, that is, relating to the mandible. It is a bilateral ellipsoidal projection found on the superior portion of the mandible's ramus, and it articulates with the glenoid fossa. The condyle sits atop the condylar neck. The combination of the condyle and the condylar neck is referred to as the condyloid process or condylar process.

condylectomy: Surgery to remove the mandibular condyle.

condylotomy: Intended surgical cut through the neck of the condyloid process for the purpose of removing the condyle. Also used in reference to the intended surgical excision of a portion of the articulating surface of the mandibular condyle (known as a condylar shave).

cone beam computed tomography (CBCT): (syn): Helical cone beam computed tomography, Spiral cone beam computed tomography. Imaging technique that uses a cone-shaped X-ray beam to acquire multiple images of a patient. Images are captured on flat panel detectors or image intensifiers. Volume data can be acquired in a single rotation of the beam and the detector, at reduced radiation exposure. It can be used for the treatment planning of dental implants with software-based planning. Machines are often classified as large volume (20 cm height and 15 cm diameter cylinder) and small volume/limited view (40×40 mm^2 or 60×60 mm^2) based on the exposure area. See: Software-based planning.

configuration: Specific size and shape of a dental implant or component.

confirmation jig: See: Verification jig.

congenital: Present at birth.

conical abutment: A transmucosal abutment used in the fabrication of a screw-retained prosthetic reconstruction.

connecting bar: See: Bar, Bar splint.

connection, abutment: See: Abutment connection.

connective tissue: Tissue of mesodermal origin consisting of various cells (e.g., fibroblasts and macrophages) and interlacing protein fibers (e.g., collagen) embedded in a chiefly carbohydrate ground substance that supports, ensheaths, and binds together other tissues. Includes loose and dense forms (e.g., adipose tissue, tendons, ligaments, and aponeuroses) and specialized forms (e.g., cartilage and bone). See: Fibrous connective tissue.

connective tissue attachment: The mechanism of attachment of the connective tissue to a tooth or dental implant. Around the latter, the connective tissue fibers are generally parallel and circumferential to the implant surface and constitute the apical part of the biologic width.

connective tissue graft: Soft tissue augmentation procedure adopted from periodontal surgery using connective tissue harvested from a palatal donor site. See: Subepithelial connective tissue graft.

connector: In fixed dental prosthodontics, the portion of a fixed dental prosthesis that unites the retainer(s) and pontic(s).

connector, intramobile: See: Intramobile connector.

conoscopic holography: A method to determine the 3D geometry of real-world objects. In this method, the light/laser reflected from the object is split into separate beams using a crystal that possesses different refractive indices. After the two beams exit the crystal, an interference pattern that depends on the distance from the light's source is generated. This interference pattern can be used to construct a 3D image of the object.

consensus: General agreement or concord.

consolidation period: Final phase of distraction osteogenesis. Once the alveolar segment has been repositioned, the device is maintained in a static mode to act as a fixation device for a given amount of time. See: Alveolar distraction osteogenesis.

consultation: The joint deliberation, usually for explanatory or diagnostic purposes, between a patient and practitioner, or two or more practitioners.

contact osteogenesis: The formation of new bone directly on a dental implant, following the migration of osteogenic progenitor cells through the fibrin clot matrix to the implant surface. See: Distance osteogenesis.

contact scanner: Scanners that probe the subject through physical touch, while the object is in contact with or resting on a precision flat surface plate, ground and polished to a specific maximum surface roughness. Where the object to be scanned is not flat or cannot rest stably on a flat surface, it is supported and held firmly in place by a fixture. It is used to scan objects in 3D.

contact surface: The area on the proximal surface of a tooth that touches an adjacent tooth.

contagious: Communicable by contact; spreading from one to another.

continuous bar connector: A metal bar arising from terminal rests of key abutments resting on the cingulums of the mandibular anterior teeth so that it aids in their stabilization and functions as an indirect retainer in a free end distal extension dental prosthesis.

continuous beam: A beam that spans over three or more abutments and resists bending when a load or force is applied.

continuous suture: A suture made with a single strand of suture material, that is begun in the same way as a simple interrupted suture. However, it consists of a series of stitches that are not individually knotted. They are typically used when the wound is in a visible part of the body and thus the stitches will not be readily apparent.

continuous wave mode (cw-mode): Type of operation in which the laser emits radiation energy as a constant, uninterrupted stream.

contraction: **Isometric c.**: An increase in muscular tension at the same muscle length, as in clenching teeth. **Isotonic c.**: Steady muscle tension generated by a shortening muscle against a load. Work rate (power output) remains constant during an isotonic contraction. **Postural c.**: Maintenance of muscular tension (usually isometric) sufficient to maintain posture.

contracture: A shortening of a muscle that is permanent and is a consequence of fibrosis.

contraindication: Any condition of the patient (i.e., medical, psychological, or social) that makes a surgical procedure inadvisable.

contralateral: Relating to or pertaining to or occurring on the opposite side. The working of the opposite side in concert with similar parts on the primary side of interest; the opposite of ipsilateral.

contrast, radiographic image: The visible differences in photographic or film density produced on a radiograph by the structural composition of the object or objects radiographed. Radiographs made with higher kilovoltage (e.g., 90 kV) have a longer scale contrast and appear dull by comparison with those made at lower voltages, but they have improved image character for interpretation.

contrast resolution: The ability to distinguish between differences in intensity in an image. The measure is used in medical imaging to quantify the quality of acquired images. It is a difficult quantity to define, because it depends on the human observer as much as the quality of the actual image.

control group: A group of subjects which receives a placebo instead of the experimental treatment but is treated in all other respects in the same way as the experimental group. See: Case–control study, Experimental group.

conventional tomography: Film tomography. Outdated in medicine, this imaging technique is of great interest in implant dentistry because it can be applied in private practice. The X-ray tube is rigidly fixed with a bar to the image receptor to move around a fixed axis.

When a patient is properly positioned, objects located in this axis are projected on the same region in the image receptor and are clearly imaged. Objects located outside this axis are blurred. Thus, cross-sectional views can be obtained, for instance, of the maxilla and mandible to determine the width of the bone. Compare: Computed tomography (CT) scan.

convergence angle: 1. The taper of a crown preparation. 2. The angle, measured in degrees, formed between opposing axial walls when a tooth or teeth are prepared for crowns or fixed dental prostheses. Usage: this term is best described as the total occlusal convergence.

conversion prosthesis: See: Transitional prosthesis.

coolant: A fluid used as an irrigating solution to reduce heat generated during drilling.

coordination: Smooth, controlled, symmetrical movement.

cope: 1. The upper half of any flask used in casting; the upper or cavity side of a denture flask used in conjunction with the drag or lower half of the flask. See: Drag. 2. To dress, cover, or furnish with a cope; to cover, as if with a cope or coping.

coping: In fixed prosthodontics, the metal substrate on which porcelain is applied in fabrication of a metal-ceramic restoration. Also used to describe the initial thin layer of wax on a die or a thin covering or crown.

coping design: Specific coping shape or pattern, or the method by which it is made or planned. The coping is designed specifically for use within an implant system.

coping impression: An impression, usually encompassing an entire dental arch, that uses metal or resin copings placed on prepared teeth. The copings are repositioned before the pouring of a working cast.

coping pick-up impression: See: Coping impression.

coping prosthesis: See: Overdenture.

coping screw: Prosthetic component (i.e., screw) incorporated as part of the anchorage by means of engaging threads so as to maintain the position of a coping (e.g., impression coping). A one-piece element can also serve as the coping, which is threaded directly into the anchorage component. See: Prosthetic retaining screw.

copolymer resin: Polymer formed from more than one type of molecular repeat unit.

copper band: A cylinder made from copper and used as a matrix for making an impression.

coral-derived   hydroxyapatite: Ca_2CO_3 skeleton of naturally occurring corals converted via a hydrothermic process to a non-biodegradable porous hydroxyapatite.

coralliform: Possessing the form of coral; coral-like in its branching; usually with reference to various types of implant materials made from hydroxyapatite.

coralline: A form of ceramic from the calcium carbonate skeleton of coral, used as a bone substitute. See: Alloplast, Porous coralline hydroxyapatite.

core-binding factor alpha 1 (CBFα1): An essential transcription factor for osteoblast differentiation and subsequent bone formation. Also called runt-related transcription factor 2 (runx2). See: Bone morphogenetic protein (BMP).

co-registration: (syn): Registration.

coronal: 1. Of or relating to a corona or crown. 2. Relating to any longitudinal plane or section that passes through a body at right angles to the median plane. 3. Pertaining to the crown of a tooth.

coronal plane: Aligning in the direction of the coronal suture, the plane that separates the front from the back of the body.

coronally positioned flap: A flap sutured in a direction coronal to its original presurgical position. See: Apically positioned flap.

coronoidectomy: Surgical excision of the coronoid process.

corrective soft tissue surgery: Plastic surgery procedure aimed at correcting either an inherited or acquired soft tissue defect. The surgery may include augmentation with a soft tissue graft (either connective tissue or free gingival graft) or correction of previous surgical scarring.

correlation coefficient: Number between -1 and $+1$ which measures the degree to which two variables are linearly related. -1 indicates perfect linear negative relationship between two variables, $+1$

indicates perfect positive linear relationship and 0 indicates lack of any linear relationship.

corrode: 1. To deteriorate or oxidize a metal as a result of electrochemical reaction within its environment. 2. Gradual deterioration, usually by chemical action.

corrosion: 1. The deterioration of a material by electrochemical reaction with the environment. The term corrosion usually refers to oxidation of metals, known as *rusting*, which results in a layer of oxide or salt on the surface. The deterioration often affects properties of the material, such as strength, appearance, and permeability. Corrosion can also occur in other materials, such as ceramics or polymers. 2. The action, process, or effect of corroding; a result of corroding. 3. The loss of elemental components to the bordering environment.

corrosion resistance: Surface passivity rather than intrinsic unreactivity.

corrosive: Tending or having the power to corrode.

corrugation: Addition of parallel folds or grooves to a surface so as to increase the relative surface area or the stiffness of the material.

cortical bone: The outer layer of osseous tissue. Cortical bone is one of the two categories of osseous tissue that make up bone. Cortical bone, the outer layer, is dense, in contrast to the inner layer, called cancellous bone, which is much less dense. Also known as compact bone. See: Bone, Bone remodeling.

cortical bone graft: Graft consisting of compact bone. See: Cancellous bone graft, Corticocancellous bone graft.

cortical perforation: See: Decortication.

corticocancellous bone: Graft derived from donor sites with both cortical and cancellous components, such as the symphysis or iliac crest. Autogenous origin of this type of bone graft is ideal because of the mechanical stability, the inherent supply of bone morphogenetic proteins (BMPs) in cortical bone, and the osteogenic potential of cancellous bone.

corticocancellous bone graft: See: Bone graft.

corticosteroid: Any of the steroid hormones produced by the adrenal cortex or their synthetic equivalents. They are involved in a wide range of physiologic systems such as stress response, immune response and regulation of inflammation, carbohydrate metabolism, protein catabolism, blood electrolyte levels, and behavior. See: Glucocorticoid.

corticotomy: Any surgical cut in bone that involves the cortex, typically made in a horizontal or vertical orientation. Can be utilized to enhance bleeding sites. Also called decortication and utilized in periodontally accelerated osteogenic orthodontics.

cortisone: An oral, intramuscular, and intravenous glucocorticoid with a short half-life. See: Glucocorticoid.

Corynebacterium matruchotii: A gram-positive, nonmotile, facultatively anaerobic bacterium commonly found in dental plaque. Capable of forming calcium hydroxyapatite and contributing to dental calculus formation. Formerly named *Bacterionema matruchotii.*

cosmetic periodontal surgery: Surgical periodontal procedures to improve gingival esthetics and achieve an ideal soft tissue–teeth relationship. It includes treatment of gingival recession, gingivectomy, and gingivoplasty.

cost analysis: Investigation and examination of factors related to value.

cost-benefit analysis (CBA): Study designed to assess all outcomes based on monetary costs and benefits. All study results are conveyed in dollars or euros. An economic conversion is used to give a monetary amount to intangible results.

cost-effectiveness analysis (CEA): Study comparing two or more therapies on the bases of monetary costs and clinical effectiveness. Results are usually reported in units of dollars or euros per clinical outcome. The outcome of therapies to be compared with CEA must be expressed in the same units.

coumadin: An anticoagulant that inhibits the hepatic synthesis of the vitamin K-dependent coagulation factors.

countersink: To enlarge with a specific drill the coronal part of an osteotomy, to accommodate the neck of a dental implant.

countersink drill: Drill used to enlarge the coronal part of an osteotomy.

countersinking: Bone preparation of the crestal area using special countersinking drills to allow an apical implant placement resulting in a subcrestal position of the implant shoulder or platform.

coupling: A device that serves to link or connect the ends of adjacent parts or objects.

cover screw: Screw with head design to fit over the implant and seal the occlusal surface of the implant prior to wound closure in a two-stage surgical implant procedure. See: Closure screw, Healing screw.

cover screw mill: Instrument or device used to remove excess bone growth over a cover screw.

coxsackievirus: An enterovirus occasionally found in association with ulcerative oral lesions.

CP-Ti (abbrev.): Commercially pure titanium.

cranial bone: Any of the bones surrounding the brain, comprising the paired bones (i.e., parietal and temporal) and the unpaired bones (i.e., occipital, frontal, sphenoid, and ethmoid). Also called calvarial bone.

cranial bone harvest: Bone taken from any of the bones surrounding the brain.

craniofacial implant: See: Percutaneous implant.

craniofacial implant prosthesis: See: Craniofacial prosthesis.

craniofacial prosthesis: Extraoral restoration replacing a portion of the cranium or face and retained by skin-penetrating implants or adhesives. See also: Maxillofacial prosthetics.

crater: A saucer-shaped defect of soft tissue or bone, often seen interdentally. See: Bony defect.

craterization: See: Pericervical saucerization.

crazing: Multiple superficial cracks or loss of surface integrity that may or may not progress into complete fractures.

creep: Property of a material, usually metal, to deform or elongate under pressure that is either cyclic or constant.

creeping substitution: See: Bone remodeling.

crepitation: A snapping or grating noise and/or sensation in a joint during movement; related to the temporomandibular joint, a crackling sound made when one opens and closes the jaw; the noise made when the ends of fractured bone rub together.

crepitus (crepitation): A crackling or grating noise in a joint during movement.

crest: A projection. Usually refers to the most coronal portion of an edentulous ridge. See: Alveolar crest.

crest of the ridge: The highest continuous surface of the residual ridge, not necessarily coincident with the center of the ridge.

crestal: Pertaining to the crest or the most coronal portion of the ridge.

crestal bone loss: Bone resorption of the most coronal aspect of the ridge around the neck of the implant. See: Atrophic alveolar bone.

crestal implant placement: The placement of a dental implant with the edge of its platform at the crest of bone. 1. Subcrestal implant placement: the placement of a dental implant with the edge of its platform apical to the crest of bone. 2. Supracrestal implant placement: the placement of a dental implant with the edge of its platform coronal to the crest of bone.

crestal incision: An incision made at the crest of the edentulous ridge. See: Midcrestal incision, Mucobuccal fold incision, Paracrestal incision.

crestal lamina dura: The layer of compact bone at the alveolar crest. See: Lamina dura.

crevicular epithelium: Epithelial lining of the gingival crevice, sulcus, or periodontal pocket; generally, a stratified squamous epithelium. Also called sulcular epithelium: the nonkeratinized epithelium of the gingival crevice.

crevicular fluid: The fluid that is typically produced in the presence of inflammation and seeps through the crevicular epithelium; it can serve as a defense mechanism against infection by carrying antibodies and other substances into the sulcus. Also known as sulcular fluid and gingival fluid. See: Gingival crevicular fluid (GCF).

cribriform: Perforated like a sieve, for example, the cribriform plate of the ethmoid sinus.

cribriform plate: In dentistry, the alveolar bone proper. Another example is the horizontal plate of bone of the ethmoid sinus, which is perforated by numerous foramina that allow passage of nerves through the bone.

critical bending moment: The moment at which the external nonaxial load applied overcomes screw joint preload, causing loss of contact between the mating surfaces of the dental implant screw joint components.

critical-size(d) defect (CSD): Smallest osseous defect that does not completely heal by spontaneous bone regeneration. Its size varies by anatomic location and species.

Crohn's disease: Also known as regional enteritis, a chronic, granulomatous disease of unknown cause involving any part of the gastrointestinal tract, but commonly involving the terminal ileum. Oral lesions may be granulomatous in nature.

cross-arch balanced articulation: The simultaneous contact of the buccal and lingual cusps of the working side maxillary teeth with the opposing buccal and lingual cusps of the mandibular teeth, concurrent with contact of the nonworking side maxillary lingual cusps with the mandibular buccal cusps.

cross-arch stabilization: Resistance against dislodging or rotational forces obtained by using a partial removable dental prosthesis design that uses natural teeth on the opposite side of the dental arch from the edentulous space to assist in stabilization.

cross-bite: A dental condition where a mandibular tooth is located facial to the opposing tooth. Normal dentition locates the mandibular dentition lingual to the maxillary dentition. **Anterior c.**: One or more maxillary incisors positioned on the lingual side of the mandibular incisors when the jaws are closed. **Posterior c.**: One or more maxillary posterior teeth positioned in a palatal relationship with the mandibular teeth when the jaws are closed.

cross-bite occlusion: Occluding tooth contact in which the natural or artificial mandibular teeth overlap the maxillary teeth. Also called reverse articulation.

cross-sectional slice: A thin, reformatted section of computed tomography scan data representing the alveolar process perpendicular to a panoramic curve of the patient's mandible or maxilla. See: Axial slice, Panoramic reconstitution.

cross-sectional study: A type of study that involves the observation of a defined population at a single point in time or time interval.

crowding: Discrepancy between tooth sizes and arch length and/or tooth positioning that results in malalignment and abnormal contact relationships between teeth.

crown: 1. Highest part of an object, such as with the normally exposed part of a natural tooth covered by enamel, or an artificial restoration replacing part or all of the coronal portion of a tooth or implant abutment for esthetic and functional purposes. See: Acrylic restoration, Ceramic restoration. 2. To place on the head, as to place a crown on a tooth, dental implant or tooth substitute. Usage: implies fabrication of a restoration for a tooth on a natural tooth, dental implant and/or dental implant abutment.

crown exposure: This procedure is used in an otherwise periodontally healthy area to remove enlarged gingival tissue to provide an anatomically correct gingival relationship with the anatomic crowns. In some instances, removal of supporting bone (ostectomy) may be required.

crown height space (CHS): Distance from the crest of bone to the plane of occlusion in the posterior region and to the incisal edge of the same arch in the anterior region, available for a prosthesis.

crown lengthening: A surgical procedure designed to increase the extent of supragingival tooth structure, primarily for restorative purposes, by apically positioning the gingival margins with or without the removal of supporting bone. See: Anatomic crown exposure.

crown-implant ratio: the ratio determined by measuring the total height of the restoration and implant.

crown-root ratio: The ratio determined by measuring the total height of the tooth above alveolar bone compared with the height of the tooth's root within alveolar bone; it is typically evaluated by radiograph.

cryosurgery: Destruction of tissue by extreme cold. Usually achieved with liquid nitrogen or carbon dioxide.

cryotherapy: Extraorally, the postsurgical application of cold dressings to reduce inflammation and pain. Intraorally, the freezing of tissue with a cold device.

crypt: 1. A chamber wholly or partly underground. 2. In anatomy, a pit, depression or simple tubular gland.

CSD (abbrev.): Critical-size(d) defect.

CT (abbrev.): Computed tomography, Connective tissue.

C-telopeptide cross-linked collagen type 1: syn. C-terminal telopeptide of type 1 collagen. Fragment of collagen released during bone remodeling and turnover. It is a biochemical marker in a variety of osseous metabolic diseases such as osteoporosis.

CTx (abbrev.): C-telopeptide test for type 1 collagen.

culture: The propagation of microorganisms or living tissue cells in special media conducive to their growth.

cumulative success rate: Estimate of the proportion of successful implants based on a predefined set of criteria, from baseline to time of interest. See: Life table analysis, Success rate.

cumulative survival rate: Estimate of the proportion of successful implants that have not led to tooth or implant loss, from baseline to time of interest. See: Life table analysis.

cuneiform: Wedge-shaped.

curative: Tending to overcome disease and promote recovery.

curet or curette: Instrument used to debride tissue. In periodontics, a curette is used for scaling and planing of tooth roots or implant surfaces and for debridement (also called curettage) of periodontal pockets and bone.

curettage: Scraping, cleaning, or debriding biological material or debris from the walls of a defect or surface by means of a curette. **Apical c.**: Surgical removal of tissue or foreign material surrounding the apex of a tooth. Also known as periapical curettage. **Gingival c.**: The process of debriding the soft tissue wall of a periodontal pocket. **Open c.**: A surgical procedure involving the debridement of tooth roots and removal of infected sulcular epithelium (granulation tissue) after flap reflection. **Surgical c.**: Elimination of tissue or biological debris contiguous to a tooth by the reflection of a flap. See: Bone curettage.

curette, periodontal: A periodontal instrument with a fine blade used primarily for removing the inner lining of pocket walls and epithelial attachment. Also used for removing periodontal fibers from walls of osseous defects and removing calculus fragments.

curtain procedure: A procedure designed to retain the marginal portion of the facial and interproximal gingiva for esthetic purposes in the surgical treatment of periodontal pockets, usually in the maxillary anterior region.

curve of Spee: Curved line produced by connecting the tip of the natural mandibular canine with the buccal cusps of the premolars and molars and extended to the anterior border of the mandibular ramus. This anatomic observation was first made by F.G. Spee in the 19th century. In the absence of natural teeth, this curve is developed to compensate for condylar path influence on occlusal contacts in the creation of a balanced occlusion, hence the term compensating curve.

cusp: Cone-shaped protuberance on the crown of a tooth that forms the occlusal surface.

cusp inclination: Relative cusp height of artificial teeth; affects the loading pattern of a supporting dental implant.

cuspid guidance: See: Canine protection.

custom abutment: A custom component created for a specific clinical situation, which can be generated by casting a waxed castable abutment or by CAD/CAM.

custom tray: A personalized impression tray prepared from a cast derived from a preliminary impression. The custom tray is used in making the final impression.

cuticle: A thin, acellular, organic structure overlying the enamel surface; proteinaceous, and may contain tissue components.

cutis: See: Skin.

cutting cone: See: Bone remodeling unit (BRU), Basic multicellular unit (BMU).

cutting resistance analysis (CRA): The energy (J/mm^3) required for a current-fed electric motor in cutting off a unit volume of bone during implant surgery, used to assess bone density.

cutting torque: Turning or twisting force produced by a rotary device (i.e., dental handpiece) to cut through a material such as bone.

cyanoacrylate: A single-component, moisture-activated, thermoplastic group of adhesives characterized by rapid polymerization and excellent bond strength.

cyclosporine: An immunosuppressant and antifungal agent used to prevent rejection in organ transplant recipients. It can be associated with gingival overgrowth.

cylinder implant: An endosseous, root-form, press-fit dental implant, with parallel-sided walls.

cylinder-to-transmucosal element: See: Gold cylinder attachment.

cylinder wrench: Device that fits on top of a dental implant and is used to tighten the implant after its placement. It can also be used to place an implant into its osteotomy.

cylindrical implant: An endosseous, root-form dental implant, with parallel-sided non-threaded walls. One such design, determined either in cross-section or three-dimension, follows the shape of a cylinder for an endosteal implant.

cyst: A pathologic cavity lined by epithelium and usually containing fluid or semi-solid material. **Apical periodontal c.**: The most common odontogenic cyst, involving the apex of a root and resulting from the inflammatory reaction to a nonvital pulp. **Calcifying cystic odontogenic tumor**: An odontogenic cyst found most often in the mandibular canine and premolar region; has distinct microscopic features including basal epithelial cells that resemble ameloblasts. **Dentigerous c.**: Forms around the crown of an unerupted tooth or odontoma. **Gingival c.**: Found within the gingiva, most commonly in the mandibular canine-premolar region. Believed to be derived from epithelial rests of the dental lamina. **Keratocystic odontogenic tumor**: Developmental odontogenic cyst of the dental lamina in which the epithelial cells produce keratin, known for its aggressive nature and high recurrence rate. **Mucocele**: A cyst or cyst-like structure that contains mucous glycoproteins. A mucocele is an extraductal extravasation of mucus into surrounding stroma. **Odontogenic c.**: A class of cysts derived from odontogenic epithelium, such as primordial, dentigerous, and lateral periodontal cysts. **Primordial c.**: An odontogenic cyst resulting from degeneration of the enamel organ of a developing tooth bud. The vast majority of all primordial cysts are odontogenic keratocysts upon histopathologic examination. **Radicular c.**: A cyst along the root of a tooth. Also known as an apical periodontal cyst. **Ranula**: Forms in the floor of the mouth as a result of trauma or blockage of a salivary gland duct. It may be lined with epithelium. A ranula is mucus extravasation occurring in the floor of the mouth and usually associated with a sublingual gland. **Residual c.**: A cyst in the maxilla or mandible that remains after the associated tooth has been removed. **Retention c.**: Caused by retention of glandular secretion.

Simple bone c.: Benign, empty or fluid-filled space within bone that is lacking an epithelial lining. Also known as hemorrhagic bone cyst or traumatic bone cyst. **Traumatic (hemorrhagic bone) c.**: A radiolucent lesion in the bone without a radiopaque border; a cavity of disputed cause, lined by extremely thin or no tissue, which may contain fluid (blood or serum). It is assumed to have been caused by trauma. Teeth, if present, are vital. Not a true cyst.

cytokine: Any of several regulatory proteins, such as the interleukins and lymphokines, that are released by cells of the immune system and act as intercellular or intracellular mediators in the generation of an immune response, e.g., platelet-derived growth factor (PDGF), insulin growth factors (IGFs), transforming growth factor beta 1 (TGF-β1), bone morphogenetic proteins (BMPs), and epidermal growth factor (EGF).

cytomegalovirus (CMV): A DNA virus, genetically distinct from other herpesviruses, that grows more readily in fibroblasts than in epithelial and lymphoid cells; causes cytomegalic inclusion disease and mononucleosis, and is secreted in renal transplant patients.

cytotoxic: Having the ability to kill cells.

cytotoxin: An agent that inhibits or prevents the function of cells.

D

dark-field microscopy: A technique utilizing a microscope modified by a special condenser that allows light to enter only peripherally so that objects such as microorganisms are obliquely illuminated and glow against a dark background.

DBM (abbrev.): Demineralized bone matrix.

debridement: Removal of inflamed, devitalized, or contaminated tissue or foreign material from or adjacent to a lesion.

debris: An accumulation of foreign material on the teeth and adjacent structures.

decalcification: The process of removing the mineral content from a hard tissue, such as bone or tooth, with the aid of acids.

decay: Demineralization of tooth structure leading to decomposition and destruction of tooth structure and then cavitation. See: Caries.

deciduous dentition: See: Dentition, Primary dentition.

decoronation: A conservative method to treat an ankylosed tooth for preservation of width and height of the alveolar process.

decortication: Intraoperative preparation of the recipient bone bed by making numerous small perforations into the cortex to induce bleeding from the marrow cavity. This technique is routinely used in combination with onlay block grafts or guided bone regeneration (GBR) procedures.

decreased occlusal vertical dimension: A reduction in the distance measured between two anatomic points when the teeth are in occlusal contact.

deep bite: See: Vertical overlap.

deepithelialize: To remove the epithelial layer of soft tissue, exposing the underlying connective tissue.

deep sedation: A drug-induced depression of consciousness during which patients cannot be easily aroused but respond purposefully following repeated or painful stimulation. The ability to independently maintain ventilatory function may be impaired.

defect: An imperfection, failure, or absence. See: Alveolar defect, Ridge defect.

definitive cast: A replica of the tooth surfaces, residual ridge areas, and/or other parts of the dental arch and/or facial structures used to fabricate a dental restoration or prosthesis. Also called final cast.

definitive prosthesis: The final prosthetic reconstruction. Any dental or maxillofacial prosthesis that will not require any further modification. Such prostheses are designed and intended for long-term use.

deflective occlusal contact: 1. The slide encountered from the initial point of tooth contact during mandibular closure causing a deviation in the mandible. 2. An undesirable contact that displaces a tooth, deters the mandible from its anticipated arc of closure, and/or dislodges a removable denture from its intended position. Also known as occlusal prematurity.

dehisce: To open at definite places; to split or peel down along a natural line; to rupture or discharge the contents by splitting open.

dehiscence: 1. Incomplete coverage or cleft-like absence of bone at a localized area around a tooth or a dental implant, extending

Glossary of Dental Implantology, First Edition. Khalid Almas, Fawad Javed and Steph Smith.
© 2018 John Wiley & Sons, Inc. Published 2018 by John Wiley & Sons, Inc.

for a variable distance from the crest. See: Fenestration. 2. Premature opening of a primary soft tissue closure.

delayed loading: Refers to the time of applying occlusal forces to a dental implant after its initial placement. A prosthesis is attached or secured after a conventional healing period. See: Early loading.

delivery: See: Placement.

delta E: Total color difference computed by use of a color difference equation. It is generally calculated as the square root of the sums of the squares of the chromaticity difference and the lightness difference.

demineralization: 1. Loss of minerals (as salts of calcium) from the body. 2. In dentistry, decalcification, usually related to the dental caries process.

demineralized bone matrix (DBM): Bone matrix, usually allogeneic in origin, that may induce bone formation via release of growth factors and bone morphogenetic proteins (BMPs) from the matrix, occasionally after osteoclastic breakdown. Osteoinductive potential may vary, dependent on method of preparation and degree of demineralization.

demineralized freeze-dried bone allograft (DFDBA): By demineralization, the mineral phase of freeze-dried bone allografts is partly or completely removed so that the collagen and noncollagenous matrix are exposed, thereby making growth factors available.

denervation: Resection of or removal of the nerves to an organ or part.

dens in dente: A developmental abnormality in tooth formation resulting from invagination of the epithelium associated with coronal development into the area that was destined to become the pulp space.

dental articulation: The contact relationships of the occlusal surfaces of the maxillary and mandibular teeth when moved against each other (gliding occlusion).

dental biomechanics: The relationship between the biologic behavior of oral structures and the physical influence of a dental restoration. Also called dental biophysics.

dental cast: A reproduction; a positive copy of segments or parts of the oral cavity.

dental casting investment: Combination of silica phosphate and gypsum bonding material used in dentistry to enclose wax or plastic patterns during the casting process in the laboratory fabrication of dental crowns and bridges. For lower casting temperatures, a gypsum bonding material is used, and for higher casting temperatures, phosphates or silica materials are used.

dental dysfunction: Atypical functioning of masticatory physiology; a disorder or functional impairment of the chewing or masticatory system.

dental dysplasia: See: Dysplasia.

dental element: Vernacular for a dental prosthesis that achieves a portion of its retention from one or more dental implants.

dental history: A complete record of all relevant aspects of an individual's oral and general health.

dental hygienist: A licensed dental auxiliary who is both an oral health educator and clinician and who uses preventive, educational, and nonsurgical therapeutic methods to control oral disease.

dental implant: 1. A device placed beneath the soft tissue layer upon (eposteal), within (endosteal), or through (transosteal) the bone to retain or support a dental prosthesis. 2. A device used to retain or support a dental abutment.

dental implant abutment: The part of a dental implant that functions to retain and/or support a removable or fixed dental prosthesis. Frequently, endosteal dental implants have a temporary or preliminary abutment before a definitive dental abutment and prosthesis is placed. Preliminary abutments are called interim (dental implant) abutments. The final abutment that supports the definitive (final) prosthesis is called a definitive (final) dental implant abutment. Dental implant abutments are often identified by their descriptive form (i.e., cylindrical, barrel), material (i.e., titanium, ceramic, zirconia ceramic), or special design factors (i.e., external/internal hex lock, Morse taper, or spline).

dental implant analog: A duplication of the entire dental implant used in the dental laboratory to assist in making a temporary or definitive prosthesis; not intended for human implantation.

dental implant attachment: The biochemical/mechanical connection between the dental implant and the hard and soft tissues to which it is attached.

dental implant loading: The process of placing often intentional axial or oblique force(s) upon a dental implant. This process is usually associated with the purposeful exposure of the dental implant at the time of surgical placement or subsequent surgical exposure. Forces may be generated from a range of causes, including habitual, deliberate, and/or unintentional.

dental implant system: Dental implant kit designed for the placement of the dental implant(s) and subsequent attachments of abutments that facilitate the retention of the dental prosthesis. The term can denote a specific concept, inventor(s), or patent(s).

dental impression: An imprint made within the oral cavity to produce a replica of the structure of interest used to make a record or to manufacture a dental restoration or prosthesis.

dental impression wax: A thermoplastic material used for making a dental impression.

dental malalignment: The displacement of a tooth from its normal position in the dental arch.

dental plaster: A slightly hydrated powder of beta calcium sulfate made from gypsum that forms a quick-setting paste when mixed with water. Used in dentistry to make casts. The beta form of calcium sulfate is an aggregate of irregularly shaped porous fine crystals. Also known as plaster of Paris.

dental prosthesis: A fixed or removable appliance used to replace one or more missing teeth and/or associated dental/alveolar structures.

dental senescence: The deterioration of teeth or other structures within the oral cavity associated with the aging process.

dental stone: A slightly hydrated powder of alpha calcium sulfate that forms a dense stone-like material when mixed with water. Used in dentistry to make casts. The alpha form of calcium sulfate is denser and superior to the beta form because it contains pieces and crystals in the form of rods or prisms.

dentate: Having teeth or pointed conical projections.

denticle: (pulp stone): A calcified mass of dentin, which may be free within the pulp, attached to the pulpal wall, or embedded in the dentin.

dentifrice: A pharmaceutical formulation commonly prepared as a paste, gel, powder or liquid which is used to clean and/or polish teeth. Active ingredients to prevent caries and plaque accumulation or to desensitize teeth may be included.

dentin: The chief substance or tissue forming the body of the teeth. It surrounds the pulp and is covered by coronal enamel and radicular cementum.

dentinal sensitivity: The short, exaggerated, painful response elicited when exposed dentin is subjected to thermal, mechanical, or chemical stimuli, often after marginal soft tissue recession has occurred. Also known as root hypersensitivity.

dentinoenamel junction: The area of union of the dentin and enamel. See: Junction.

dentition: Collective teeth in the dental arches. **Natural d.**: Normal living teeth that erupt into the oral cavity. **Permanent d.**: Natural teeth that succeed the primary teeth as the primary teeth are shed. Called also succedaneous dentition. **Primary d.**: Earliest natural teeth that erupt into the dental arches of the oral cavity normally during childhood. Also called deciduous dentition.

dentofacial orthopedics: The branch of dentistry that deals with the prevention and correction of abnormal jaw and tooth relationships, often by surgery.

dentoform: Having the likeness of a tooth; a tooth-like substitute.

dentulous: 1. Possessing natural teeth. 2. A condition in which natural teeth are present in the mouth. (syn): Dentate.

denture: A prosthetic device used to replace one or more teeth. A fixed partial denture may be bonded or cemented on adjacent teeth or implants and cannot be removed by the patient. A removable overdenture, partial denture, or full denture may rest on remaining teeth, retained roots, implants, or completely on soft tissue for support and stability. See: Fixed prosthesis, Removable prosthesis.

denture adhesive: A material used to adhere a denture to the oral mucosa.

denture base: The gingiva-colored portion of the denture that is supported by the underlying soft tissue and holds the denture teeth.

denture base material: The substance used to make the gingival (pink) portion of a removable plate or frame that supports artificial teeth.

denture border: 1. The periphery of the denture base at the point where the polished surface and the intaglio surface meet. 2. The facial, lingual, and posterior periphery of a denture base.

denture characterization: Alteration of the texture and color of the denture base and teeth to create a more natural appearance.

denture curing: The procedure used to polymerize and harden the acrylic materials that form a denture.

denture design: The intended outline form used when fabricating a removable dental prosthesis for the purpose of replacing natural teeth with artificial teeth in a way that meets the clinician's and patient's requirements.

denture esthetics: The appearance of a dental prosthesis worn by the patient. The goal is a prosthesis that is proper and attractive for the patient.

denture flange: The portion of the denture base that extends into the soft tissue vestibule. It runs from the cervical ends of the prosthetic teeth to the edge of the denture's border.

denture foundation: The soft tissue oral structures that support a dental prosthesis that replaces missing natural teeth with artificial teeth.

denture occlusal surface: The designated chewing portion of a dental prosthesis with artificial teeth that make contact with the opposing dentition.

denture prognosis: An attempt by a clinician or laboratory technician to predict the success of a denture.

denture prosthesis: A generic term for the long-standing concept of artificial replacement of natural teeth and related structures, most commonly a removable device. The term is also used to denote its distinctness from an implant-supported or a craniofacial prosthesis.

denture prosthetics: The science of replacing natural teeth in a complete arch with an artificial substitute that is both functional and cosmetically pleasing.

denture resin packing: The placement of a denture base material with pressure into a mold positioned in the refractory flask.

denture retention: 1. The resistance in the movement of a denture away from its tissue foundation, especially in a vertical direction. 2. A quality of a denture that holds it to the tissue foundation and/or abutment teeth. See: Denture stability.

denture service: The clinical practices provided in the diagnosis, assembly, and maintenance of dentures.

denture space: 1. The three-dimensional area of the mouth that is or may be occupied by maxillary and/or mandibular dentures. 2. The space once occupied by teeth, alveolar bone, and surrounding soft and hard tissues but is now available for a complete or partial denture.

denture stability: 1. The resistance of a denture to movement on its tissue foundation, especially to lateral (horizontal) forces as opposed to vertical displacement (termed denture retention). 2. A quality of a denture that permits it to maintain a state of equilibrium in relation to its tissue foundation and/or abutment teeth. See: Denture retention.

denture supporting structures: The remaining alveolar ridges or teeth that serve as foundational support for a removable partial or full denture.

denturist: 1. Any nondentist who makes, fits, and repairs removable dentures directly for the public. 2. A nondentist licensed to provide complete dentures directly to the public.

denudation: The process of removing the covering from any surface. In periodontics, often refers to removal of all soft tissue overlying the bone.

deosseointegration: The loss of a previously achieved osseointegration of a dental implant due to periimplantitis, occlusal overload, or other factors.

deoxyribonucleic acid (DNA): A nucleic acid that constitutes the genetic material of all cellular organisms and the DNA viruses.

depassivation: Loss or removal of the surface oxide layer of a metal. See: Passivation.

deprogrammer: Any device that alters reflexive proprioceptive behavior during mandibular closure.

deproteinized bovine bone material: See: Anorganic bovine bone matrix (ABBM).

depth gauge: Graduated instrument with markings designed to measure the vertical extent of an osteotomy preparation.

dermal graft: Tissue graft from a human or animal cadaver, which has undergone a process of deepithelialization and decellularization, leaving an immunologically inert avascular connective tissue.

desensitize: To diminish or abolish sensation of pain or sensitivity, as in dentin.

design (implant): The three-dimensional structure of a dental implant or component, with all the elements and characteristics that compose it: form, shape, configuration, surface macrostructure, and microirregularities.

desktop optical scanner: A device that uses light/laser to scan and digitize objects (impressions, casts). This device is stationary and cannot be used for intraoral scanning.

desquamation: Exfoliation; the process of shedding surface epithelium; the loss of surface epithelial cells.

detoxicant: A chemical that degrades a toxic agent.

detrusion: Distraction (downward movement) of the mandibular condyle.

developmental anomaly: Aberration in the normal sequence of events associated with growth and development. This process could result over time in distortion of the face and jaws, abnormality of tooth formation or position, and irregularity of function.

developmental dysmorphia: Anomalous growth related to or induced by interference from neighboring structures.

developmental dysplasia: An abnormal growth pattern at the cellular or organ level.

developmental hyperplasia: Excessive growth of tissue or organ system.

developmental hypoplasia: Less than normal growth of tissue or organ system.

devest: Removal of investing material to retrieve a casting or prosthesis.

deviation: With respect to movement of the mandible, a discursive movement that ends in the centered position and is indicative of interference during movement.

device: Something developed by the application of ideas or principles that are designed to serve a special purpose or perform a special function. See: Restoration.

device orientation: The direction in which a distraction device is positioned, usually relative to the anatomical axis of the bone segments to be distracted.

devitrification: The process by which glassy substances change their structure to crystalline solids. This phenomenon may occur partially in dental ceramics if a ceramic restoration is fired too often, and it is typically associated with an opacified appearance.

DEXA (abbrev.): Dual-energy X-ray absorptiometry.

dexamethasone: A long-acting synthetic glucocorticoid used as a potent antiinflammatory drug. It may be administered intramuscularly, orally, or intravenously. See: Glucocorticoid.

DFDBA (abbrev.): Demineralized freeze-dried bone allograft.

diabetes mellitus (DM): Syndrome characterized by disordered metabolism and abnormally high blood sugar resulting from insufficient levels of the hormone insulin. In implant dentistry, good diabetic control is a prerequisite to achieving and maintaining osseointegration. See: Glycosylated hemoglobin A1c test.

diagnose: To identify or define a disease or unwanted pathological condition by study of and deliberation on the signs and symptoms the patient presents with.

diagnosis: 1. The art and science of detecting and distinguishing deviations from health and the cause and nature thereof. 2. The determination of the nature, location, and causes of a disease or disorder. **Clinical d.**: Determination of a condition based on history and physical examination without use of laboratory or microscopic tests. **Laboratory d.**: Diagnosis based on the examination of fluids or tissues in the laboratory. **Periodontal d.**: The process (or opinion derived from the process) of identifying the nature and cause of a disease of the periodontium; relevant information used in this process typically includes medical and dental histories, clinical and radiographic examination.

diagnostic: Relating to or used in determining the nature of a disease or condition.

diagnostic cast: A static replica of a part or parts of the oral cavity and/or facial structures for the purpose of diagnosis and development of a treatment plan. See: Cast.

diagnostic denture: A provisional removable dental prosthesis constructed for the purposes of functional and esthetic evaluation of the intended final therapy.

diagnostic imaging: Visual representation of a body part made for diagnostic and/or treatment planning purposes. Such procedures include radiography, computed tomography (CT), magnetic resonance imaging (MRI), ultrasound, and digital volume tomography.

diagnostic index: See: Prosthodontic diagnostic index.

diagnostic mounting: See: Mounting.

diagnostic occlusal prosthesis: A removable dental prosthesis, usually made of acrylic resin, that includes an overlay of the occlusal surfaces, designed to evaluate a patient's response to extensive restorative intervention.

diagnostic radiation: The radiation a patient receives when radiographs are used for the purpose of determining the nature of a disease.

diagnostic set-ups: See: Tooth arrangement.

diagnostic splint: See: Occlusal device.

diagnostic study cast: See: Diagnostic cast.

diagnostic tooth preparation: Alterations performed on a dental cast before actual tooth preparation so the proposed tooth preparation can be evaluated and changed as needed before actually cutting the intended tooth.

diagnostic waxing: Waxing of proposed restorative forms on dental casts for the evaluation and planning of intended restorations.

diagnostic wax-up: Laboratory procedure in which teeth are created in wax according to the planned restoration. It may be used to evaluate the feasibility of a proposed plan and to fabricate a radiographic template, a surgical guide, or laboratory guides. See: Tooth arrangement.

diapedesis: The outward passage of cells through intact blood vessels.

diarthrodial joint: A freely moving joint.

diarthrosis: A specific articulation permitting more or less free movement; a bone articulation that permits free movement in a joint. Structurally, it is a synovial joint.

diastema: A space between two adjacent teeth in a dental arch.

diathermy: Tissue resistance-generated heat resulting from high-frequency electric current.

diatoric: A canal placed in denture teeth to provide mechanical retention of the teeth in a denture base of a chemically different material.

diazepam: A benzodiazepine anxiolytic, Schedule IV controlled substance having antianxiety, sedative-hypnotic, amnesic, anticonvulsant, skeletal muscle relaxant, and drug dependence properties. Used in the management of short-term anxiety disorders.

DICOM (abbrev.): Digital imaging and communications in medicine. Standard for handling, storing, printing, and transmitting information in medical imaging. It includes a file format definition and a network communications protocol. DICOM enables the integration of scanners, servers, workstations, printers, and network hardware from multiple manufacturers into a picture archiving and communication system (PACS).

die: The positive reproduction of the form of a prepared tooth in any suitable substance.

die spacer: An agent applied to a die to provide space for the luting agent in the finished casting.

dietary analysis: The evaluation of a diet on the basis of its content, quality, and nutrients in order to determine any imbalance or deficiency that might contribute to a disease process.

differential diagnosis: The distinguishing of a disease or pathological condition from others presenting similar signs.

digital denture: A complete denture created by or through automation using CAD, CAM, and CAE in lieu of traditional processes. A digital denture is achieved when the final shape of the denture is manufactured through automation to ensure there are no conventional errors from pouring, investment casting, or injecting the material as done in traditional denture fabrication.

digital imaging: Computer-based digital technology allowing the dentist to create true-to-life photographs of the dentition, as if the recommended procedures had already been completed.

digital print/printing: Method of printing from a digital-based image directly to a variety of media. It usually refers to professional printing where small-run jobs from desktop publishing and other digital sources are printed using large-format and/or high-volume laser or inkjet printers or 3D printers.

digital sculpting: The use of software that offers tools to push, pull, smooth, grab, pinch or otherwise manipulate a digital object as if it were made of a real-life substance such as clay. When creating 3D models in an application, this includes manipulating vertices and edges to get the desired look. While this works, it can be hard to get the fine detail often required, especially in organic models. Digital sculpting works around this issue by allowing the user to create a 3D mesh in much the same way as a traditional sculptor would. By interactively pushing and pulling areas of the model, one can create details like texture, pits, and sharp transitions (e.g., the cementoenamel junction) without having to select an edge or vertex.

digital volume tomography (DVT): See: Cone beam computed tomography.

digital workflow: Any workflow that occurs primarily through the use of converting physical or "analog" structures into a digital format to be manipulated using CAD software. Often, the digital process resembles the analog process in steps, but is accomplished virtually on a computer until the design is machine fabricated through automated milling or 3D printing methods.

dilaceration: 1. A tearing apart. 2. In dentistry, a condition due to injury of a tooth during its development and characterized by a band or crease at the junction of the crown and root, or alternatively by tortuous roots with abnormal curvatures.

dimensional stability: The capacity of a material or substance to maintain its shape and size when subjected to various environmental changes, including moisture, temperature, and stress.

dimensions of color: The three-dimensional system describing color developed by Munsell. The dimensions are (1) hue (color family), (2) value (lightness/darkness), and (3) chroma (strength).

diphosphonate: See: Bisphosphonate.

direct bone impression: A negative likeness of bone produced through a flap reflection of overlying tissues and direct impression. Usually, it is the initial part of the two-stage surgical impression technique for subperiosteal implant construction.

direct impression: See: Open-tray impression.

direct retainer: The unit of a removable dental prosthesis that engages an abutment tooth to resist movement of the prosthesis away from the basal seats. The unit consists of an extracoronal clasp assembly or intracoronal retainer, for example, precision attachment.

direct retention: Retention obtained in a partial removable dental prosthesis by the use of clasps or attachments that resist removal from the abutment teeth.

direct sinus graft: See: Lateral window technique, Sinus graft.

direction indicator: Device inserted into an osteotomy in order to assess its orientation or position relative to adjacent teeth and anatomic structures. Also used to verify and assist in achieving parallelism in the preparation of multiple osteotomies.

disarticulation: The separation of two articulated structures at their joint parts.

disc: Variant spelling of disk.

discectomy: Removal of the intraarticular disk. It typically refers to removing the meniscus or intraarticular cartilage in a joint.

disclosant: A tablet or solution that when rinsed in the oral cavity visibly stains dental plaque colonies. It is often used as an adjunct in oral hygiene instructions because it helps the patient identify the areas of plaque accumulation that can potentially induce hard and soft tissue damage.

disclusion: See: Disocclusion.

disease: A pathologic condition that presents a group of clinical signs, symptoms, and laboratory findings peculiar to it and setting the condition apart as an abnormal entity differing from normal or other pathologic conditions.

disinfectant: Typically, a liquid agent that is applied to surfaces of objects for the purpose of destroying or inhibiting disease-producing microorganisms or other harmful substances.

disjunctor: A component of artificial prosthesis that allows movement between two or more parts.

disk: A thin, flat, circular object or plate. See: Disk, articular.

disk, articular: Fibrous connective tissue that separates temporomandibular joint cavity into two compartments. Also called the meniscus. Fibrous connective tissue between two bony structures to reduce abrasion and friction located in a joint cavity.

disk degeneration: Progressive degenerative changes in the temporomandibular joint articular disk; the breakdown of the joint articular disk through degenerative disease.

disk derangement: A misalignment of the articular disk between the condyle, fossa,

and/or the bony eminence that often results in pain, swelling, and/or difficulty with mastication.

disk detachment: A separation of the disk from its capsule, ligament, or bony surface.

disk displacement with reduction: Disk dislodgment where the temporomandibular joint disk has shifted in an anterior-medial direction when at rest but returns to its proper position with mandibular movement. It frequently has an associated clicking sound.

disk displacement without reduction: Disk dislodgment where the temporomandibular joint disk has shifted in an anterior-medial direction when at rest but does not return to its proper position with mandibular movement.

disk implant: An endosseous dental implant consisting of a plate, neck, and abutment. The implant is inserted laterally into the edentulous ridge.

disk interference: Restriction of mandibular movement because of pathology or dysfunction of the disk; a dysfunction of the normal articular disk movement that often results in pain and normal mandibular movement.

disk locking: A dysfunction of the disk's normal position and/or function in the temporomandibular joint in which it cannot return to normal position or function.

disk perforation: A bounded hole or tear in the center of the temporomandibular joint's articular disk that is the result of deterioration associated with habitual increased compressive forces. The opening allows for communication between the superior and inferior joint spaces. The attachment associated with the capsule, ligaments, or bone is not altered.

disk prolapse: Rotation of the temporomandibular disk downward and forward on the face of the condyle eminence.

disk space: The space that is typically occupied by the intraarticular disk between the mandibular condyle and the articular fossa that is represented on a temporomandibular joint radiograph as a radiolucency.

disk thinning: Reduced thickness of the intraarticular disk as a result of an autoimmune degenerative process, chronic pressure during function, or the combination of both.

dislocated fracture: A break of a bone associated with displacement of the fractured segment from its intended joint.

dislocation: Pathologic displacement of a bone out of the natural anatomic boundaries of its fossae. It is frequently associated with pain, reduced range of motion of the affected bone, and ligament or cartilage pathosis. It may be chronic or recurrent. See: Condylar d., Functional d., Mandibular d., Partial d.

disocclude: Progressive separation of occluding teeth from maximum intercuspation position during jaw movements due to tooth guidance, occlusal interferences, or occlusal adjustment.

disocclusion: Separation of opposing teeth during eccentric movements of the mandible.

displacement of the mandible: A position or movement of the mandible beyond its normal anatomic boundaries.

distal: Remote; farther from the point of reference; away from the median sagittal plane of the face following the curvature of the dental arch.

distal extension: Edentulous space posterior to the most distal tooth or implant abutment.

distal extension partial denture: The boundaries of a removable partial denture distal to the terminal tooth. A removable partial denture prosthesis that does not have a natural abutment tooth at the distal aspect either on one or both sides; rather, the distal tooth at the distal aspect is an artificial tooth provided by the prosthesis. See: Extension base partial removable dental prosthesis.

distal extension prosthesis: As seen in the median sagittal plane, a prosthesis addition posterior to the most distal tooth or implant abutment. The extension can be uni- or bilateral and in the form of an artificial tooth or teeth, a cantilever for a fixed prosthesis, or a denture base segment for a removable partial denture. See: Partial denture.

distal wedge: A periodontal surgical intervention at the distal area of a terminal tooth in an arch. The goal is to remove excessive tissue, reduce periodontal pocket depth, and facilitate oral hygiene at the area. See: Proximal wedge.

distance osteogenesis: A gradual process of bone healing from the edge of an osteotomy toward a dental implant. Initially, bone does not grow directly onto the implant surface. See: Contact osteogenesis.

distocclusion: The clinical situation where at maximum intercuspation, the mandibular teeth have a distal relationship to the maxillary teeth as in an Angle's Class II occlusion.

distoversion: A deviation or positioning towards the distal. Any deviation along the median sagittal plane directed from the incisors to the retromolar pads.

distraction: See: Distraction osteogenesis.

distraction axis: The direction in which the bone segment is distracted during distraction osteogenesis.

distraction device: An appliance that allows gradual incremental movement of bone segments away from each other. See: Distraction osteogenesis.

distraction of the condyle: Dislocation of the condyle in an inferior direction; the clinical condition where the condyle is inferiorly displaced and typically associated with pain.

distraction osteogenesis (DO): (syn): Osteodistraction. The gradual and controlled distraction of two vascularized bone segments created by an osteotomy. Formation of new soft tissue and bone between vascular bone surfaces created by an osteotomy and separated by gradual and controlled distraction. It begins with the development of a reparative callus. The callus is placed under tension by stretching, which generates new bone. Distraction osteogenesis consists of three sequential periods. 1. Latency period: the period from bone division (i.e., surgical separation of bone into two segments) to the onset of traction, which represents the time allowed for callus formation. 2. Distraction period: the time when gradual traction is applied to bone segments and new tissue (regenerate tissue) is formed. 3. Consolidation period, also called fixation period: consolidation and corticalization of the distraction regenerate after traction forces and segment movement are discontinued.

distraction parameters: Biological and biomechanical variables that affect the quality and quantity of bone formed during distraction osteogenesis.

distraction period: See: Distraction osteogenesis.

distraction protocol: The sequence and duration of treatment events during distraction osteogenesis.

distraction rate: Distance of distraction per day. Ideal rate depends on the ability of the soft tissue to respond with expansion and regeneration. Periodontal status of adjacent teeth may also limit the transport rate. In general, a rate of 0.4 mm per day is sufficient to allow the soft tissue to respond while avoiding premature consolidation (i.e., fusion) across the vertical osteotomy components prior to completion of the transport process. If the distraction rate is too slow, the risk for premature consolidation is increased. See: Distraction osteogenesis (DO).

distraction regenerate: Newly regenerated tissue between the transported section and the surgically cut base achieved following distraction osteogenesis. See: Alveolar distraction osteogenesis.

distraction rhythm: The number of increments per day into which the rate of distraction osteogenesis is divided.

distraction vector: The final direction and magnitude of traction forces during distraction osteogenesis.

distraction zone: Zone between the transported segment and its surgically cut base.

distractor: Device used for distraction osteogenesis.

distribution force: Pattern in which applied forces are distributed throughout a structure, i.e., pattern of load distribution throughout an implant-supported fixed cantilever prosthesis.

disuse atrophy: Diminution in dimension and/or density of bone, resulting from inadequate loading by physiologic forces. See: Atrophy, disuse.

divergence: 1. A drawing apart as a surface extends away from a common point. 2. The reverse taper of walls of a preparation for a restoration – divergency.

divergence angle: The sum of the tapered angles for the divergent opposing walls of a tooth preparation.

DM (abbrev.): Diabetes mellitus.

DO (abbrev.): Distraction osteogenesis.

documentation, periodontal: Diagnostic, radiographic, and therapeutic dental charting records of a patient's soft and hard tissue support for the teeth.

dolder bar: One of many bar attachments that splint teeth or roots together while acting as an abutment for a partial removable dental prosthesis. The bar is straight with parallel sides and a round top and comes in assorted sizes.

donor site: The part of the body from which an autogenous graft is obtained. Examples include skin, mucosa, connective tissue, and bone.

double wire clasp: A wire circumferential clasp with back-to-back retentive arms.

dovetail: A widened portion of a prepared cavity used to increase retention and/or resistance.

dowel: A post usually made of metal that is fitted into a prepared root canal of a natural tooth. When combined with an artificial crown or core, it provides retention and resistance for the restoration. See: Post.

dowel pin: A metal indexing pin used in stone casts that permits removal of the die section and its precise replacement in the original position.

doxycycline: Semi-synthetic broad-spectrum antibacterial of the tetracycline group, administered orally. This antibiotic is often used to treat periodontal and periimplant disease. Low-dose formulations also possess inhibitory effects on matrix metalloproteinase (MMP) enzymes responsible for destroying connective tissues and bone.

drag: The inferior or lower side of a refractory denture flask. It fits precisely with the upper (cope) side of the denture flask.

draw: For a crown or restorative preparation, the taper or convergence of the opposing walls.

drill: A cutting instrument used to create holes by rotary motion.

drill extender: Intermediate handpiece or wrench component used to lengthen the shaft of an instrument connected to a rotary drill or implant mount.

drill/drilling guide: A template, sleeve, other device, or system used to direct/control a rotary cutting instrument when preparing an implant osteotomy site. See: Stereolithographic guide, Surgical guide.

drill stop: Device attached to a drill to control the depth of an osteotomy.

drilling sequence: The use of drills in a specific order to gradually prepare and increase the diameter of an osteotomy prior to dental implant insertion.

dross: 1. The solid scum produced from oxides, impurities, or waste materials on the surface of a metal when melted. 2. Waste matter, refuse.

drug: Any chemical that alters the physiologic processes of living systems.

drug agonist: Chemicals that react with a receptor and initiate a cellular reaction. This reaction is similar to that of an endogenous hormone or neurotransmitter.

drug antagonist: Chemicals that prevent reaction of a drug agonist with its receptor. The antagonist drug competes for the available receptors.

drug efficacy: The ability of a chemical or a drug to produce a biological effect.

dry processing/dry milling: A manufacturing process where a material is machined without the need for liquid for cooling and lubrication. Dry processing is applied mainly with respect to zirconium oxide blanks with a low degree of presintering.

dry socket: Localized osteitis of the alveolus following tooth extraction due to infection or loss of the blood clot.

dual-energy X-ray absorptiometry (DXA, DEXA): Test measuring bone mineral "density" (BMD). Two low-dose X-ray beams with differing energy levels are aimed at the patient's bones. By subtracting the soft tissue absorption, the BMD can be determined from the absorption of each beam by bone.

dual scan: Digital technique where two scans, containing different data sets, are combined together into one file. An example of a dual scan is a CBCT scan combined with an intraoral scan. The resultant file contains the surface data captured by the intraoral scan and the 3D slices of the underlying hard tissue from the CBCT scan.

ductility: The ability of a material to withstand permanent deformation under a tensile load without rupture; ability of a material to be plastically strained in tension. A material is brittle if it does not have appreciable plastic deformation in tension before rupture.

duplicate denture: A second denture that is identical in all aspects to the in-use or functioning denture.

durometer: An instrument that measures the hardness of a material.

DXA (abbrev.): Dual-energy X-ray absorptiometry.

dynamic loading: Situation in which the loading of an implant is continually changing, as would happen during occlusal function. Both the magnitude and direction of applied force are in constant flux.

dynamic relations: Relations of two objects involving the element of relative movement of one object to another, as the relationship of the mandible to the maxillae.

dysesthesia: An abnormal and unpleasant sensation that is either spontaneous or evoked. Dysesthesia includes paresthesia but not vice versa.

dysfunction: To not function properly or normally as a cell or within an organ. In dentistry, a dysfunction means any abnormality between the physical nature of the teeth, bones, or joints within the oral cavity and their function as mediated through muscles or nerves affecting the oral cavity and causing abnormal functioning.

dysgeusia: Any change, disturbance or distortion in the sense of taste.

dyskinesia: Impairment of the power of voluntary movement resulting in fragmentary or incomplete movement. See: Incoordination.

dyslalia: Defective articulation due to faulty learning or to abnormality of the external speech organs and not due to lesions of the central nervous system.

dysmasesis: Difficulty in chewing (mastication).

dysostosis: Imperfect ossification resulting in abnormal bone development.

dysphagia: Difficulty in or lack of complete swallowing, which slows the movement of food from the mouth into the stomach.

dysphonia: Disorder of the voice caused by the inability to make voice sounds through the vocal cords, resulting in hoarseness or difficulty in speaking.

dysplasia: Abnormality of development; in pathology, alteration in size, shape, and organization of cells. **Dentinal d.**: A hereditary disorder affecting the teeth and characterized by abnormal dentin, defective root formation, and a tendency for periapical pathosis. **Ectodermal d.**: An inherited condition characterized by fine, scanty, blond hair, depressed bridge of the nose, and a partial or complete absence of sweat glands and teeth. **Periapical cemental d. (cementoma)**: A process of unknown origin in which the periapical bone of vital teeth is replaced first by a fibrous type of connective tissue, and then by an osseocementoid tissue. During its early stages, this abnormality appears radiolucent and with time the center becomes opaque. It is classified as an odontogenic tumor.

dystonia: A neurologic disorder resulting in sustained, acute, irregular, tonic muscular spasms causing twisting and repetitive motions that affect movement of the tongue, jaw, eyes, neck, and sometimes the entire body.

dystrophy, periodontal: Degeneration of the periodontium caused by changes in bone mechanics and circulation, that results in abnormal physiological function.

E

ear prosthesis: Fixed/removable artificial replacement for all or part of a human ear. Called also auricular prosthesis.

early implant failure: (syn): Primary implant failure. The failure of a dental implant due to the failure to establish osseointegration. See: Late implant failure.

early implant loss: Loss of an implant that occurs prior to implant osseointegration.

early implant placement: Early implant placement takes place 4–8 weeks following tooth extraction, providing sufficient time for soft tissue healing. This approach is often used by clinicians in esthetic sites, where implant placement often requires a simultaneous guided bone regeneration (GBR) procedure and primary soft tissue closure is critical. It helps to reduce the risk of postrestorative soft tissue complications.

early loading: Placing of an implant into function or a load-bearing situation following a reduced period of healing after the initial placement. It is generally considered to be loading more than 48 hours but less than 3 months after implant placement. See: Delayed loading.

early-onset periodontitis: See: Periodontitis.

EBM (abbrev.): Electron beam melting.

eccentric: l. Not having the same center. 2. Deviating from a circular path. 3. Located elsewhere than at the geometric center. 4. Any position of the mandible other than that which is its normal position.

eccentric jaw record: See: Eccentric interocclusal record.

eccentric jaw relation: Any relationship between the jaws other than centric relation.

eccentric occlusion: An occlusion other than centric occlusion.

eccentric position: See: Eccentric relation.

eccentric record: See: Eccentric interocclusal record.

eccentric relation: Any relationship of the mandible to the maxilla other than centric relation. See: Acquired e.r.

ecchymosis: The extravasation and collection of blood into the subcutaneous tissues, which appears as a yellow to bluish mark on the mucous membrane or skin.

ECM (abbrev.): Extracellular matrix.

ecology: The study of the relationships of organisms with other organisms and the surrounding environment.

ectodermal dysplasia: See: Dysplasia, ectodermal.

ectopic: Occurring in an unusual position, manner, or form, as in ectopic eruption.

ectopic eruption: Eruption of a tooth outside the expected or usual location or in a displaced position.

edema: A condition of abnormally large fluid volume or abnormal swelling subsequent to the collection of fluid in a tissue or part.

edentulate: Lacking teeth.

edentulism: Oral condition of being without one or more teeth, completely (i.e., complete edentulism) or in segments of a dental arch (i.e., partial edentulism).

edentulous: Without teeth.

Glossary of Dental Implantology, First Edition. Khalid Almas, Fawad Javed and Steph Smith.
© 2018 John Wiley & Sons, Inc. Published 2018 by John Wiley & Sons, Inc.

edentulous site: See: Edentulous space.

edentulous space: Area previously occupied by a tooth or teeth.

edge to edge articulation: Articulation in which the opposing anterior teeth meet along the incisal edges when the teeth are in maximum intercuspation.

edge to edge bite: See: Edge to edge articulation.

edge to edge occlusion: See: Edge to edge articulation.

EDM (abbrev.): Electric discharge method.

effector cell: Cell that becomes active in response to stimulation. In immunology, a differentiated lymphocyte capable of mounting a specific immune response, e.g., antibody production, lymphokine production or helper, suppressor, or killer function. Called also effector lymphocyte.

EGF (abbrev.): Epidermal growth factor.

Eikonella corrodens: Gram-negative, nonmotile, microaerophilic, rod-shaped bacteria found primarily in subgingival plaque. Also associated with sinusitis, meningitis, pneumonia, and endocarditis.

elastic modulus: Measure of elasticity; relative stiffness of a material within the range of elastic deformation (below the point of plastic deformation). Called also modulus of elasticity or Young modulus. Elastic modulus = Stress/Strain or $E = \sigma/\varepsilon$.

elasticity: The quality that allows a structure or material to return to its original form on removal of an external force.

elastomer: A polymer whose glass transition temperature is below its service temperature (usually room temperature). These materials are characterized by low stiffness and extremely large elastic strains. *Adj:* Elastomeric.

elastomeric impression material: A polymer that has weak intermolecular forces with characteristics of viscosity and elasticity; compared with other materials it has a low Young's modulus and high failure strain. The term originates from *elastic polymer*, which is also known as rubber.

electric discharge method (EDM): syn. Spark erosion. A precision metal removal process, using a series of electrical sparks, to erode material from a workpiece in a liquid medium under carefully controlled conditions.

electrode: A solid electric conductor that allows for current to enter or leave a medium or electrolytic cell.

electromyographic biofeedback: A process using instruments to help patients learn how to control tension in muscles that are normally under automatic control.

electromyography: The graphic display and record of the electrical potential of muscle(s). See: Nocturnal e.

electron accelerator: An instrument designed to increase the energy level of electrons in radiation therapeutics.

electron beam melting (EBM): Additive manufacturing for metal parts. EBM is often classified as a rapid manufacturing method. The technology manufactures parts by melting metal powder layer by layer with an electron beam in a high vacuum. Unlike some metal sintering techniques, the parts are fully dense, void free, and extremely strong.

electron beam therapy: The use of high-energy electrons for therapy, such as with a betatron.

electroplating: The process of covering the surface of an object with a thin coating of metal by means of electrolysis.

electropolishing: The electrolytic removal of a thin layer of metal to produce a bright surface.

electrosurgery: Division of tissues by high-frequency electrical current applied locally with a metal instrument or needle.

elements: When used in reference to dental implants, component parts of a dental implant structure such as the dental implant, dental implant abutment, and abutment screw.

elevator: Surgical instrument. A luxating elevator is used to luxate teeth during extraction. A periosteal elevator is used to elevate a full-thickness or mucoperiosteal flap.

elevator muscle: One of the contracting muscles that raises or closes the lower jaw.

ELISA (abbrev.): Enzyme-linked immunosorbent assay.

elongation: l. Deformation as a result of tensile force application. 2. The degree to which a material will stretch before breaking. 3. The overeruption of a tooth.

embolus: A blood clot, air, or other foreign material that travels in the bloodstream until it obstructs a blood vessel.

embouchure: The manner in which people position and use their mouth (teeth, lips, and tongue) when playing a wind instrument.

embrasure: l. The space formed when adjacent surfaces flare away from one another. 2. In dentistry, the space defined by surfaces of two adjacent teeth; there are four embrasure spaces associated with each proximal contact area: occlusal/incisal, mesial, distal, and gingival.

EMD (abbrev.): Enamel matrix derivative from porcine material.

emergence angle: The incline created by a dental implant's transitional shape as determined by the correlation of the long axis of the implant body to the implant abutment or prosthesis. See also: Emergence profile.

emergence profile: The part of the axial contour of a tooth or prosthetic crown that extends from the base of the sulcus past the free soft tissue margin. The emergence profile extends to the height of contour of the crown, producing a straight or convex profile in the apical third of the axial surface. Control of this surface is important in achieving acceptable esthetics and maintaining soft tissue health. See also: Emergence angle.

EMG (abbrev.): Electromyogram.

eminence: The projecting prominent part of an object, especially on the surface of a bone.

emphysema: 1. A pathological swelling caused by accumulation of air or gas in tissue spaces. In the oral cavity and facial region, it may be initiated by the unintentional introduction of air into a tooth socket or gingival crevice with an air syringe, an air-driven dental handpiece, a continuous positive airway pressure or bilevel positive airway pressure machine, coughing, or nose blowing. 2. A chronic respiratory disease in which there is a perpetual dilation of the respiratory alveoli in the lung, causing a reduction in lung function and frequently breathlessness.

empty mouth movement: Voluntary or involuntary changes of the mandible's position when the jaws are not engaged in incising or chewing.

enamel: In dentistry, the hard, thin, translucent layer of calcified material that covers the coronal portion of a tooth. It protects the dentin located directly underneath it and is known to be the hardest substance in the body. Called also adamantine layer.

enamel matrix derivative (EMD): Sterile protein aggregate from enamel matrix, amelogenins, the precursor of enamel of developing teeth. The proteins are harvested from around developing pig embryo teeth, with special processing procedures (porcine derivative). EMD has been used as a periodontal regenerative treatment.

enamel pearl: A developmental abnormality that results in a small localized mass of enamel formed apical to a tooth's cementoenamel junction. It is frequently found in the bifurcation of molar teeth.

enamel projection: An apical extension of a tooth's enamel that is often found at the root furcation.

enameloplasty: See: Occlusal reshaping.

enarthrosis: A joint in which the rounded (ball-like) head of one bone fits into the socket form of another bone (e.g., hip joint).

endemic: Present in a community at all times. Occurring continuously.

endocarditis: Exudative and proliferative inflammation of the endocardial surface of the heart. Infective endocarditis is a bacterial infection of the endocardial surface of the heart, most often involving the heart valves. Previously was categorized as acute, subacute, or chronic bacterial endocarditis but is now categorized by the offending microorganism (i.e., streptococcal infective endocarditis).

endochondral ossification: Formation of long bones on the basis of a cartilaginous model. Longitudinal growth takes place both in growth plates and in the articular cartilage. At the growth plates, chondral ossification takes place. Cartilage cells calcify, serving as a basis for bone formation, and bone is deposited; cartilage is then replaced by bone.

endocrine: Transfer of chemical compounds such as hormones and growth factors from secreting glands via blood to cells.

endodontic-endosseous implant: See: Implant, oral.

endodontic endosteal dental implant: A smooth and/or threaded pin implant that extends through the root canal of a tooth into periapical bone and is used to stabilize a mobile tooth; sometimes called an endodontic stabilizer.

endodontic implant: (syn): Endodontic pin, endodontic stabilizer. A pin placed into a root canal of a tooth and extending beyond its apex, into the bone.

endodontic pin: A metal pin that is intentionally placed through the apex of a mobile tooth and into the surrounding apical bone for stabilization. See: Endodontic implant.

endodontic stabilizer: Tapered post made of a biocompatible alloy that is cemented into a natural tooth, extending beyond the apex into the surrounding bone, on the assumption that it would stabilize the tooth. Called also endodontic pin. See: Endodontic endosteal dental implant.

endogenous: 1. Growing from within. 2. Developing or originating within an organism or arising from causes within an organism.

endoscope: An instrument with a flexible or rigid thin tube used for examining the interior of a canal, hollow space, or structure.

endosseous: (syn): Intrabony, intraosseous. Within the bone.

endosseous blade implant: See: Blade endosteal dental implant.

endosseous distractor: (syn): Intraosseous distractor. A distraction device placed into the edentulous ridge and/or basal bone of the maxilla or mandible used in distraction osteogenesis.

endosseous implant: (syn): Endosteal implant. A device placed into the alveolar and/or basal bone of the maxilla or mandible and used to support a prosthesis. See: Endosteal dental implant and Implant, oral.

endosseous provisional implant: See: Provisional implant.

endosseous ramus implant: Single- or multiple-piece implant in which the endosseous elements are placed in the symphysis area and into the anterior portion of bilateral mandibular rami. The transmucosal element extends from the endosseous portion that supports a mesostructure. The mesostructure can consist of a bar that follows the general outline of the residual mandibular bone. It is U-shaped as viewed from the occlusal.

endosteal dental implant: A manmade device positioned into the alveolar and/or basal bone of the mandible or maxilla that transects a cortical plate. It is made up of an endosteal dental implant body that provides anchorage when positioned and integrated within the bone and the endosteal dental implant abutment that retains the prosthesis. Multiple adjectives are used to describe the endosteal dental implant. It can be described by its shape (e.g., cylinder, screw, conical, blade, or basket) or by the materials from which the implant is constructed (e.g., titanium, titanium alloy, or ceramic).

endosteal dental implant abutment: The part of the implant that passes through the oral mucosa and allows for the connection between the body of the implant and the restorative prosthesis. The abutment is often referred to as an implant element. It attaches to the body of the dental implant with screws, thread/screw interfacing, and a male/ female Morse taper fit. The purpose of an abutment is to support and/or retain a fixed or removable dental prosthesis or a maxillofacial prosthesis. The dental implant abutment may be for interim (provisional) or definitive use. Description of the dental implant abutment is based on number of pieces (one piece joined to implant body, two piece, or three piece), fabrication technique (stock, stock-adjusted, or custom), angulation (straight or angled), and material from which it is made (titanium, titanium alloy, gold, or ceramic).

endosteal dental implant abutment element: A dental implant component used to attach the dental implant body to the prosthesis or the prosthetic attachment.

endosteal implant: See: Endosseous implant.

endosteum: Thin, vascular membrane that lines the inner aspect of cortical bone surrounding the medullary cavity of bone. This delicate connective tissue is composed of vessels, lining cells, and osteoprogenitor cells and has a marked osteogenic potential.

endothelial progenitor cell: Adherent cell obtained from peripheral blood-derived or bone marrow-derived mononuclear cells demonstrating low-density lipoprotein (LDL) uptake and isolectin-binding capacity. These cells may be used as a potential therapy for a variety of vascular diseases. The number of circulating endothelial progenitor cells is reduced in patients with cardiovascular disease and may be a surrogate marker for this disease risk.

endothelium: Epithelium of mesoblastic origin composed of a single layer of thin, flattened cells that line the cavities of the heart, the lumina of blood and lymph vessels, and the serous cavities of the body.

endotoxin: Potentially toxic, natural compound found inside pathogens such as bacteria. Unlike an exotoxin, it is not secreted in soluble form by live bacteria but is a structural component in the bacteria that is released mainly when bacteria are lyzed. Endotoxin is associated with the outer membranes of certain gram-negative bacteria, and its main active ingredient is the lipopolysaccharide (LPS) or lipooligosaccharide (LOS) complex. It can be cytotoxic or pyogenic, has been shown to induce and/or amplify inflammation, and has been implicated in the etiologies of periodontitis. For most purposes, the terms endotoxin and LPS are used interchangeably. See: Lipopolysaccharide (LPS).

engaging: Feature of a dental implant or prosthetic component that incorporates an antirotation mechanical design. See: Nonengaging.

enostosis: Denotes a concentration of mature compact (cortical) bone within the cancellous bone (spongiosa) and can be referred to as condensing osteitis. This benign lesion may be located anywhere in the skeleton but has a predilection for the long bones and pelvis. It is probably congenital in nature and suggests failure of resorption during endochondral ossification. See: Osteitis, condensing.

enteral administration: Any technique of administration in which the agent is absorbed through the gastrointestinal (GI) tract or oral mucosa (i.e., oral, rectal, sublingual).

entrance port: The area on the surface of a patient where a radiation beam is incident.

enucleate: To remove an organ or lesion in its entirety without rupture. Often used to describe the removal of a benign odontogenic cyst from the jaws.

envelope flap: Flap that is elevated from a horizontal linear incision, parallel to the free gingival margin, with no vertical incision, creating an envelope or pouch; most often used in combination with connective tissue grafts. It may be sulcular or submarginal.

enzyme: A catalytic protein formed by living cells and having a specific action in promoting a chemical change.

enzyme-linked immunosorbent assay (ELISA): Enzyme-linked immunosorbent assay wherein an enzyme-antibody complex binds to an agent thought to be present in a sample. Typically, an enzyme-activated dye is used to detect the presence of bound immunoglobulin-enzyme.

epidermal cell: Any of the cells making up the epidermis, the outer layer of the skin covering the exterior body surface. Epidermis comprises, from within, five epithelial layers: the basal layer (stratum basale), the spinous layer (stratum spinosum), the granular layer (stratum granulosum), the clear layer (stratum lucidum), and the cornified layer (stratum corneum).

epidermal growth factor: Mitogenic polypeptide that promotes growth and differentiation, is essential in embryogenesis, and is important in wound healing.

epinephrine: A catecholamine neurohormone produced by the adrenal medulla and secreted into the blood supply, whereupon it is circulated throughout the body and may stimulate receptors that initiate sympathomimetic effects; used in local anesthetic solutions for its activation of alpha receptors, which induces vasoconstriction.

epiphysis: End of a bone shaft, consisting of trabecular bone covered by a thin cortex.

epithelial apical migration: Migration of gingival sulcular and junctional epithelia in the apical direction as a result of periodontitis progression. During the healing process after periodontal therapy, the epithelial cells migrate apically, attaching to the root or oral implant surface and preventing connective tissue cell attachment.

epithelial attachment: The mechanism of attachment of the junctional epithelium to a tooth or dental implant, i.e., hemidesmosomes. See: Junctional epithelium.

epithelial cell: Cell that lines hollow organs and glands and makes up the outer surface of the body. Arranged in single or multiple layers, depending on the type, they help protect or enclose organs. Some produce mucus or other secretions, and others have tiny hairs called cilia, which help remove foreign substances, for example from the respiratory tract.

epithelial cuff: A term that describes the intimate relationship between the gingival mucosa and the dental implant. The use of this term implies a close adherence, and suggests a lack of true biochemical connection or attachment between the implant and mucosa.

epithelial implant: See: Mucosal insert.

epithelialization (epithelization): 1. The growth of epithelium over connective tissue during the healing process. 2. The process, either pathologic or part of normal healing, whereby an area of the oral cavity is covered by or converted to epithelium.

epithelial pegs: Oral epithelium connects to the underlying connective tissue by ridge-like projections of epithelium (rete ridges). The epithelial projections appear as pegs in cross-section.

epithelium: Anatomy term used to describe the surface layer or lining of an organ. In the mouth, it is used to describe the mucosal tissue serving as the lining of the intraoral surfaces. See: Crevicular epithelium, Junctional epithelium.

epithelium, oral: The tissue serving as the lining of the intraoral surfaces. The junctional form is nonkeratinized, is single or multiple layered, and adheres to the tooth surface at the base of the gingival crevice. The epithelium in the oral cavity is either keratinized or nonkeratinized depending on its location.

eposteal dental implant: A dental implant that obtains its principal support through sitting on top of the edentulous areas of the alveolar bone. Supplementary retaining screws that enter directly into the bone for the purposes of securing this implant framework to the alveolar bone are referred to as an endosteal dental implant component. If the eposteal framework should become submerged and covered by the alveolar bone, then it may be described as having become an endosteal dental implant; an eposteal dental implant's support system is also known as the implant frame, implant framework, or implant substructure.

eposteal implant: Device that receives its primary bone support by means of resting upon bone. See: Subperiosteal implant.

epoxy resin: A strong, yet flexible, chemically resistant, dimensionally constant resin of epoxy polymers; frequently used as a denture base material in dentistry.

epoxy resin die: A reproduction or model produced with/in epoxy resin.

Epstein–Barr virus (EBV): Herpes DNA virus that causes Burkitt's lymphoma in which the human peripheral blood leukocytes are transformed into lymphoblast-like cells with an indefinite life span.

e-PTFE (abbrev.): Expanded polytetrafluoroethylene.

epulis: A nonspecific word for any inflammatory cellular proliferation or a tumor-like growth or lump of the gingiva.

epulis fissuratum: Overgrowth of intraoral tissue as the result of chronic irritation such as that caused by the overextended flange of a denture.

equalization of pressure: The act of evenly distributing a load.

equilibrate: To bring or to place in balance or equilibrium.

equilibration: The action or process of creating a state of balance or equilibrium.

equilibration, occlusal: 1. The process of bringing patients' teeth when closed into a state of balance by selectively grinding premature or excessive opposing tooth contacts. 2. The equalization of occlusal stress by modifying the chewing surfaces of a tooth or teeth that results in the formation of proper occlusal contacts or harmonizing cuspal relations. See: Occlusal adjustment.

equilibrium: 1. A state of even adjustment between opposing forces. 2. That state or condition of a body in which any forces acting on it are so arranged that their product at every point is zero. 3. A balance between active forces and negative resistance.

erosion: 1. An eating away; a type of ulceration. 2. In dentistry, the progressive loss of tooth substance by chemical processes that do not involve bacterial action, producing defects that are sharply defined, wedge-shaped depressions often in facial and cervical areas. Compare: Abfraction, Abrasion, Attrition.

eruption, dental: The emergence of a tooth into the oral cavity. **Active e.**: The process by which a tooth moves from its germinative position to its functional position in occlusion with the opposing arch. **Passive e.**: Tooth exposure secondary to apical migration of the gingival margin to a location at or slightly coronal to the cementoenamel junction.

Er-YAG laser: Er-YAG is an acronym for erbium-doped yttrium aluminum garnet, a compound used as the lasing medium for certain solid-state lasers. Er-YAG lasers typically emit light with a wavelength of 2940 nm, which is in the infrared range. The frequency of Er-YAG lasers is at the resonant frequency of water, which causes it to be quickly absorbed; this limits its use in surgery.

erythema: Redness of the skin or mucous membranes produced by congestion of the capillaries.

erythema multiforme: An acute dermatitis of unknown cause that may be precipitated by drug intake, herpes simplex infection, or other diseases. Characteristic erythematous "target" or "bull's eye" lesions occur on the skin; intraorally, diffuse hyperemic macules, papules, and vesicles may be seen.

erythrocyte: Mature red blood cell. The function of this nonnucleated, biconcave disk containing hemoglobin is to transport oxygen.

erythromycin: A bacteriostatic macrolide group of antibiotics that has both gram-positive and gram-negative antibacterial spectra and acts by inhibiting ribosomal protein synthesis.

erythroplasia (erythroplakia): A red, papular, or macular lesion that is frequently ulcerated and found on a mucous membrane. It is considered to be precancerous.

eschar: A scab or slough caused by a burn, by cauterization, or through application of a corrosive substance.

esthetic: 1. Descriptive of a specific creation that results from such study; objectifies beauty and attractiveness, and elicits pleasure. 2. Pertaining to sensation; variant spelling of aesthetic.

esthetic complication: Complication caused by the malposition of an implant in either the mesiodistal, coronal-apical, or orofacial direction, or by the lack of peri-implant bone or soft tissues. Such complications can be a major concern for clinicians, since removal of the implant may be required.

esthetic reshaping: Physical modification of biological surfaces, such as the teeth or face, to enhance beauty or to improve appearance.

esthetic zone: Any dentoalveolar segment visible upon full smile. The relationship of the three components involved in the smile (i.e., gingiva, lips, teeth) determines whether a particular smile will be classified as (a) an extremely high smile line; (b) a high smile line; (c) a moderate smile line; (d) a low smile line.

esthetics: 1. The branch of philosophy dealing with beauty. 2. In dentistry, the theory and philosophy that deals with beauty and the beautiful, especially with respect to the appearance of a dental restoration, as achieved through its form and/or color.

Those subjective and objective elements and principles underlying the beauty and attractiveness of an object, design, or principle.

estrogen: A generic term for naturally occurring steroid hormones containing an estrane nucleus (estrone, estradiol, estriol, etc.); secreted from the testis, ovary, and placenta; stimulates protein anabolic actions and exerts a positive effect on nitrogen balance; regulates the growth and maintenance of female accessory sex organs and secondary sex characteristics; implicated in hormonal, pubertal, and menopausal desquamative gingivitis.

etch: 1. To produce a retentive surface, especially on glass or metal, by the corrosive action of an acid. 2. To subject to such etching. 3. To delineate or impress clearly.

etchant: An agent that is capable of etching a surface.

etching: 1. The act or process of selective dissolution. 2. In dentistry, the selective dissolution of the surface of tooth enamel, metal, or porcelain through the use of acids or other agents (etchants) to create a retentive surface.

ethylene oxide: A bactericidal agent that is a toxic, flammable, colorless gas or liquid, frequently used for sterilizing or disinfecting medical instruments.

etiologic factors: The elements or influences that can be assigned as the cause or reason for a disease or lesion.

etiology: The study of the causes of disease; alternatively, the cause of a disease.

Eubacterium **ssp.**: Gram-positive, nonmotile anaerobic, rod-shaped bacteria frequently found in subgingival plaque.

Eubacterium brachii: Gram-positive, nonmotile, anaerobic, pleomorphic bacilli or coccobacilli that occur in pairs of short chains. Found in the oral cavity, they are usually part of the indigenous oral flora.

Eubacterium timidum: Gram-positive, nonmotile, anaerobic bacilli that are isolated from wounds and other infections and are associated with other anaerobes and facultative bacteria. May be involved in bacteremia and endocarditis.

evidence-based dentistry: An interdisciplinary approach for clinical decision making on the oral healthcare of each patient by integrating best current research evidence, one's own clinical expertise, the patient's preferences and needs, and other resources.

evisceration: Elimination of the viscera or contents of a cavity; extraction; removal, usually unexpected.

evulsion: Extraction; removal, usually of a sudden nature. See: Avulsion.

exacerbation: An increase in the severity of the signs or symptoms of a disease.

excision: A cutting out; removal; the process of amputating or cutting away any portion of the body.

exclusion criteria: The specific characteristics that prevent a participant from entering a clinical trial or study group. See: Inclusion criteria.

excursion: 1. A movement away from and back to the mean position or alignment; also, the distance navigated. 2. In dentistry, the movement transpiring when the mandible moves from the position of maximum intercuspation.

excursive: Constituting a digression; characterized by digression.

excursive movement: Movement occurring when the mandible and its associated teeth move away from the maximum intercuspation position with the maxillary teeth.

exenteration: Removal of an organ. For maxillofacial prosthetics, removal of the eye and surrounding contents from the orbit, called orbital exenteration; usually implies the fabrication of an orbital prosthesis.

exfoliation: 1. The sloughing of a previously attached matter or tissue from the body. 2. The sloughing of the oldest nonvital epithelial cells from the skin's outermost surface. 3. In dentistry, the physiological shedding of the primary teeth or the loss of implanted materials.

exogenous: Due to external source or cause; not developing from within the organism.

exophytic: Emergent outward; proliferation on the outside or surface of an organ.

exostosis (singular), **exostoses** (plural): A benign, bony growth projecting outward from the surface of a bone. See: Torus.

exotoxin: A toxic substance or matter formed by a bacterial species that is released to the surrounding tissues.

expanded polytetrafluoroethylene (e-PTFE): A polymer of tetrafluoroethylene, stretched to allow fluid passage but not cells, used as a nonresorbable membrane in guided bone regeneration (GBR) and guided tissue regeneration (GTR). It is used with or without titanium reinforcement to maintain its shape. It is also used as a nonabsorbable suture material.

expanded polytetrafluoroethylene (e-PTFE) **membrane**: Barrier membrane made of a polymer of tetrafluoroethylene. e-PTFE is a matrix of polytetrafluoroethylene (PTFE) nodes and fibrils in a microstructure that can be varied in porosity to address the clinical and biologic requirements of its intended applications.

experimental group: (syn): Test group. A group of subjects who receive the treatment being studied. See: Control group.

experimental study: Study in which measurements are made of one independent variable while everything else around that one variable remains constant.

exposure: 1. Dental implant: the dehiscence of soft tissue exposing the dental implant cover screw, neck, body, or threads. Colloquial term for stage two surgery. 2. Barrier membrane: the dehiscence of soft tissue exposing an occlusive membrane during the healing period. 3. In radiology, a measure of the roentgen rays or gamma radiation at a certain place based on its ability to cause ionization. The unit of exposure is the roentgen. Called also exposure dose.

extender: A surgical component used as an intermediary piece between the handpiece or wrench and another component (e.g., drill, implant mount) to increase the effective reach of the latter.

extension: 1. The movement by which the two elements of any jointed part are drawn away from each other, the process of increasing the angle between two skeletal levers having end-to-end articulation with each other. The opposite of flexion. 2. In maxillofacial prosthetics, that portion of a prosthesis added to fill a defect or provide a function not inherent in a dental restoration, e.g., palatal extension, pharyngeal extension.

extension base partial removable dental prosthesis: A removable dental prosthesis that is supported and retained by natural teeth only at one end of the denture base segment and in which a portion of the functional load is carried by the residual ridge.

external abutment connection: Interface between a transmucosal component (abutment) and the coronal surface of an implant. The implant's coronal surface may have an external hexagon, which is engaged when the transmucosal component is seated. See also: Abutment connection.

external bevel incision: Blade cut, made in an apical-coronal direction, designed to reduce the thickness of gingiva or periimplant mucosa from the external surface. See: Internal bevel incision.

external connection: A prosthetic connection interface external to the dental implant platform. The external hexagon is an example. See: Internal connection.

external hexagon: A hexagonal connection interface of the platform of a dental implant extending coronally. It prevents gross rotation of the attached component. See: Internal hexagon.

external hexagon abutment connection: See: External abutment connection, Hex.

external hex implant: See: External abutment connection, Hex.

external irrigation: Method of irrigation during the drilling of osteotomies for the placement of dental implants from an external device, whereby the cooling solution is directed at the drilling bur during preparation of the osteotomy. This method delivers the cooling solution at the entrance of the osteotomy. The cooling solution may be delivered through tubing connected to the handpiece and drilling unit, or it may be from a hand-held system. See: Internal irrigation.

external oblique ridge: A smooth edge or ridge on the buccal surface of the body of the mandible that ranges from the anterior border of the ramus, with lessening prominence, downward and forward to the region of the mental foramen. This edge or ridge remains unchanged in size and direction for the most part throughout life. It is where the buccinator muscle attaches and affords a consistent landmark for the construction of dentures and subperiosteal implants.

external sinus graft: See: Lateral window technique, Sinus graft.

extirpate: 1. To deliberately pull up or out. 2. To completely annihilate or destroy. 3. To surgically remove – extirpation.

extirpation: The complete surgical elimination or removal of a tissue or organ.

extracapsular ankyloses: Immobility and consolidation of a joint due to rigidity of any structure external to the joint capsule resulting from disease, injury, or surgery.

extracapsular disorder: Pain and dysfunction associated with the masticatory apparatus, which is caused by etiologic factors located outside the temporomandibular joint capsule.

extracellular matrix (ECM): Material produced by cells and excreted to the extracellular space within the tissues. It takes the form of both ground substance and fibers and is composed chiefly of fibrous elements, proteins involved in cell adhesion, glycosaminoglycans, and other space-filling molecules. It serves as a scaffold for holding tissues together, and its form and composition help determine tissue characteristics. The matrix may be mineralized to resist compression (as in bone) or dominated by tension-resisting fibers (as in tendon).

extracoronal: That which is outside or external to the crown portion of a natural tooth, e.g., an extracoronal preparation, restoration, partial, or complete crown.

extracoronal attachment: Any prefabricated attachment for support and retention of a removable dental prosthesis. The male and female components are positioned outside the normal contour of the abutment tooth. See: Intracoronal attachment, Precision attachment.

extracoronal retainer: That part of a fixed dental prosthesis uniting the abutment to the other elements of a prosthesis that surrounds all or part of the prepared crown.

extracortical: Outside the cortical plate of the bone or bone cortex.

extraction: Removal of a tooth or teeth.

extraction socket: Open socket or alveolar space in the alveolar process following removal of a tooth.

extraction socket graft: See: Bio-Col technique.

extraoral (external) distraction device: A device that is located outside the oral cavity and used in distraction osteogenesis. The bone segments are usually attached via percutaneous pins connected externally to device fixation clamps.

extraoral tracing: A recording of mandibular movements made with a stylus on a recording plate that extends outside the oral cavity. A tracing made outside the oral cavity.

extraosseous distractor: Jack-like device attached lateral to maxillary or mandibular basal bone for the purpose of creating incremental separation between jaw segments planned for distraction. See: Distraction osteogenesis (DO).

extraversion: See: Labioversion.

extrinsic: External, extraneous, as originating from or on the outside.

extrinsic coloring: Shading from without; color applied to the exterior surface of a prosthesis.

extrusion: 1. The overeruption or movement of teeth outside the desired occlusal plane that may be accompanied by a similar movement of their supporting tissues. 2. Squeezing out of material through the application of pressure, such as denture acrylic escaping from the invested flask as hydraulic pressure is applied to it.

exudate: A fluid produced as a result of injury to tissue and/or to a blood vessel. The secreted material can be made of serum, fibrin, white blood cells, and/or red blood cells that escape from blood vessels into a superficial lesion or area of inflammation. The content of the fluid is dependent upon the *in situ* environment. Serum can be predominant if the exudate is fabricated by the contraction of a fibrin plug in the damaged space that releases serum into the area, or the exudate composition could be primarily made of polymorphonuclear leukocytes as in the case of pus formation at an injury site. **Fibrinous e.**: Characterized by an abundance of fibrinogen resulting in subsequent fibrin formation at the site of injury. **Hemorrhagic e.**: Characterized by an abundance of red blood cells. **Purulent e.**: Characterized by an abundance of polymorphonuclear leukocytes, resulting in pus formation at the site of injury. **Serous e.**: Characterized by an abundance of serous fluid of high protein content.

F

fabrication: The building, making, or constructing of a restoration.

facebow: A caliper-like instrument used to record the spatial relationship of the maxillary arch to some anatomic reference point or points and then transfer this relationship to an articulator; it orients the dental cast in the same relationship to the opening axis of the articulator. Customarily, the anatomic references are the mandibular condyles transverse horizontal axis and one other selected anterior point. Called also hinge bow.

facebow fork: Component attached to the facebow that transfers the maxillary arch position to the facebow, thus orienting the occlusal table of the dentition to the center of rotation of the condylar joints of the mandible to a selected anterior point on the face (e.g., the infraorbital fossa).

facebow record: The registration obtained through the use of a facebow and facebow fork using three points of orientation (center of rotation of both condylar joints and an arbitrary point on the face) that have been locked into place in relation to each other.

facebow transfer: The process of conveying the recorded facebow three-deminsional correlation of the maxillary dental arch and additional anatomic orientation point(s) to the articulator.

face form: The outline shape of the face from the frontal view, designated by shape as square, tapering, ovoid, or a blend of these shapes. Facial shape may be used to choose tooth shapes for a dental restoration to be in harmony with the facial form, creating a more natural and pleasing esthetic effect.

facet: A small, flat visible surface on any hard body created by function. Specifically, a facet on a tooth may indicate wear, usually on the occlusal or incisal surface of a tooth, which has been caused by wearing against an opposing tooth. The observation of facets of wear on teeth can be clues to parafunctional habits or disharmony of the occlusion of opposing teeth due to malocclusion.

facial: The surface of a tooth or other oral structure approximating the face (including both the lips and cheeks).

facial augmentation implant prosthesis: A maxillofacial prosthesis made of implantable biocompatible material generally onlayed upon an existing bony area beneath the skin tissue to fill in or selectively raise portions of the overlaying facial skin tissues to create acceptable contours. Although some forms of premade surgical implants are commercially available, the facial augmentation implant prosthesis is usually custom made for surgical implantation for each individual patient due to the irregular or extensive nature of the facial deficit. Also called a facial implant.

facial form: Anterior view of the facial outline.

facial moulage: Impression of facial soft tissues and bony contours to obtain a working cast for the fabrication of an extraoral prosthesis.

facial profile: The outline form of the face from a lateral view.

Glossary of Dental Implantology, First Edition. Khalid Almas, Fawad Javed and Steph Smith.
© 2018 John Wiley & Sons, Inc. Published 2018 by John Wiley & Sons, Inc.

facial prosthesis: A maxillofacial prosthetic device that restores a portion of the face that is congenitally absent or altered due to surgery or trauma. Also called an extraoral prosthesis or prosthetic dressing.

facial prosthetic adhesive: A substance used to retain a facial prosthesis in its proper position.

facial symmetry: Mutually balanced relationship of facial parts relative to size, arrangement, or measurements.

facing: A veneer of a restoration on a natural tooth or prosthetic device to alter, duplicate, or improve upon the appearance of a natural tooth.

facultative: 1. Voluntary; possessing the power to do or not to do a thing. 2. Capable of existing under different conditions, as a microorganism that can exist in either aerobic or anaerobic conditions.

failed implant: A dental implant that is mobile (has not achieved or has lost osseointegration), or that is symptomatic in spite of osseointegration.

failing implant: General term for a dental implant that is progressively losing its supporting bone anchorage. It may exhibit increased probing depth or purulence, but is still clinically stable. See: Periimplantitis.

failure rate: The percentage of failures in a study or clinical trial, of a procedure or device (e.g., dental implant), according to defined criteria.

familial: A condition that occurs in members of a family. See: Congenital.

fatigue: The breaking or fracturing of a material caused by repeated cyclic or applied loads below the yield limit; usually viewed initially as minute cracks followed by tearing and rupture; also termed brittle failure or metal fracture.

fatigue failure: A structural failure caused by multiple loading episodes when all loads lie below the structure's ultimate strength. Typically, such failures occur after multiple loading episodes.

fatigue fracture (failure): Structural failure caused by repetitive stresses, which cause a slowly propagating crack to cross the material.

FDBA (abbrev.): Freeze-dried bone allograft.

FEA (abbrev.): Finite element analysis.

feature locating object (FLO): A general term used to describe a digital implant physical marker used in laboratory scanning, providing for the digital capture of the implant fixture/platform position. See: Fiducial marker.

Feldkamp back projection: Standard method algorithm used with most CBCT for constructing slice sets.

feldspar: 1. Any one of a group of minerals, principally aluminosilicate of sodium, potassium, calcium, or barium, that are essential constituents of nearly all crystalline rocks. 2. A crystalline mineral of aluminum silicate with sodium, potassium, barium, and/or calcium; a major constituent of some dental porcelains.

fenestrate: To puncture or perforate with one or several openings.

fenestration: A hole or opening in a body part, for example, a hole in alveolar bone or the soft tissue that covers the root of a tooth. See: Dehiscence.

ferrule: l. A metal band or ring used to fit the root or crown of a tooth. The ferrule is to be on sound tooth structure and ideally 2 mm or more in height. 2. Any short tube or bushing for making a tight joint.

ferrule length: The occlusal-apical height of tooth structure apical to a foundation restoration that is engaged by a full coverage restoration.

festoon: Contour of the soft tissues covering the roots of the teeth that tends to follow the cervical lines. Specifically, in prosthodontics, a carving in the base material of a denture that simulates the contours of the natural tissues being replaced by the denture.

festoons, gingival: The contours of the gingiva and oral mucosa over the roots of the teeth that tend to follow the cervical lines. These are prominent in the presence of a thin alveolar process.

fetor oris: Foul or unpleasant odor from the oral cavity; breath odor. See: Halitosis.

FGF (abbrev.): Fibroblast growth factor.

FHA (abbrev.): Fluorohydroxyapatite.

fiber: A filament or strand-like structure. **Alveolar crest f.**: Attaches to the cementum just apical to the cementoenamel junction and runs apically and laterally to insert into the surface of the alveolus. **Alveolar gingival f.**: Collagenous fiber that radiates from the bone of the alveolar crest into the lamina propria of the free and attached gingiva. **Apical f.**: Radiates from the cementum around the apex of the root to the adjacent bone. **Circular f.**: Collagenous fiber bundles within the gingiva that encircle the tooth in a ring-like fashion. **Collagen f.**: elastic, soft, white fibers containing protein collagen fibril bundles that are the most representative component of all connective tissue. **Dentogingival f.**: Numerous collagenous fibers that extend from cervical cementum to the lamina propria of the free and attached gingiva. **Dentoperiosteal f.**: Fibers running from the cementum over the periosteum of the outer cortical plates of the alveolar process where they insert into the alveolar process or muscle in the vestibule of the floor of the mouth. **Gingival f.**: Collagen fibrils organized into bundles, or fibers, provide the major structural component of the connective tissue matrix of gingiva. Type I and type III collagens are most abundant in the gingiva. **Horizontal f.**: Located just apical to the alveolar crest group, these fibers run perpendicular to the long axis of the root from cementum to bone. **Interradicular f.**: Found between the roots of multirooted teeth, these fibers run from the cementum into the crestal bone of the interradicular septum. **Muscle f.**: Skeletal or heart muscle cells. **Nerve f.**: The slim axonal process of a nerve cell. **Oblique f.**: The most numerous collagenous fiber group of the periodontal ligament; run from the cementum outwardly and coronally to insert into the bone. **Periodontal f.**: Typically, a collection of collagenous or elastic connective tissue. **Principal f.**: The major fiber groups of the functioning periodontium. **Reticular f.**: Immature connective tissue fibers. **Transseptal f.**: Collagenous fibers that run interdentally from the cementum just apical to the base of the junctional epithelium of one tooth over the alveolar crest to insert into a comparable region of an adjacent tooth.

fiberotomy: See: Gingival fiberotomy.

fibrin clot: Clump that results from coagulation of the blood after a sequential process by which the multiple coagulation factors of the blood interact in the coagulation cascade. Essentially composed of fibrin, this insoluble protein is formed from fibrinogen by the proteolytic action of thrombin. Called also a blood clot.

fibrinolysis: enzymatic process of dissolution of fibrin. Plasmin, the main enzyme involved, degrades the fibrin mesh, leading to the production of circulating fragments that are cleared by other proteinases or organs.

fibrin-rich matrix: Provisional matrix provided by the fibrin clot and fibronectin at the first phase of wound healing. It helps monocytes, fibroblasts, and epidermal cells migrate into the healing area.

fibroblast: The principal connective tissue cell; a flattened, irregularly branched cell with a large, oval nucleus that functions in the production and remodeling of extracellular matrix.

fibroblast growth factor (FGF): Family of growth factors with mitogenic properties for fibroblasts and mesoderm-derived cell types. They have important roles in angiogenesis, neurogenesis, wound healing, and tumor growth. In humans, more than 20 proteins have been identified as members of the FGF family. FGF-2, or basic FGF (bFGF), has been the most studied member of the FGF family for therapeutic purposes in regenerative treatments, notably soft tissue healing.

fibrointegration: See: Fibrous integration.

fibroma: Fibrous connective tissue that is a benign neoplasm; peripheral. **Ossifying f.**: A fibroma, normally of the gingiva, presenting with areas of calcification or ossification.

fibromatosis: Group of tumor-like lesions that have an infiltrative nature and can be locally aggressive, making them difficult to remove completely. They can recur following surgery but do not metastasize to other parts of the body. Fibromatoses have also been known to undergo spontaneous regression and completely disappear.

fibronectin: Adhesive glycoprotein with a high molecular weight (450 kD), composed of two disulfide-linked polypeptides. Functional domains of the molecule have an affinity for cells and the extracellular matrix components. It is found on cell surfaces, in connective tissues, blood, and other body fluids. Fibronectins are important in connective tissue, where they cross-link to collagen, promote cellular adhesion and/or migration, and are involved in aggregation of platelets.

fibroosseous (fibro-steal) integrated implant: See: Implant, oral.

fibroosseous integration: Direct attachment of bone to fibrous tissue without a definable intervening tissue. Compare: Osseointegration. See: Fibrous integration, Integration.

fibrosis: A subsurface collagenous soft tissue replacement that occurs as a result of chronic inflammation. The tissue appears and feels thick and dense. Fibrosis may occur as a result of chronic inflammation around dental implants that support prosthetic crowns. The tissue becomes thick and enlarges with collagen deposition in the surrounding gingival tissue. There is usually no bleeding on probing of the surrounding sulcus. The collagenous deposition may occur interproximally at supporting implants that fill the embrasure space to mimic interdental papillae.

fibrous: Composed of or containing fibers.

fibrous adhesion: A fibrous band or structure by which parts not normally connected adhere to each other.

fibrous ankylosis: Decreased movement of a joint due to proliferation of fibrous tissue.

fibrous encapsulation: Layer of fibrous connective tissue formed between a dental implant and surrounding bone. See also: Fibroosseous integration, Fibrous encapsulation.

fibrous integration: The existence of a sheet of interfering fibrous connective tissue membrane found between a dental implant body and the contiguous bone.

fibrous integration of implant: interposition of healthy dense collagenous tissue between implant and bone. See: Fibrous encapsulation.

fibula free flap: Graft used in oral and maxillofacial surgery for jaw reconstruction following tumor resection. It provides a long segment of bone and can include a large fasciocutaneous component. Flap harvested as osteocutaneous or purely osseous.

fibular bone graft with free flap: See: Fibula free flap.

fiducial marker: An object used in the field of view of an imaging system which appears in the image produced, for use as a point of reference or a measure. It may be either something placed into or on the imaging subject, or a mark or set of marks in the reticule (or reticle) of an optical instrument.

filiform papilla: See: Papilla.

final impression: The impression that represents completion of the registration of the surface or object.

finger-joint replacement: Artificial replacement for human finger-joints, including the thumb.

finish: To put a definitive covering or surface on; the enhancement of a form before polishing.

finish junction: The marginal adaptation of tooth and restoration.

finish line: 1. A delineation line determined by two points. 2. The marginal extension of a tooth preparation. 3. The prearranged seam of dissimilar materials. 4. The end portion of the prepared tooth.

finite element analysis (FEA): Science of creating computer simulations of mechanical or clinical situations. It is used to predict properties of structures and for structural design.

finite element model: Structural simulation generated by computer programming.

firing: The method of porcelain fusion; in dentistry, purposely to fabricate porcelain restorations.

first stage dental implant surgery: The initial surgical procedure in dental implant placement. For eposteal dental implants, this refers to the reflection of the oral mucosa, the impression made of the surgically exposed bone and usually an interocclusal record made to fabricate the implant body followed by surgical closure. For an endosteal implant, this refers to the reflection of the oral mucosa and investing tissues, preparation of the implantation site (i.e., removal of alveolar bone and, occasionally, tapping), placement of the dental implant body, and surgical closure of the overlying investing soft tissues. Compare: Second stage dental implant surgery.

Fisher exact test: Statistical test used in medical research, testing independence of rows and columns in a 2×2 contingency table (with two horizontal rows crossing two vertical columns, creating four places for data) based on exact sampling distribution of observed frequencies.

fissure: A general term for a cleft or groove.

fistula: A pathologic or atypical passage that is the result of poor healing; an unintended or unwanted pathway between differing internal structures or one that connects an internal structure to the (external) surface of a body; usually named according to the body parts it connects. **Oroantral f.**: An abnormal opening between the maxillary sinus and the mouth. **Orofacial f.**: An abnormal opening between the cutaneous surface of the face and mouth. **Oronasal f.**: An abnormal opening between the nasal cavity and the mouth.

fit: 1.To conform correctly to the shape or size of something. 2. To insert or adjust until correctly in place; to make or adjust to the correct size or shape, i.e., to adapt one structure to another, as the adaptation of any dental restoration to its site, in the mouth.

fixation, bicortical: See: Bicortical stabilization.

fixation period: See: Distraction osteogenesis, Consolidation period.

fixation screw: A mechanical device used to stabilize block grafts, membranes, and other devices by fixation to the alveolar bone.

fixation tack: Element designed to resemble a simple tack. It is used to retain a membrane over augmentation material during ridge augmentation surgery.

fixed: Firmly placed; immovable and stable in one place, does not move.

fixed bridge: See: Fixed dental prosthesis.

fixed dental prosthesis (FDP): A replacement of one or more missing teeth that cannot be readily removed by the patient or dentist; it is fixed or bonded to natural teeth, roots, or implants which furnish the primary support to the prosthesis.

fixed dental prosthesis retainer: The portion of a fixed dental device that joins the abutment(s) to the other parts of the device.

fixed-detachable: Prosthesis fixed to a dental implant or implants, only removable by the dentist. See: Fixed prosthesis.

fixed hybrid prosthesis: Nonremovable hybrid prosthesis. See: Hybrid prosthesis.

fixed movable bridge: A fixed partial denture having one or more nonrigid connectors.

fixed partial denture: Nonremovable partial prosthesis supported by teeth and/or implants. See: Fixed dental prosthesis.

fixed prosthesis: Dental or maxillofacial prosthesis supported and retained by natural teeth, tooth roots, or dental implants, not readily removed by the patient. Synonym for bridge. See: Hybrid prosthesis, Implant-supported prosthesis (ISP), Provisional prosthesis.

fixed prosthodontics: Subdivision of prosthodontics concerned with the replacement of teeth with dental implants and/or replacement of tooth crowns with restorations fixed in place (nonremovable).

fixed-removable: Prosthesis fixed to an implant or implants, only removable by the dentist. See: Fixed prosthesis.

fixture: An endosteal dental implant. Term coined to define an endosteal dental implant, root form, blade, ramus frame, that are embedded and integrated or fixed in the bone for stabilization of the superstructured prosthetics. See: Endosseous implant.

flabby tissue: Excessive movable tissue.

flange: A rim used for strength, for directing or connecting to another segment of an object. The portion of denture material protruding into the buccal, lingual, or labial tissue area of a denture.

flange contour: The design of the extension of a denture shape or form of a protuberance or extension of a denture tissue surface.

flank angle: The angle made by the flank of a screw thread with a line perpendicular to the axis of the screw.

flap: A loosened section of tissue separated from the surrounding tissues except at its base. **Coronally positioned f.**: surgical flap that is moved to a new position coronal to its previous position. **Double papilla pedicle f.**: The use of the papillae on the mesial and distal of a tooth as laterally positioned flaps sutured together over the tooth root. **Envelope f.**: A flap retracted from a horizontal linear incision, as along the free gingival margin, with no vertical incision. **Gingival f.**: A flap that does not extend apical to the mucogingival junction. **Modified Widman f.**: A scalloped, replaced, mucoperiosteal flap, accomplished with an internal bevel incision, that provides access to the root for root planing. **Mucogingival f.**: A flap that includes both gingiva and alveolar mucosa. **Mucoperiosteal (full thickness) f.**: A mucosal flap (usually gingiva and alveolar mucosa) that includes the periosteum. **Papillary pedicle f.**: A laterally rotated flap employing the gingival papilla. **Partial, thickness (split thickness) f.**: A surgical flap of mucosa and connective tissue that does not include the periosteum. **Pedicle f.**: A surgical flap with lateral releasing incisions. See: Sliding flap. **Positioned f.**: A surgical flap that is moved or advanced laterally, coronally, or apically to a new position. **Replaced f.**: A flap replaced in its original position. **Repositioned f.**: See: Replaced flap. **Sliding f.**: A pedicle flap moved to a new position.

flapless implant surgery: Surgical technique where no soft tissue flaps are raised or when a circular piece of tissue is removed to permit placement of a dental implant.

flapless surgery: Implant placement performed without the elevation of a flap.

flask: A container used in investing procedures, usually a metal case or tube.

flask closure: A process by which two halves, or parts, of a flask are brought together.

flasking: Before the final molding preparation of the denture, this process is the act of investing the wax replica of the anticipated form into a flask.

flat panel detectors: A square or rectangular amorphous plate with a scintillator that replaces film, used in cone beam computed tomography.

fleece, collagen: See: Collagen fleece.

flipper: A prosthesis that is usually considered to be temporary in design. It traditionally has one tooth attached to an acrylic base typically without clasps, although wrought wire clasps may be used for additional retention. See: Interim prosthesis, Provisional prosthesis.

FLO (abbrev.): Feature locating object.

flow cytometry: Measures the physical and chemical characteristics of individual cells as they move past optical or electronic sensors; can be used to detect and characterize specific cells in a mixed population; used to determine the effects of drugs, hormones, chemicals.

flowing composite resin: Compared with a conventional composite resin, this type of resin has less filler and less viscosity but improved wettability.

fluoride-modifying surface treatment: Implant treatment that exposes the surface to a cleansing bath of hydrofluoric acid following treatment with etching or blasting. This technique has been shown to improve biomechanical anchorage and bone integration when compared to control implants treated without the hydrofluoric acid bath.

fluorochrome: Fluorescent substance used as a stain or label for biologic specimens. In implant dentistry, it is used in research to evaluate the kinetics of osteogenesis and osseointegration on implant surfaces.

fluorohydroxyapatite: (FHA): Pyrolytical segmentation of natural algae and hydrothermal transformation of the calcium carbonate ($CaCO_3$) skeleton of algae into FHA ($Ca_5(PO_4)_3OHxF1-x$). Particles consist of a pore system (mean diameter 10 μm), periodically separated (mean interval 30 μm) and interconnectedly microperforated (mean diameter of perforations 1 μm).

fluorosis: Condition that occurs because of excessive intake of fluoride either through naturally occurring fluoride in the water, water fluoridation, toothpaste, or other sources.

focal sclerosing osteomyelitis: A diffuse radiopaque lesion believed to represent a localized bony reaction to a low-grade infection of the pulp. It is usually seen at the apex of a tooth (or its extraction site) that has experienced chronic inflammation.

foliate papilla: See: Papilla.

follow-up: Periodic monitoring of patient health after medical or surgical treatment, including that of clinical study or trial participants.

Food and Drug Administration (FDA): Agency of United States Department of Health and Human Services that regulates testing of experimental drugs and devices. The FDA clears new drugs and medical products based on evidence of safety and efficacy.

food impaction: The forceful wedging of food into the interproximal space by chewing pressure (vertical impaction) or the forcing of food interproximally by tongue or cheek pressure (horizontal impaction).

foramen: A natural opening or passageway, specifically into or through a bone.

force: Vector of load application creating acceleration or deformation along the direction of its application. See: Biting force, Closure force, Distribution force, Pullout force. **Axial f.**: Force directed axially or through the long axis of an object. **Lateral f.**: In dentistry, forces other than axial in direction. **Pullout f.**: Force applied to dislodge an implant along its long axis and opposite from its direction of placement. See: Pullout strength.

force vector: Force applied through direction and magnitude.

Fordyce's granules: A developmental anomaly characterized by ectopic sebaceous glands appearing as minute, yellowish papules on the oral mucosa.

foreign body: A nonnative substance in the tissues or body cavities.

foreign body reaction: A granulomatous reaction around a foreign material within a tissue or organ, often characterized by giant cells. This may present as acute or chronic gingival inflammation and may produce tattoos or red, red/white or suppurative lesions.

fornix: Any arch-shaped structure or vault-like space created by that structure, such as the vestibular fornix.

forward protrusion: An anterior or front-ward protuberance of the centric position.

FOSS, F/OSS (abbrev.): Free and open-source software.

fossa: A shallow anatomic pit, concavity, depression, groove, or depression or hollow area.

foveae palatinae: Two depressions found in the posterior portion of the palatal mucosa, one on each side of the midline, either at or in close proximity to the place where the soft and hard palates meet.

fracture: 1. Failure caused by growth of a crack. 2. To result in a fracture; to split up, rupture, or tear.

fracture strength: Strength at a fracture based on the original dimensions of the specimen.

framework: 1. An interior or imbedded, openwork or structural frame used to support some other object or objects. 2. The skeletal portion of prosthesis (usually metal, sometimes ceramic) around which and to which are attached the remaining portions of the prosthesis to produce a finished restoration. For dental prostheses, the framework may be any metal or combination of metals or ceramic material, with various forms including designed slots, incorporated corrective angulation patterns, etc. which provide rigidity to a dental prosthesis. Such a framework can be made in whole or made of component parts. Frequently used to anchor a prosthesis to natural teeth (by cementation) or dental implant abutments (by cementation, mechanical undercuts, screws) or both.

framework misfit: Contacting surface discrepancy between an accurately fitting framework and one which does not fit accurately.

free and open-source software (F/OSS, FOSS): Software that is liberally licensed to grant users the right to use, copy, study, change, and improve its design through the availability of its source code.

free gingiva: That part of the gingiva that surrounds the tooth and is not directly attached to the tooth surface.

free gingival graft: Soft tissue graft taken from the patient's palate that includes the epithelium.

free gingival groove: See: Gingival groove.

free gingival margin: The unattached gingiva surrounding the teeth in a collar-like fashion and demarcated from the attached gingiva by a shallow linear depression, termed the free gingival groove.

free mandibular movement: 1. Any mandibular movement made without interference. 2. Any uninhibited movement of the mandible.

free soft tissue autograft: (syn): Gingival graft.

free-standing implant: A dental implant that is not connected to a natural tooth or splinted to adjacent teeth or implants.

freeway space: The space between the maxillary and mandibular teeth when the mandible is suspended in the postural position. See: Interocclusal rest space.

freeze-dried bone allograft (FDBA): Most commonly used allograft, which is frozen and freeze-dried (lyophilized). It may form bone or participate in new bone formation by osteoinduction or osteoconduction. It is effective when used with barrier membranes. The freezing and freeze-drying process essentially lowers the antigenicity.

freeze-drying: Method of tissue preparation in which a tissue specimen is frozen and then dehydrated at a low temperature under high-vacuum conditions. In this process, the frozen water in material is sublimated directly from solid phase to gas. See: Lyophilization.

fremitus: A vibration that can be observed visibly or is perceivable on palpation; in dentistry, the movement of a tooth that is felt when the teeth come into contact.

frenectomy: Surgical detachment and/or excision of a frenulum from its attachment into the mucoperiosteal covering of the alveolar process, especially the release of ankyloglossia.

frenulectomy: The surgical excision of a frenulum. Indicated for either orthodontic or mucogingival issues involving the frenum. Also known as frenectomy.

frenulum: A small strip or fold of integument or mucous membrane that restricts the movements of an adjacent structure.

frenuluma: Connecting fold of membrane serving to support or retain a part.

frenum: A fold of mucous membrane tissue that attaches the lips and cheeks to the alveolar mucosa (and/or gingiva) and underlying periosteum. See: Frenulum. **Abnormal f.**: Aberrant insertions of labial, buccal, or lingual frenula capable of retracting gingival margins, creating diastemata, and limiting lip and tongue movements. **Labial f.**: The fold of mucous membrane connecting the lip and the alveolar process in the midline of both the maxilla and mandible. **Lingual f.**: The fold of mucous membrane connecting the tongue with the floor of the mouth and the mandibular alveolar process.

friction retained pin: A metal dowel placed into a hole drilled by the clinician in the dentin to enhance retention of a restoration; it is retained exclusively by the elasticity of the tooth's dentin.

frictional attachment: A precision or semi-precision attachment that achieves retention by metal to metal contact, without springs, clips or other mechanical means of retention. See: Precision attachment.

friction-fit: Component retained and/or stabilized through frictional contact with another component.

friction-retained: Use of intimate fit of parts for the retention of an abutment or a prosthesis (e.g., spark erosion prosthesis).

frontal plane: Any plane passing longitudinally through the body from side to side at right angles to the median plane. It divides the body into front and back parts.

fulcrum line: 1. A theoretical line passing through the point around which a lever functions and at right angles to its path of movement. 2. An imaginary line, connecting occlusal rests, around which a partial removable dental prosthesis tends to rotate under masticatory forces. The determinants for the fulcrum line are usually the cross-arch occlusal rests located adjacent to the tissue-borne components.

full-denture prosthetics: 1. Substitution of the natural teeth in the arch and the related parts by manmade alternatives, including but not limited to acrylics, alloys, and porcelain. 2. The discipline of rebuilding an edentulous mouth.

full-thickness graft: Transfer of skin or gingival epithelium in full thickness with little or no attached subcutaneous tissue.

full veneer crown: See: Complete crown.

fully adjustable articulator: An articulator that permits simulation and duplication of the three-dimensional movements of recorded mandibular motion. See: Class IV articulator.

fully adjustable gnathologic articulator: An articulator that permits simulation and replication of the three-dimensional mandibular movements with the added benefit of providing documented timing of the mandibular motion; also called a Class IV articulator.

functional ankylosis: Concept developed by Andre Schroeder in 1981 to describe the junction between an implant and surrounding bone. Elasticity of bone makes contact and connection a functional unit in which contact between implant and bone is maintained. See: Osseointegration.

functional articulation: The occlusal contacts of the maxillary and mandibular teeth during mastication and deglutition.

functional dislocation: Displacement of the temporomandibular joint's articular disk during function due to derangement of the disk–condyle complex.

functional jaw orthopedics: Application of muscle forces to influence changes in jaw position and tooth alignment by removable appliances.

functional loading: Load applied to teeth or implant-supported prosthesis during normal chewing function.

functional mandibular movements: All normal, proper, or characteristic movements of the mandible made during speech, mastication, yawning, swallowing, and other associated movements.

functional occlusal harmony: The highest degree of masticatory efficiency in all ranges of motion without functional strain or trauma.

functional occlusal splint: Any device that works to control the plane and range of mandibular movement.

functional occlusion: Position of the working contacts of the maxillary and mandibular teeth during mastication and deglutition.

functional record: The recording of the envelope of motion of the mandible for measurement or duplication in a prosthetic device.

functional side: The side of the body towards which the mandible moves in lateral excursion.

functionally generated path: The path of motion dictated and constrained by the morphology and position of the teeth, joint anatomy, and muscles of mastication.

fungi: A eukaryotic (nucleated) group of microbes. A phylum of plants whose members are devoid of any pigment capable of photosynthesis; they are unable to synthesize protein or other organic material from simple compounds, and are therefore parasitic or saprophytic.

fungiform papilla: See: Papilla.

furcation: The anatomic area of a multirooted tooth where the roots diverge.

furcation invasion: The extension of periodontitis or pulpitis into a trifurcation area.

fused teeth: Two or more teeth that are structurally united. See: Gemination.

fusiform: A term to describe the morphology of certain types of bacteria, indicating a spindle or cigar shape; reflective in the genus *Fusobacterium*.

Fusobacterium nucleatum: Gram-negative, nonmotile, anaerobic, rod-shaped bacterium commonly associated with periodontal and periimplant disease.

G

gag: 1. An involuntary contraction of the muscles of the soft palate or pharynx that results in retching. 2. A surgical device for holding the mouth open.

galvanic stimulation: Excitation of muscle fibers by applying mild electrical current.

galvanism: Induction of an electrical current between two materials with different electronegativities. This can produce nerve or muscle stimulations. An accelerated oxidization of a metal from an electrical interaction with a more noble metal in a corrosive electrolyte. The consequential current flow can create nerve stimulation, an electric shock-like experience, or a disagreeable taste.

gamma ray: Part of electromagnetic radiation with the smallest wavelengths and thus the most energy of any wave in the electromagnetic spectrum.

gamma-linolenic acid (GLA): See: Osteocalcin.

gangrene: Death of a mass of tissue, generally associated with loss of vascular (nutritive) supply and followed by bacterial invasion and putrefaction.

gap: See: Edentulous space.

gap distance: syn. Jumping distance. The space between the bony walls of an osteotomy or an extraction socket and a dental implant at stage one surgery. The dimension of the gap and type of implant surface influence the level of the first bone-to-implant contact.

GBR (abbrev.): Guided bone regeneration.

gemination: Teeth that are structurally united and have developed from the same tooth germ. See: Fused teeth.

gene: A segment of a DNA molecule coded for the synthesis of a single polypeptide; a unit of genetic information.

gene therapy: Treatment of human disease by the transfer of genetic material into specific cells. **Nonviral g. t.**: method of gene therapy that uses nonviral vectors to deliver genetic material into target cells, i.e., plasmid DNA and synthetic vectors (e.g., lipoplexes, polyplexes). **Viral g. t.**: method of gene therapy that uses viruses as gene delivery vectors; viruses have a portion of their genome replaced by a therapeutic gene. The most widely used viruses are adenovirus, adeno-associated virus, lentivirus, and retrovirus.

gene transfer: Introduction of genes into cells. The viral particle binds to specific cellular receptors and is taken up by endocytosis. Acidification of the endosome results in release to the cytoplasm and partial disassembly of the viral particle. Transport through the nuclear pore is by viral proteins. Once in the nucleus, the DNA remains extra-chromosomal, and transcription and translation are by the host cell's own protein synthetic machinery. See: Gene therapy.

general anesthesia: A drug-induced loss of consciousness during which patients are not arousable, even by painful stimulation. The ability to independently maintain ventilatory function is often impaired.

genial: Relating to the chin.

genial tubercles: Bony projections at the midline on the lower lingual surface of the mandible to which the genioglossus

Glossary of Dental Implantology, First Edition. Khalid Almas, Fawad Javed and Steph Smith.
© 2018 John Wiley & Sons, Inc. Published 2018 by John Wiley & Sons, Inc.

muscle attaches above and the geniohyoid muscle below.

genioplasty: 1. A surgical procedure performed to alter the contour of the mandibular symphysis. 2. Plastic surgery of the chin.

genome: The complete chromosomal set derived from one parent.

genomics: The study of the genes and their interrelationships in order to recognize the combined effect on the growth and development of the organism.

genotype: The genetic composition of an individual or defined population.

geographic tongue (benign migratory glossitis): A chronic condition characterized by desquamation of the superficial epithelium of the dorsum of the tongue, which migrates continuously.

germicide: A disinfectant that kills germs, especially pathogenic microorganisms.

germination: Two teeth that are joined and have developed from the same tooth bud.

gingiva: That part of the masticatory mucosa covering the alveolar process and surrounding cervical portion of teeth. This fibrous connective tissue, covered by keratinized epithelium, is contiguous with periodontal ligament and mucosal tissues of the mouth. See: Attached gingiva, Keratinized gingiva, Marginal gingiva, Free gingiva.

gingival: Relating to the gingiva.

gingival abscess: Localized purulent infection involving the marginal gingivae or interdental papillae.

gingival cleft: A fissure in the gingival tissues. Vertical fissure in gingiva occurring over a dehiscence of bone covering a root.

gingival crater: Saucer-shaped defect of interproximal gingiva.

gingival crevice: The envelope formed between the gingival cuff and the tooth or implant, coronal to its epithelial attachment. See: Gingival sulcus, Periodontal pocket.

gingival crevicular fluid (GCF): Serum ultrafiltrate tissue fluid that seeps into the gingival sulcus from gingival connective tissue and vasculature through thin sulcular epithelia. GCF is increased in the presence of inflammation and contains multiple mediators

involved in inflammation, connective tissue homeostasis, and host response.

gingival curettage: Process of debriding the soft tissue wall of a periodontal pocket. See: Curettage.

gingival denture contour: Portions of a prosthesis that mimic the soft tissue surrounding a tooth or teeth. Syn: Pink porcelain, pink acrylic.

gingival diseases: The pattern of observable signs and symptoms of different disease entities that are localized to the gingiva. **g. enlargement**: An overgrowth or increase in size of the gingiva. **g. exudate**: An exudate that escapes into the oral cavity via the gingival crevice. **g. festoon**: See: Festoons, gingival. **g. fibromatosis**: A diffuse, fibrous overgrowth of the gingiva; can be idiopathic, hereditary, or associated with drug administration. **hereditary g. f.**: A genetically derived fibrotic gingival enlargement. **g. hyperplasia**: An enlargement of the gingiva due to an increase in the number of cells. **g. hypertrophy**: An enlargement of the gingiva due to an increase in the size of cells. **g. pocket**: A pathologically deepened gingival crevice that does not involve loss of connective tissue attachment. Frequently observed when there is gingival enlargement. **g. recession**: See: Recession, gingival.

gingival diseases of fungal origin: Fungal infection that affects the gingival tissues either as a result of local infection or a manifestation of a systemic condition.

gingival diseases of specific bacterial origin: Conditions induced by specific local or systemic bacterial pathogens.

gingival diseases of viral origin: Acute manifestations of viral infections of the oral mucosa, characterized by redness and multiple vesicles that easily rupture to form painful ulcers affecting the gingiva. They may be accompanied by fever, malaise, and regional lymphadenopathy.

gingival displacement: The movement or retraction of the marginal gingiva, the gingiva located at the buccal, labial, lingual, and palatal areas of the teeth, away from a tooth.

gingival embrasure: Area of the gingiva, usually having a V shape in the maxilla and an inverted V shape in the mandible, that fills the space between adjacent teeth that lies cervical to the interproximal contact area.

gingival fiberotomy: A circumferential crevicular incision through all gingival and periodontal fibers coronal to the crest of the alveolar bone.

gingival fluid: Tissue fluid that seeps through the crevicular and junctional epithelium. It is increased in the presence of inflammation.

gingival enlargement: Increase in size of the gingiva. Gingival enlargement may result from systemic drug use. Drugs commonly associated with this condition include calcium channel blockers, cyclosporine, the anticonvulsant phenytoin, and dilantin. Called also gingival overgrowth.

gingival exudate: A cellular fluid that filters into the oral cavity via the gingival crevice.

gingival flap: A flap that does not extend apical to the mucogingival junction.

gingival graft: (syn): Free soft tissue autograft. Surgical procedure performed to establish an adequate amount of keratinized tissue around a tooth or dental implant, or to increase the quantity of tissue of an edentulous ridge.

gingival groove: A shallow linear depression on the gingival surface that demarcates the free gingiva from the attached gingiva.

gingival margin: See: Marginal gingiva.

gingival massage: The application of frictional, compressional, rubbing, and stroking forces to the gingiva.

gingival overgrowth: See: Gingival enlargement.

gingival papilla: Portion of the gingiva that occupies interproximal spaces; interdental or interimplant extension of the gingiva.

gingival porcelain: Porcelains (usually pink in color) used to blend the cervical portions of the gingival margins between the prosthetic and the oral cavity.

gingival recession: Location of gingival margin apical to the cementoenamel junction or implant connection. Marginal tissue recessions were classified by Miller in four classes according to predictability of root coverage. **Class I**: Recession does not extend to the mucogingival junction and there is no tissue loss in the interproximal area. **Class II**: Recession extends to or beyond the mucogingival junction. There is no periodontal loss in the interproximal area. **Class III**: Recession extends to or beyond the mucogingival junction. Bone or soft tissue loss is present in the interdental area, or there is malpositioning of the teeth which prevents total root coverage. **Class IV**: Recession extends to or beyond the mucogingival junction. The bone or soft tissue loss in the interdental area and/or malpositioning of teeth is so severe that root coverage cannot be anticipated.

gingival retraction: See Gingival displacement.

gingival stippling: Pitted, orange-peel appearance frequently seen in attached gingiva. Although it is commonly seen in healthy gingiva, it is not a requirement for gingival health.

gingival sulcus: Shallow space coronal to attachment of the junctional epithelium. It is bound by tooth and sulcular epithelium on either side. The coronal extent of gingival sulcus is the gingival margin. See: Gingival crevice.

gingivectomy: Excision of a portion of the gingiva, usually performed to reduce the soft tissue wall of the periodontal pocket or to remove excess tissue in the condition of gingival enlargement.

gingivitis: Gingival inflammation. See: Periodontitis. **Ascorbic acid deficiency g.**: An inflammatory response of the gingiva to microbial plaque, aggravated by chronically low ascorbic acid levels, resulting in inadequate collagen synthesis, gingival edema, hemorrhage, and ulceration. **Desquamative g.**: A nonspecific term describing erythema, and ulceration of the free and attached gingiva. It reflects diffuse inflammation of the gingiva with sloughing of the surface epithelium. It can be a manifestation of one or more vesiculoerosive lesions. **Diabetes mellitus-associated g.**: Inflammatory response of the gingiva to plaque modified by poorly controlled plasma glucose levels. **Drug-influenced g.**:

Inflammatory response of the gingiva to plaque and drug(s). **Leukemia- associated g.**: Inflammatory response of the gingiva to plaque, modified or accentuated by the presence of leukemia, resulting in increased bleeding and enlargement which may be partially due to leukemic cell infiltration of the gingiva. **Menstrual cycle-associated g.**: A pronounced inflammatory response of the gingiva to microbial plaque, modified or accentuated by hormonal alterations during the menstrual period. **Necrotizing ulcerative g.** (NUG): An inflammatory disease of the gingiva which reflects an impaired host response, with signs and symptoms including pain, interdental papillary necrosis, and a tendency toward spontaneous bleeding. **Nonplaque-induced g.**: An inflammation of the gingiva with an etiology other than dental plaque, such as gingival diseases of specific bacterial, viral, fungal, or genetic origin, or due to systemic conditions, trauma and foreign body reactions. **Oral contraceptive-associated g.**: Inflammatory response of the gingiva to microbial plaque, modified or accentuated by oral contraceptives. **Plaque-induced g.**: Inflammation of the gingiva resulting from microbial plaque. **Pregnancy-associated g.**: Inflammatory response of the gingiva to microbial plaque, modified or accentuated by hormonal changes which occur most often during the second and third trimesters of pregnancy; typically reversible at parturition. **Puberty-associated g.**: Inflammatory response of the gingiva to microbial plaque, modified or accentuated by hormonal changes during the circumpubertal period.

gingivoplasty: A resective gingival surgical procedure performed to reshape and recontour the gingiva.

gingivosis: Former nomenclature for desquamative gingivitis.

gingivostomatitis: Inflammatory process involving the gingiva and mucosa. The term is a compound word derived from the Greek word *stoma*, which means mouth. The term encompasses any intraoral inflammatory process located within the oral cavity.

Herpetic g.: An infection of the oral soft tissues caused by the herpes simplex virus and characterized by redness, formation of multiple vesicles, painful ulcers, fever, and lymphadenopathy.

ginglymoarthrodial joint: A joint that involves hinging and gliding movement during function; it has a ginglymus and arthrodial form.

ginglymus joint: Joint involving hinging movements during function.

GLA protein (abbrev.): Gamma-linolenic acid protein. See: Osteocalcin.

glass ceramic: Ceramic of silicon dioxide or similar materials that solidify from molten state without crystallizing. See: Ceramic.

glaze: 1. To cover with a glossy, smooth surface or coating. 2. The attainment of a smooth and reflective surface. 3. The final firing of porcelain in which the surface is vitrified and a high gloss is imparted to the material. 4. A ceramic veneer on a dental porcelain restoration after it has been fired, producing a nonporous, glossy or semi-glossy surface.

glenoid fossa: The concavity in the temporal bone at the root of the zygomatic arch that receives the mandibular condyle.

glossalgia: Pain in the tongue.

glossectomy: Partial or total resection of the tongue.

glossitis, migratory: See: Geographic tongue.

glossodynia: Painful or burning sensation in the tongue.

glossoplasty: Plastic or altering surgery of the tongue.

glossopynia: Painful or burning tongue.

glucocorticoid: A class of steroid hormones characterized by an ability to bind with the glucocorticoid receptor. Their main therapeutic use in dentistry is as an antiinflammatory and immunosuppressant agent.

glucose tolerance test: A laboratory test that denotes a patient's ability to regulate blood sugar level after carbohydrate intake. One of the best laboratory tests (in terms of reliability) for detecting diabetes mellitus.

glycoprotein: Conjugated protein in which the nonprotein group is generally a carbohydrate.

It can contain one or more covalently linked carbohydrate residues. Called also glucoprotein.

glycosaminoglycan: A polysaccharide that is important in tissue repair, hydration, and joint health. Also known as mucopolysaccharide.

glycosylated hemoglobin A1c test (HbA1c test): (syn): Glycated hemoglobin A1c test. Laboratory test which reveals average plasma glucose concentration over a period of 3 months. Specifically, it measures the number of glucose molecules attached to hemoglobin. Results are expressed as a percentage, with 4–6% considered normal.

gnathic: Relating to the anatomy or function of the maxilla or mandible.

gnathion: A reference point commonly used in orthodontic evaluation (especially radiographically) of the skull, which designates the most inferior and outward point of the bony chin as measured at the midsagittal plane.

gnathodynamometer: An instrument used to measure maximal bite force and masticatory efficiency. Also known as an occlusometer.

gnathology: The science of relating tooth position, anatomy, and function to the exact movements of the temporomandibular joints bilaterally, in an attempt to define ideal masticatory function and stability. Also known as neuromuscular dentistry.

gold cylinder: See: Prefabricated cylinder.

gold cylinder attachment: Attachment element comprising part of a prosthetic component. This term specifically refers to the alloy used in fabrication of the element. Called also cylinder-to-transmucosal element. See: Attachment element.

Golden Proportion: A mathematical progression of numeric expressions thought to have ideal esthetic value. It describes the ideal dimensions and visual relationships of the human dentition, as well as human facial dimensions. Dr Eddy Levin, of London, England, found that by applying the Golden Proportion to the eight maxillary anterior teeth (1st bicuspid to 1st bicuspid), ideal esthetics could be achieved. The ratio is 1.618 to 1. It has been accepted that the Golden Proportion exists in natural dentitions as observed from the labial surfaces, the ratio of the widths of cuspids to lateral incisors as well as central incisors to lateral incisors. The four front teeth, from central incisor to 1st bicuspids, are the most significant part of the smile and are in Golden Proportion to each other. Also, the combined width of the central incisors compared with their height follows the Golden Proportion.

gothic arch tracer: A device rarely used in contemporary dental practice that determines an accurate, verifiable, and reproducible centric relation position and the proper occlusal vertical dimension.

gothic arch tracing: See: Central bearing tracing.

graft: 1. Any tissue or organ transferred to a patient. 2. Any tissue or organ from a donor or a second site in the recipient used for implantation or transplantation into the recipient at the required site. 3. A piece of viable (living) tissue positioned in contact with injured tissues to afford a scaffold for repairing a defect or correcting a deficiency. 4. To stimulate closure between separate tissues. **Allograft**: A graft between genetically dissimilar members of the same species. **Alloplast**: A synthetic graft or inert foreign body implanted into tissue. See: Implant, oral. **Autogenous g.**: See: Graft, Autograft. **Autogenous bone g.**: An osseous autograft. **Autograft**: Tissue transferred from one position to another within the same individual. **Block g.**: An autogenous or allogeneic bone graft in a block form used for augmentation of deficient bony ridges. **Connective tissue g.**: An autogenous graft of connective tissue completely or partially detached from its original site and placed in a prepared recipient bed. Indicated for root coverage or ridge augmentation procedures around natural dentition, pontics and implants. **Double papilla pedicle g.**: See: Flap, Double papilla pedicle. **Heterograft**: A graft taken from a donor of another species. **Homograft**: See: Allograft. **Iliac g.**: Bone graft material obtained from the iliac crest. **Isograft**: A graft between genetically identical individuals, usually between identical twins.

Papillary pedicle g.: See: Flap, Papillary pedicle. **Pedicle g.**: See: Flap, Pedicle. **Soft tissue (gingival) g.**: An autogenous graft of masticatory mucosa or collagenous tissue completely or partially detached from its original site and placed in a prepared recipient bed. **Xenograft**: A heterograft.

graft consolidation (bone): The vascularization and integration at the cellular level of a graft with its recipient site. It involves the formation of a graft-woven bone complex that remodels into lamellar bone and further adapts based on loading.

graft healing: The restoration of implanted living tissue to its original integrity. Bone graft healing has two different routes: either it fails to incorporate and gradually disappears, or it becomes incorporated as a mechanically functioning part of the host bone. Osteoblasts or osteoprogenitor cells may be transferred to the recipient site. Via resorption of bone graft, various growth factors are released from the noncollagenous part of bone matrix.

grafting material: A substance, natural or synthetic, used to enhance or repair a tissue defect or deficiency.

gram negative: Pertaining to bacteria that counterstain pale red with Gram stain. These bacteria have a lipopolysaccharide (endotoxin) layer exterior to a thin peptidoglycan layer in the cell walls.

gram positive: Pertaining to bacteria that stain deep purple with Gram stain. These bacteria have a thick peptidoglycan layer but no lipopolysaccharide in their cell walls.

gram stain: A method for classifying bacteria into two groups on the basis of their cell wall composition, which causes them to stain either purple (positive) or pale red (negative).

granulation tissue: Healing tissue that forms in response to any injury or surgical insult of soft tissue and consists of fibroblasts, capillary buds, inflammatory cells, and edema.

granulocytopenia: See: Agranulocytosis.

granuloma: A reactive nodule consisting of modified macrophages resembling epithelial cells surrounded by a rim of mononuclear cells, usually lymphocytes, and often containing giant cells. **Apical g.**: Circumscribed granulomatous tissue adjacent to the apex of a tooth. **Central giant cell g.**: Usually restricted to the jaw bones, this lytic lesion displays loose fibrillar connective tissue, numerous capillaries, and multinuclear giant cells, and a histologic appearance similar to the bony lesions of hyperparathyroidism. **Peripheral giant cell g.**: Reactive proliferation of osteoclasts arising from the periosteum or superficial periodontal ligament possibly in response to local irritation or trauma. **Pregnancy-associated pyogenic g.**: A pyogenic granuloma resulting from dental plaque and hormonal changes during pregnancy; often regresses following parturition. Also known as pregnancy tumor. **Pyogenic g.**: A reactive overgrowth of exuberant granulation tissue possibly in response to local irritation or trauma. This vascular mass often is ulcerated and may be smooth or lobulated and pedunculated or sessile.

granulomatous tissue: A distinctive morphologic pattern of inflammation consisting of histiocytes that have been transformed into epithelioid cells that are surrounded by mononuclear cells, usually lymphocytes.

gray (Gy): A unit of absorbed radiation dose equivalent to 100 rad.

grinding, selective: Alteration of the occlusal forms of teeth to improve occlusal function and to decrease or redirect occlusal forces to the teeth.

grinding-in: A term used to denote the act of correcting occlusal disharmonies by grinding the natural or artificial teeth (GPT-1). See: Occlusal reshaping.

grit-blasted implant surface: Modification of an implant or other surface through the application of sand, aluminum oxide, or other abrasive material by intense air pressure.

grit blasting: Delivery to a dental implant surface of a high-velocity stream of abrasive particles propelled by compressed air, designed to increase surface area.

groove: A long narrow channel or depression, such as the indentation between tooth cusps or the retentive features placed on tooth surfaces to augment the retentive characteristics of crown preparations. **Palatal g.**:A developmental, anomalous groove usually found on the palatal aspect of maxillary central and lateral incisors.

group function: Multiple contact relations between the maxillary and mandibular teeth in lateral movements on the working side whereby simultaneous contact of several teeth acts as a group to distribute occlusal forces.

growth factor: Diverse group of polypeptides with important roles in the regulation of growth and the development of a variety of organs. These factors control key aspects involved in wound repair, including cellular mitogenesis, matrix biosynthesis, chemotaxis, and differentiation.

growth hormone: Protein hormone of about 190 amino acids that is synthesized and secreted by cells called somatotrophs in the anterior pituitary. It is a major participant in control of several complex physiologic processes, including growth and metabolism.

GTR (abbrev.): Guided tissue regeneration.

guard: See: Occlusal guard.

guidance: The process of controlling or directing an object on a predetermined course or track. **Canine g.**: Guidance provided by maxillary canine teeth that permits posterior disocclusion during lateral mandibular movements. **Condylar g.**: The path the condyles travel during normal mandibular movement, measured in degrees relative to the Frankfort horizontal plane. **Incisal g.**: The influence on mandibular movements exerted by the palatal surfaces of the maxillary anterior teeth.

guide: See: Radiographic template, Stereolithographic guide, Surgical guide.

guide drill: Round-shaped or pointed drill used to mark the site of an osteotomy by making an initial entry into cortical bone.

guide pin: 1. Device placed within a dental implant osteotomy to assist in determining the location and angulation of the site relative to adjacent teeth, implants or other landmarks. 2. Extended occlusal or abutment screws used during prosthesis fabrication in the laboratory.

guide plane: 1. The plane developed in the occlusal surfaces of the occlusion rims (i.e., to position the mandible in centric relation). 2. A plane which guides movement (GPT-4).

guide stent: See: Surgical template.

guided bone regeneration (GBR): Bone regenerative technique that uses physical means (e.g., barrier membranes) to seal off an anatomic site where bone is to be regenerated. The goal is to direct bone formation and prevent other tissues (e.g., connective tissue) from interfering with osteogenesis.

guided cylinder: (syn): Guided sleeve.

guided sleeve: (syn): Guided cylinder. Round metal cylinder usually 5 mm in length and available in various diameters, which is incorporated into a surgical or stereolithographic guide to precisely position the drill and subsequently the dental implant during surgery.

guided surgery: The capability of performing virtual surgery based on the use of medical/dental imaging files (DICOM, STL, vrml, obj, etc.) using computer software. The results are used to develop digitally manufactured guides or navigation directions for robotic guidance for surgery.

guided tissue regeneration: (GTR): Surgical procedure aimed at regenerating lost periodontal attachment. Creation of a secluded space favoring angiogenic and osteogenic cells, protecting the vascular and cellular elements while probably supporting accumulation of growth factors. True periodontal regeneration must include new cementum formation, periodontal ligament, and alveolar bone on a previously diseased root surface. GTR follows the principle of maintaining a surgically created space around teeth via a barrier membrane, thus allowing the slower proliferating periodontal ligament cells, bone cells, and possibly cementoblasts to populate the root surface. This term is not to be confused with guided bone regeneration (GBR), which describes a similar principle for isolated bone defects following tooth loss and concerns the regeneration or augmentation of bone only.

guided tissue (bone) regeneration: Procedures attempting to regenerate lost periodontal structures through differential tissue responses. Guided bone regeneration typically refers to ridge augmentation or bone regenerative procedures; guided tissue regeneration typically refers to regeneration of periodontal attachment. Barrier techniques, using materials such as expanded polytetrafluoroethylene, polyglactin, polylactic acid, calcium sulfate and collagen, are employed in the hope of excluding epithelium and the gingival corium from the root or existing bone surface in the belief that they interfere with regeneration.

guiding occlusion: Used in the sense of designating contacts of teeth in motion.

guiding planes: Vertically parallel surfaces on abutment teeth or/and dental implant abutments oriented so as to contribute to the direction of the path of placement and removal of a removable dental prosthesis.

gustation: The act of perceiving taste.

gypsum: See: Medical-grade calcium sulfate.

H

H (abbrev.): Hounsfield unit.

HA (abbrev.): Hydroxyapatite.

habit: An act that has become a repeated performance, almost automatic, such as bruxism or tongue thrusting.

hader bar: A rigid bar that connects two or more abutments designed for the retention of a restoration(s). The removable restoration contains housings that are machined to clip over the bar.

Haemophilus: Genus of gram-negative, nonmotile, microaerophilic, pleomorphic bacilli and coccobacilli.

hairy leukoplakia: A corrugated, white plaque of the oral mucosa, primarily on the lateral borders of the tongue, that contains the Epstein–Barr virus. Most patients with confirmed hairy leukoplakia are infected with the human immunodeficiency virus (HIV).

half-life (drug): The amount of time for plasma concentration of a drug to be reduced by 50%.

halitosis: Malodorous breath often offensive to others. Halitosis results from a variety of causes, such as bacteria on the tongue, periodontal disease, poor oral hygiene, systemic disorders, and consumption of some food types. Also known as fetor ex ore, fetor oris, and stomatodysodia.

Hanau Quint: Five factors involved in developing a balanced articulation for removable complete dentures: incisal guidance, condylar guidance, cusp height, plane of occlusion, and compensating curve. First described by Rudolph Hanau in 1926 and incorporated in the design of a semi-adjustable articulator (Hanau H) that provided for horizontal condylar guidance to be set using an intraoral protrusive interocclusal record. Lateral condylar guidance (L) can then be calculated using the Hanau formula, $L = H/8 + 12$, where H is the recorded horizontal condylar guidance.

handpiece motion tracker: An array of active emitters or passive reflectors that are attached to a surgical instrument to enable their localization within the operative field by an overhead detector.

hand prosthesis: Artificial substitute for a human hand.

hapten: A relatively small, lipophilic, non-protein molecule that is able to elicit an immune response (contact or delayed hypersensitivity) only when bound to a carrier protein. Any chemical, drug, or its metabolite that combines with tissue protein to form a complete antigen; most allergenic drugs are haptens.

haptic technology (haptics): A tactile feedback technology that takes advantage of the sense of touch by applying forces, vibrations, or motions to the user.

hard palate: Bony partition separating the oral and nasal cavities.

hard tissue graft: See: Bone graft, Bone replacement graft.

harvest: Procurement of a graft from a donor site.

Haversian canal: Freely anastomosing channels within cortical (dense) bone containing blood and lymph vessels, and surrounded by concentric bone lamellae.

Glossary of Dental Implantology, First Edition. Khalid Almas, Fawad Javed and Steph Smith.
© 2018 John Wiley & Sons, Inc. Published 2018 by John Wiley & Sons, Inc.

Hawley appliance: A removable orthodontic palatal retainer made of acrylic and wire often modified to allow for minor tooth movement or tooth position stabilization.

hazard ratio: The risk of an event occurring in one group compared with another when the primary response variable is the time to event. A hazard ratio of 1 indicates that neither group is more at risk for the event than the other. If the hazard ratio is, for example, 5, then one group is five times more likely to experience the event than the other.

HbA1c test (abbrev.): Glycosylated hemoglobin A1c test.

HBOT (abbrev.): Hyperbaric oxygen therapy.

healing: Regeneration or repair of injured, lost or surgically treated tissue. See: Healing by first (primary) intention, Healing by second (secondary) intention.

healing abutment: Implant component placed at stage two surgery to guide periodontal soft tissue healing prior to definitive prosthetic restoration. Typical cross-sectional design is cylindrical. See: Anatomic healing abutment, Interim endosteal dental implant abutment.

healing by first (primary) intention: syn. Primary closure. Healing of a wound in which the edges are closely reapproximated. Union or restoration of continuity occurs directly with minimal granulation tissue and scar formation.

healing by second (secondary) intention: syn. Secondary closure. Healing of a wound in which a gap is left between its edges. Union occurs by granulation tissue formation from the base and the sides. This requires epithelial migration, collagen deposition, contraction, and remodeling during healing.

healing by third intention: Also known as delayed primary closure or tertiary wound healing. A method to manage heavily infected or contaminated wounds in which the wound is left open for several days following tissue injury.

healing cap: A cover for an implant fixture that guides gingival healing and gingival cuff formation. See: Healing abutment.

healing collar: See: Healing abutment.

healing component: See: Interim endosteal dental implant abutment.

healing period: (syn): Healing phase. The time allocated for healing following a surgery, before the next procedure is performed at the same site.

healing phase: See: Healing period.

healing screw: The cover for an implant fixture that protects the fixture during the healing phase after surgical placement of the implant body. The purpose of the healing screw is to ensure access to the internal threaded cavity for later use. See: Cover screw.

health: The condition of a patient when there is normal function without evidence of disease or abnormality.

hearing aid: See: Bone-anchored hearing aid (BAHA).

heat-curing resin: Resin requiring external heat to activate polymerization.

heat necrosis: Cell death due to effectively prolonged exposure of bone to elevated temperature, such as during osteotomy preparation.

heel: The distal end of a denture.

height of contour: A line encircling a tooth and designating its greatest circumference at a selected axial position determined by a dental surveyor; a line encircling a body designating its greatest circumference in a specified plane.

helical cone beam computed tomography: See: Cone beam computed tomography (CBCT).

HEMA (abbrev.): Hydroxyethyl methacrylate.

hemangioma: A benign blood vessel neoplasm; may occur as capillary or cavernous; soft, painless, red to purple, blanches on pressure.

hematoma: A confined gathering of extravasated blood, usually clotted, that presents as a mass in a tissue, organ, or space.

hematopoietic stem cell: Progenitor or precursor cells found in the bone marrow from which all blood cell types of both the myeloid and lymphoid lineages are derived.

hemidesmosome: An ultrastructural feature located on the basal surface of some epithelial cells forming the position of attachment between the basal surface of the cell and the basement membrane, or the conditioning film of a dental implant.

hemi-maxillectomy: Partial surgical removal of the maxilla.

hemisection: The surgical separation of a multirooted tooth, especially a mandibular molar, through the furcation in such a way that a root and the associated portion of the crown may be removed.

hemiseptum: See: Periodontal bony defects.

hemorrhage: Escape of blood from the circulatory system; often excessive and may be uncontrollable.

hemostasis: The arrest of bleeding, either physiologically, surgically, or mechanically.

hemostat: An agent, apparatus, or instrument that may be used to stop hemorrhage.

hemostatic agent: Any compound, such as aluminum chloride or ferric sulfate, that stops or decreases hemorrhage. Oftentimes, these agents are used to control bleeding during impression taking, restoration delivery, and surgical procedures.

heparin: A glycosaminoglycan that is attached to a core protein found in mast cells; anticoagulant activity; serves as a catalyst for antithrombin attachment to thrombin.

heparin sulfate: A glycosaminoglycan found on the surface of most mammalian cells and in the extracellular matrix.

hepatitis: Inflammation of the liver caused by various disease states, drug reactions, and viruses. Common systemic signs include fever, jaundice, and an enlarged liver. **Hepatitis A (HAV)**: An acute infectious disease of the liver caused by the hepatitis A virus. Commonly spread by fecal–oral contamination. It usually occurs in children and young adults and follows a mild course. Immunization is available. **Hepatitis B (HBV)**: An infectious inflammatory disease of the liver caused by the hepatitis B virus. It can be transmitted in the healthcare environment. Has an insidious onset. Features include anorexia, malaise, nausea, vomiting, abdominal pain, and jaundice. **Hepatitis C: non-A, non-B, HCV. Hepatitis D (Delta h.)**: An infection of the liver dependent on the presence of the hepatitis B virus for clinical expression. It may occur as a co-infection with acute hepatitis B or as a superinfection in a hepatitis B carrier.

hereditary gingival fibromatosis: See: Gingival diseases.

herpes: herpes can affect both men and women but most of the time there are no symptoms. **Herpes labialis**: A form of HSV-1 recurrent infection found on the vermillion border of the lips. Commonly called cold sores or fever blisters**. Herpetic gingivostomatitis (*H. simplex*)**: An acute infection of the oral mucosa by the herpes simplex virus (usually Type 1) that is characterized by redness and multiple vesicles that easily rupture to form painful ulcers. It may be accompanied by fever, malaise, and regional lymphadenopathy. See: Gingivostomatitis. **Intraoral recurrent herpes**: Rarely presents with vesicles. The lesions begin as red macules which cave-in to create small depressed ulcerations. Also known as intraoral recurrent herpetic gingivostomatitis and intraoral recurrent herpes simplex.

herpes simplex viruses type I, type II: Herpesviruses are the most ubiquitous, communicable, infectious viruses in humans. They are double-stranded DNA viruses with icosahedral nucleocapsids. Herpes simplex viruses cause acute infection or latent and recurrent infection of human tissues. Herpes simplex virus type I usually causes oral lesions, while type II usually causes genital lesions.

herpetiform: Lesions that resemble herpetic (herpes) lesions.

herpetiform aphtha: Characterized by clusters of multiple, shallow ulcers throughout the oral cavity. Almost continuous in nature.

Hertwig's epithelial root sheath: An extension of the enamel organ (cervical loop). Determines the shape of the roots and initiates dentin formation during tooth development. Its remnants persist as epithelial rests of Malassez in the periodontal ligament.

heterogeneous graft: See: Xenograft.

heterograft: A tissue graft where the species of the donor and recipient are different. Also known as a xenograft.

heterotopic pain: Pain felt in a site distant from the site of origination. See: Referred pain.

hex: The hexagonal shape of a connection interface.

hexed: A component or a dental implant with a hexagonal connection interface.

high lip line: The greatest height to which the inferior border of the upper lip is capable of being raised by muscle function.

high noble metal alloy: A dental casting alloy composed of a minimum of 60% noble metal (gold, platinum, palladium, rhodium, ruthenium, iridium, osmium) by weight with at least 40% gold as classified by the American Dental Association.

high-water prosthesis: See: Hybrid prosthesis.

hinge axis: An imaginary line created by rotation of the mandible through the sagittal plane.

hinge joint: A joint that allows movement in only one plane, such as a door hinge. See: Ginglymus joint.

hinge movement: See: Transverse horizontal axis.

hinge position: Orientation of parts allowing hinge movement between them.

histamine: A low molecular weight, bioactive amine that causes smooth muscle contraction of bronchioles, increased capillary permeability, and increased secretions by the nasal and bronchial mucous glands. Released primarily from mast cells and basophils.

histiocyte: A large phagocyte (macrophage) in the connective tissue derived from circulating monocytes. It has additional functions including antigen processing and immunoregulation.

histology: That part of anatomic study that deals with the minute structure, composition, and function of the tissues.

histomorphometry: The quantitative study of the microscopic organization and structure of a tissue (e.g., bone, soft tissue, and vascularity, from histologic specimens; involves a large range of measurements, including numbers, length, surface area,

volume, angles, and curvature), especially by computer-assisted analysis of images acquired from a microscope.

histopathology: The study of pathological changes within the structures of tissues at the microscopic level.

HIV: See: Human immunodeficiency virus.

hollow basket implant: A root-form dental implant with a central internal channel penetrating the implant body from/at its apical aspect.

hollow cylinder: See: Implant basket.

homograft: (syn): Homogeneous graft, homologous graft. A graft taken from one human subject and transplanted into another. See: Allograft.

homologous graft: See: Homograft, Allogeneic bone graft.

horizontal mattress suture: See: Mattress suture.

horizontal osteotomy: Horizontal surgical cut in bone.

horizontal overlap: Overjet. The projection of the maxillary anterior or posterior teeth beyond their antagonists in a horizontal direction. See: Overbite.

horizontal plane: Any plane passing through the body at right angles to both the median and frontal planes, thus dividing the body into upper and lower parts; in dentistry, the plane passing through a tooth at right angles to its long axis.

hormone: Chemical messenger secreted into the bloodstream by specialized cells capable of synthesizing and secreting them in response to specific signals.

host modulation: Therapy designed to alter the host response to bacteria by reducing the destructive aspects of the inflammatory response.

host modulation therapy: A drug such as low-dose doxycycline that reduces the clinical signs and symptoms and the progression of periodontitis by modifying a key element or pathway of the host response to the infection.

host resistance: The host defensive mechanisms preventing pathogens from invading the tissues. These defense mechanisms include physical and biochemical barriers such as the skin, enzymes in secretions (e.g., tears), immunoglobulins, gastric acid, cilia, and mucus.

host response: A reaction of the host immune system directed against infectious organisms.

host site: See: Recipient site.

Hounsfield scale: Named after Sir Godfrey Newbold Hounsfield, it is a quantitative scale for describing radiodensity on CT images; however, due to the inconsistency of contrast, it does not apply to CBCT.

Hounsfield unit (H): A unit of X-ray attenuation used for computed tomography scans as a measurement of bone density. Each pixel is assigned a value on a scale on which air is 1000, water 0, and compact bone +1000.

Hounsfield unit scale: A linear transformation of the original linear attenuation coefficient measurement into one in which the radiodensity of distilled water at standard temperature and pressure (STP) is defined as zero Hounsfield units (HU), while the radiodensity of air at STP is defined as -1000 HU.

Howship lacuna: Small pit or groove formed by resorbing osteoclasts on the surface of bone undergoing resorption. See: Osteoclast.

hue: Often referred to as the basic color, hue is the quality of sensation according to which an observer is aware of the varying wavelengths of radiant energy. The dimension of color dictated by the wavelength of the stimulus that is used to distinguish one family of color from another, as red, green, blue, etc. The attribute of color by means of which a color is perceived to be red, yellow, green, blue, purple, etc. White, black, and grays possess no hue.

human immunodeficiency virus (HIV): A RNA virus that exists as two major types, HIV-1 and HIV-2. The genetic material is in the form of messenger RNA and is classified as a retrovirus. The targets of infection of HIV are primarily the T4 helper (CD4+) lymphocytes.

human leukocyte antigen (HLA): The human major histocompatibility complex composed of both MHC class I and MHC class II molecules, present in all nucleated mammalian cells. Primarily responsible for graft rejection between individuals.

humoral immunity: The immune response mediated by the secretion of immunoglobulins (antibodies) produced by activated B cells (plasma cells) against antigens. Also known as antibody-dependent immunity.

hybrid denture: Slang for any modification or alteration in the usual form of a dental prosthesis.

hybrid implant: An endosseous, root-form dental implant, with different surface geometries or textures at different levels.

hybrid prosthesis: (syn): High-water prosthesis. A screw-retained, metal-resin, implant-supported, fixed complete denture. The term "hybrid" implies a combination of a metal framework with a complete denture (prefabricated resin teeth and heat-polymerized resin). The term "high-water" refers to the design of this prosthesis using long standard abutments with several millimeters of space between the prosthesis and the underlying mucosa of the edentulous ridge.

hydroxyapatite (HA): An inorganic compound, $Ca_5(PO_4)_3(OH)$, found in the mineralized matrices of bone and teeth that provides hardness to these structures. Various synthetic forms are used in ridge augmentation and intrabony defects, as well as coating of dental implants. The ceramic form is manufactured by a sintering process, in which the HA is heated to 1100 °C, whereby the crystals fuse and grow in size. See: Bovine-derived anorganic bone matrix, Hydroxyapatite implant surface, Porous coralline hydroxyapatite, Porous marine-derived coralline hydroxyapatite.

hydroxyapatite-bone grafting: Method of grafting in which granules of hydroxyapatite can be added to chips of autogenous bone to obtain the desired shape and compromise or delay resorption.

hydroxyapatite ceramic: A composition of calcium and phosphate in physiologic ratios to provide a dense, nonresorbable, biocompatible ceramic used for dental implants and residual ridge augmentation.

hydroxyapatite implant surface: Primarily insoluble or partially soluble amorphous and crystalline calcium phosphate coating applied to the surface of an implant, intended to enhance osseointegration.

hydroxyethyl methacrylate (HEMA): Alloplastic material made of hydrosoluble monomer, which can polymerize under various circumstances at low temperatures. It can be used to prepare various hydrogels to immobilize proteins or cells for grafting purposes.

hydroxylapatite: See: Hydroxyapatite (HA).

hygiene cap: (syn): Comfort cap, healing abutment, healing cap, sealing screw. Component inserted over a prosthetic abutment. Its function is to prevent debris and calculus from invading the internal portion of the abutment between prosthetic appointments.

hygienic (sanitary) pontic: A pontic (suspended crown in a fixed bridge) that is simpler to clean because it has a rounded or bullet-shaped cervical form and does not contact the edentulous ridge.

hypalgesia (hypoalgesia): Reduced sensitivity to pain that results from a raised pain threshold.

hyperalgesia: Increased pain response to a normally painful stimulus.

hyperbaric chamber: An enclosed space or tube that accommodates a patient and subjects the patient to ambient gas pressures >1 atm.

hyperbaric oxygen therapy (HBOT): Treatment modality where a patient is placed in a pressurized (hyperbaric) chamber that allows for the delivery of oxygen in high concentrations for therapeutic benefits. It is sometimes used prior to implant therapy for patients who underwent radiation therapy in the head and neck areas, to reduce the risks of osteoradionecrosis.

hyperbaric oxygen treatment (HBOT): Therapy used in irradiated cancer patients to improve wound healing and osseointegration of implants. Administration of 100% oxygen under increased atmospheric pressure (usually 2 atm or 10 m sea water). The elevated partial pressure of oxygen to tissues has been shown to improve angiogenesis, bone metabolism, and success of osseointegration. It has been recommended that patients receive several treatments in a hyperbaric oxygen chamber, both pre- and postoperatively. This therapy also has been used to treat severe anaerobic infections in the jaws.

hyperbaric oxygenation: The administration of oxygen in an enclosed space at greater than atmospheric pressure; also called hyperbaric oxygen therapy.

hypercementosis: An excessive deposition of cementum.

hyperemia: An excessive accumulation of blood in a tissue due to vascular engorgement.

hyperesthesia: A dysesthesia consisting of increased sensitivity, particularly a painful sensation from a normally painless touch stimulus.

hyperglycemia: Abnormally increased blood sugar. Usually increased or high blood glucose when typically >11.1 mmol/L; however, symptoms may not be noticeable until even higher values are reached, such as 15–20 mmol/L. A patient with a consistent range between ~5.6 and ~7 mmol/L is considered hyperglycemic, values >7 mmol/L are considered a state of diabetes. Chronic levels >7 mmol/L can produce organ damage.

hyperkeratosis: Extreme development of keratin by epithelial cells.

hypermineralization: Abnormal quantities of mineral elements in calcified tissue.

hyperocclusion: Premature or abnormal contact of opposing teeth, creating excessive or traumatic force.

hyperorthokeratosis: An abnormal increase in the thickness of the orthokeratin layer (stratum corneum) of the epithelium. The subjacent stratum granulosum may be prominent.

hyperosmia: An uncharacteristically increased sensitivity to odors.

hyperostosis: A limited overgrowth of bone in one particular area. See: Exostosis, Torus.

hyperparakeratosis: An abnormal increase in the thickness of the keratin layer of the epithelium with persistence of nuclei or nuclear remnants. The stratum granulosum is seldom seen in hyperparakeratosis. Also known as parakeratosis.

hyperparathyroidism: Physical condition created by excessive amounts of parathyroid hormone. Primary hyperparathyroidism is caused by dysfunction of the parathyroid glands. This results in oversecretion of parathyroid hormone (PTH), leading to increased bone resorption and subsequent hypercalcemia, as well as reduced renal clearance of calcium and increased intestinal calcium absorption.

hyperplasia: Excessive enlargement of a tissue or structure due to an increase in the number of cells.

hyperplastic tissue: Surplus tissue that is often caused as a response to chronic irritation that stimulates overproduction of the cells in the tissue.

hypersensitivity: An exaggerated or inappropriate immune response to a pathogen or antigen that is damaging to the host. Classified as immediate (anaphylactic), antibody dependent (cytotoxic), immune complex (Arthus), and delayed (T cell mediated).

hypertension: Persistent, sustained high blood pressure of 140/90 mmHg or above. Hypertension becomes a surgical risk factor if the condition is uncontrolled.

hypertrophy: Nontumor-associated increase in tissue or organ size related to an increase in constituent cell size. A hypertrophic response may occur as a result of a particular condition. To be distinguished from hyperplasia, which is related to an increase in cell number.

hypodontia: Congenital absence of one or more, but not all, of the normal complement of teeth.

hypoesthesia: Decreased perception of stimulation by noxious or non-noxious stimuli.

hypogeusia (hypoageusia): Reduced sense of taste, including sweet, sour, salty, and bitter substances. Called also hypogeusesthesia.

hyponasality: A speech characteristic caused by insufficient resonance of air in the nasal cavity such that the speaker sounds as though he or she has a cold. Also known as denasality.

hypophosphatasia: An inborn error of metabolism characterized by deficient alkaline phosphatase in serum and bone, resulting in the defective formation of bone and cementum.

hypoplasia: A congenital disorder that is the result of a decrease in the typical number of cells and manifests as defective or incomplete organ/tissue development.

I

IAJ (abbrev.): Implant–abutment junction.

IAN (abbrev.): Inferior alveolar nerve.

iatrogenic: An abnormal mental or physical condition induced in a patient by the effects of treatment.

ibuprofen: A nonsteroidal antiinflammatory medication that possesses analgesic and antipyretic properties. See: Nonsteroidal antiinflammatory drug (NSAID).

idiopathic: Of unknown causation.

idiopathic resorption: See: Resorption.

IGF (abbrev.): Insulin-like growth factor.

IL (abbrev.): Interleukin.

iliac bone: See: Ilium.

iliac crest: Superior part of the ilium used as a source of autogenous bone. See: Iliac graft.

iliac crest graft: Common extraoral corticocancellous autogenous bone graft used in cases where large block volumes for alveolar ridge reconstruction are required.

iliac graft: A bone graft harvested from the crest of the iliac bone. The bone can be removed from the anterior iliac crest posterior to the anterosuperior iliac spine or the posterior ilium. The graft may be cancellous, cortical, or corticocancellous.

ilium: The largest and uppermost portion of the hip bone. The hip bone is the broadest bone of the skeleton, located in the sidewall and anterior wall of the pelvis. It is made up of three bones or parts: the ilium, ischium, and pubis.

image capture: The process of 3D scanning to record digital information about the shape of an object with equipment that uses a laser or light to measure the distance between the scanner and the object.

image guidance: The use of preoperative imaging with computer-based planning tools for the diagnosis, planning, and execution of dental implant placement and prosthetic reconstruction. See: Navigation surgery, Stereolithographic guide.

image registration: The process of transforming different sets of data into one coordinate system. Data may be multiple photographs, data from different sensors, from different times, or from different viewpoints. It is used in computer vision, medical imaging, and military applications. Registration is necessary in order to be able to compare or integrate the data obtained from these different measurements.

image resolution: Umbrella term that describes the detail an image holds. Resolution quantifies how close lines can be to each other and still be visibly resolved. The term applies to raster digital images, film images, and other types of images. Higher resolution means more image detail. Image resolution can be measured in various ways. Resolution units can be tied to physical sizes (e.g., lines per mm, lines per inch), to the overall size of a picture (e.g., lines per picture height, also known simply as lines, TV lines, or TVL), or to angular subtenant.

image scaling: The process of resizing a digital image. Scaling is a nontrivial process that involves a trade-off between efficiency, smoothness, and sharpness. As the size of an

Glossary of Dental Implantology, First Edition. Khalid Almas, Fawad Javed and Steph Smith.
© 2018 John Wiley & Sons, Inc. Published 2018 by John Wiley & Sons, Inc.

image is increased, so the pixels that comprise the image become increasingly visible, making the image appear "soft." Conversely, reducing an image will tend to enhance its smoothness and apparent sharpness.

image scanner: A device that optically scans an image, printed text, handwriting, or an object, and converts it to a digital image. Hand-held scanners, where the device is moved by hand, have evolved from text scanning "wands" to 3D scanners used for industrial design, reverse engineering, test and measurement, orthotics, gaming, and other applications.

image stitching: The process of combining multiple photographic images with overlapping fields of view to produce a segmented panorama or high-resolution image.

imaging guide: Scan to determine bone volume, inclination and shape of the alveolar process, and bone height and width, which is used at the surgical site.

IME (abbrev.): Intramobile element.

immediate denture: Any removable dental prosthesis fabricated for placement immediately following the removal of a natural tooth/teeth.

immediate disocclusion: Instantaneous separation of the posterior teeth due to the anterior guidance.

immediate functional loading: Implant prosthesis is seated at the time of implant placement and immediately subjected to functional loading. See: Functional loading, Immediate occlusal loading.

immediate implant placement: Implant placement immediately following extraction of a tooth. This procedure must be combined in most patients with a bone grafting technique to eliminate periimplant bone defects.

immediate implantation: See: Immediate implant placement.

immediate insertion denture: See: Immediate denture.

immediate loading: Application of functional or nonfunctional load to an implant at the time of surgical placement or shortly thereafter, i.e., generally considered to be loading within 48 hours of implant placement. See: Immediate functional loading,

Immediate nonfunctional loading, Immediate occlusal loading, Immediate nonocclusal loading. **Orthodontics and i. l.**: Loading of temporary orthodontic implants immediately after placement, without an intervening period of unloaded healing. See: Orthodontic anchorage implant. **Tooth extraction and i. l.**: Implant placed and put into function at the time the natural tooth is extracted.

immediate mandibular lateral translation: Leaving the position described as centric relation, the nonworking-side condyle moves straight and medially, which is considered the translatory portion of lateral movement.

immediate nonfunctional loading: Implant prosthesis is seated at the time of implant placement but kept out of direct occlusal contact. Loading occurs from lip and tongue pressure and contact with food, but not from contact with the opposing teeth.

immediate nonocclusal loading: A clinical protocol for the placement of a dental implant(s) in a partially edentulous arch, with a fixed or removable restoration not in occlusal contact with the opposing dentition, at the same clinical visit. See: Nonocclusal loading.

immediate occlusal loading: A clinical protocol for the placement and application of force on dental implants, with a fixed or removable restoration in occlusal contact with the opposing dentition, at the same clinical visit. See: Occlusal loading.

immediate placement: See: Immediate implant placement.

immediate provisionalization: Fabrication and seating of provisional restoration at the time of implant placement. The provisional restoration may or may not be designed for immediate functional occlusal contact.

immediate restoration: Replacement dental prosthesis placed immediately following the removal of a natural tooth or teeth. See: Immediate provisionalization.

immediate temporization: See: Immediate provisionalization.

immobilization, tooth: Any procedure that renders a tooth fixed or nonmobile. In periodontics, it refers to splinting of teeth.

immunity: A state of host-mediated resistance defending against foreign agents or organisms encountered on or within the tissues that is capable of distinguishing between self and nonself. **Acquired i.**: An adaptive and specialized immune response with two key characteristics: memory and specificity. Long-lived lymphocytes previously primed by antigens react readily when restimulated (memory). **Innate i.**: Congenital. Nonspecific immunity present from birth. Responsible for the initial protection from infectious agents previously unseen by the host. Composed of soluble immune proteins (including complement) and phagocytes.

immunocompetence: Ability or capacity to develop a normal immune response following exposure to antigen.

immunodeficiency: A condition where elements of the immune system are defective or deficient and the individual may not be able to fight infections adequately; may be congenital (primary) or acquired (secondary).

immunofluorescent microscopy: A process in which cells or tissues are labeled with fluorescent dye-conjugated antibodies and examined with an ultraviolet light microscope. Used to identify certain structures or markers on cells.

immunoglobulin: A glycoprotein composed of "heavy" and "light" peptide chains; functions as antibody in serum and secretions. There are five major classes (IgG, IgA, IgM, IgE, and IgD), each with specialized functions.

immunologic response: Bodily defense in reaction to an invading substance (antigen, such as virus, fungus, bacteria, or transplanted organ) that produces a response, including antibody production, cell-mediated immunity, or immunologic tolerance.

immunosuppression: A reduced response of the immune system caused deliberately, by medications or radiation, or not deliberately, by malnutrition, cancer or certain diseases such as acquired immunodeficiency syndrome (AIDS).

impacted tooth (impaction): An unerupted or partially erupted tooth so positioned that complete eruption is unlikely.

impaction of tooth: Developmental disturbance in which a tooth does not fully erupt into occlusion. It may be a tooth bud or fully developed tooth surrounded by bone, either partially or fully. The most frequently impacted teeth are mandibular third molars.

impingement: An area of displacement or compression of a tissue.

implant: 1.To place a device or material into the body. 2. An alloplastic device or material that is placed into the body. See: Dental implant.

implant abutment: A part or section of an implant or that which is connected to the implant that allows for the connection to a crown, prosthesis, or other device. See: Abutment.

implant–abutment interface: The surface where the dental implant and the prosthetic abutment connect. See: Implant–abutment junction (IAJ).

implant–abutment junction (IAJ): (syn): Microgap. The external margin where the coronal aspect of a dental implant and its prosthetic abutment or restoration connect.

implant analog: See: Analog.

implant anchorage: Use of a dental implant as support for orthodontic tooth movement or arch expansion.

implant apex: Portion of a root-form dental implant that first engages an osteotomy during its insertion. It may incorporate self-tapping characteristics.

implant-assisted prosthesis: Any prosthesis that is completely or partly supported by an implant or implants.

implant basket: Design feature of an implant that has a hollow apical portion, which allows a core of bone to remain in the preparation of the osteotomy site and fit within the confines of the hollow apical portion. Called also inverted basket or hollow cylinder.

implant body: Anchorage component embedded in tissue, usually bone, by which all other components in an implant system are supported. Other components are stacked or threaded one into another.

implant–bone interface: When bone substitutes are applied, newly formed host bone creates an interface between the implant surface and alveolar bone as the implant becomes osseointegrated.

implant collar: The smooth part of a dental implant, just apical to the edge of its platform or the implant–abutment junction. Some root-form implants do not have a collar.

implant component: One of the principal portions of an implant system or one of the structural sections of a dental implant abutment.

implant configuration: Pattern or arrangement of the positions of two or more implants placed intraorally.

implant connecting bar: Slang for a device made of metal or other materials that attaches to one or more implant abutments and serves to act as a framework.

implant crown: A crown or fixed dental prosthesis is not an implantable device. The prosthesis receives support and stability from the dental implant.

implant–crown ratio: See: Crown–implant ratio.

implant dentistry: The field of dentistry relating to implants and involving all aspects of implantology from the initial planning phase to the care and maintenance oriented toward enhancing the likelihood of a long-term successful outcome.

implant denture: Slang usage: a denture is not an implantable device. Dental prostheses (fixed dental prostheses, removable dental prostheses) as well as maxillofacial prostheses can be supported and retained in part or whole by dental implants. Terminology to assist in describing the means of retention, support and dental materials should be limited to no more than four adjectives to provide clarity. Descriptive terminology (modifiers) expressed as adjectives to each dental prosthesis may include the method of retention, composition, nature of support, design characteristics, and form of anchorage.

implant design: Conceptualization of an implant form at the planning or designing stage as carried through production.

implant diameter: Length of the horizontal axis through the center of an implant body.

Anchorage components (implants) are available in various diameters and lengths, and the dimensions vary among the various implant manufacturers. The symbol used to reflect the diameter is Ø.

implant drill: Rotary cutting tool used for creating an osteotomy.

implant exposure: Postoperative condition in which an implant is not completely covered by soft tissues because of wound dehiscence. A second surgical procedure following implant placement is used to access the implant shoulder, remove the healing screw, and replace it with an abutment. This can be accomplished with a punch technique or flap elevation.

implant failure: See: Failed implant.

implant fixture: A synonym for an implant, especially an endosseous implant.

implant fracture: The breakage of a dental implant into two or more parts.

implant head: For subperiosteal or blade implants, refers to the segment of the implant above the neck and used to connect to the prosthetic reconstruction. Also called abutment.

implant infrastructure: While a dental implant may have an infrastructure, the proper geometric reference to such an area of the implant is referenced relative to the long axis of the dental implant, in this case, the inferior portion of the dental implant.

implant insertion: Mechanical act of delivering a dental implant into an osteotomy.

implant installation: See: Implant insertion, Implant placement.

implant interface: The area of contact between tissues (e.g., bone, connective tissue) and the surface of a dental implant.

implant length: The measurement in millimeters of a two-piece implant in the coronoapical direction from the edge of the platform to its apex. For a one-piece implant, the measurement in millimeters in the coronoapical direction of the surface intended for osseointegration.

implant-level impression: To record an implant platform at the tissue level, a coping is attached to the implant and an impression is made for laboratory restorative procedures. The resultant cast usually contains an elastomeric material at the implant site.

implant loading: Act of placing forces on an implant through function and/or parafunction.

implant loss: Circumstances whereby the implant is removed from the patient. See: Early implant loss, Failed implant, Late implant loss.

implant material: See: Commercially pure titanium (CPTi), Hydroxyapatite (HA), Titanium alloy, Zirconium oxide.

implant micromotion: See: Micromotion.

implant micromovement: Relative motion between an implant body and its investing tissues at the microscopic level; not clinically visible.

implant mobility: Clinically detectable motion of a dental implant. See: Macromotion, Micromotion.

implant mount: Component positioned onto the implant facilitating surgical placement of the implant into the osteotomy site. May be removed by loosening the attachment mechanism to the implant, either through removal of a screw or release of a frictional fit into the implant.

implant neck: (syn): Cervix. 1. Root-form dental implant: the most coronal aspect of a dental implant. 2. Subperiosteal or blade implant: the transmucosal segment connecting the implant to the head or abutment.

implant, oral: An alloplastic material or device that is surgically placed into the oral tissue beneath the mucosal or periosteal layer or within the bone for functional, therapeutic, or esthetic purposes. **Blade i.**: A flat, blade-shaped endosseous implant which derives its support from a horizontal length of bone. Most commonly made of metal, it can be perforated, smooth, fluted, textured, coated, wedge-shaped, and/or multiheaded. **Endosseous root- form i.**: An implant placed into the alveolar process and/or basal bone that derives its support from a vertical length of bone, and supports a prosthesis or other device. Most commonly made of titanium, it can be cylindrical or tapered. **Osseointegrated i.**: A direct structural and functional connection between ordered, living bone and the surface of an immobile, load-bearing implant as detected on a light microscopic level. **Ramus frame i.**: A full arch implant of tripoidal design consisting of a horizontal supragingival connecting bar with endosseous units placed into the two rami and symphyseal area. **Subperiosteal i.**: An implant placed on the surface of the maxillary or mandibular bone for support and attachment of a prosthesis.

implant overdenture: Complete or partial removable prosthesis that covers and is supported by dental implants, individual or splinted, and related tissue structures. **Bar-clip attachment and i. o.**: Removable prosthesis covering and supported by endosseous implants. The implants are connected by a bar, and support is provided by associated hard and soft tissue structures. The overdenture receives its retention in part by a clip embedded in the impression surface of the acrylic resin base. See: Denture.

implant periapical lesion: Radiolucency localized at the apex of a root-form dental implant. It can be asymptomatic or symptomatic. The symptoms of the acute form may include a fistula with purulent exudate and/or pain on palpation.

implant placement: Surgical steps involved in stage one or flapless surgery.

implant placement, after extraction: See: Immediate implant placement.

implant placement, in irradiated bone: Irradiated cancer patients are at higher risk for failure to achieve osseointegration. However, the use of long implants, fixed retention, and adjuvant hyperbaric oxygen therapy has resulted in a decrease of implant failures. Clearly, the clinician and patient should be aware of the considerations involving irradiated patients, and a team approach should be applied.

implant placement, with maxillary sinus floor elevation: Implants may be placed simultaneously with a sinus floor elevation when the residual bone height is sufficient for primary implant stability. Otherwise, a staged approach must be considered.

implant prosthesis: Any prosthesis (fixed, removable, or maxillofacial) that utilizes dental implants in part or whole for retention, support, and stability. Slang usage: a prosthesis is not an implantable device. Dental prostheses such as crown and other fixed dental prostheses, removable dental prostheses as well as maxillofacial prostheses can be supported and retained in part or whole by dental implants. See: Implant-supported prosthesis (ISP).

implant prosthodontics: The area of prosthodontics that deals with the replacement of maxillofacial structures (including teeth) by prostheses that attach to dental implants.

implant rejection: Failure of a dental implant to achieve osseointegration.

implant-retained prosthesis: See: Implant-supported prosthesis, Implant–tissue-supported prosthesis.

implant retention: Resistance to displacement (vertically) in the plane of placement. Dental implant(s) may be used for prosthesis retention alone or as part of a coupling system providing retention, support, and stability for the prosthesis. Rarely could implants provide retention only without simultaneously providing some degree of prosthesis stability as well.

implant root: (syn): Implant body.

implant scaler: Instrument used for plaque removal and debridement of the periimplant sulcus. A variety of nonmetallic, plastic, graphite, nylon, or teflon-coated instrument tips are recommended for titanium surfaces.

implant selection: Process of choosing the type and size of a dental implant, based on site anatomy, surgical approach, and planned prosthetic reconstruction.

implant shaft: Portion of the implant between the coronal and apical ends. See: Implant body.

implant shape: Design used to categorize the type of implant, including the overall shape such as cylinder, blade, frame, or button.

implant shoulder position: Final apicocoronal position of the implant shoulder, as determined by the surgeon, relative to the alveolar crest, i.e., supracrestal, crestal, or subcrestal.

implant site: Edentulous area in the alveolar ridge where an implant is planned for support of a restoration.

implant site development: Alveolar ridge augmentation for future implant placement; requires a staged approach. See: Alveolar ridge augmentation.

implant soft tissue management: Procedures performed to maintain periodontal health of the soft tissues surrounding oral implants, including nonsurgical procedures such as scaling, polishing, and oral hygiene instruction at defined intervals.

implant splinting: Act of connecting dental implants to each other or to natural teeth to enhance the strength, stability, and stress distribution of the supporting units. See: Splinting.

implant stability: Clinical evaluation of the degree of fixation of a dental implant.

implant stability quotient (ISQ): Measure of the stability of a dental implant (from 1 to 100, 100 being the highest degree of stability) obtained by resonance frequency testing.

implant stability quotient (ISQ): Ratio used to evaluate implant and/or abutment stability using resonance frequency analysis (RFA). See also: Resonance frequency analysis (RFA).

implant stiffness: Stiffness or rigidity of an implant body as determined by mechanical testing. Influenced by implant body design, composition, and diameter. See: Moment of inertia.

implant substructure: The metal framework of a eposteal dental implant that is embedded beneath the soft tissues, in contact with the bone, and stabilized by means of endosteal screws. The periosteal tissues retain the framework to the bone. The framework supports the prosthesis, frequently by means of dental implant abutments and other superstructure components.

implant success: Status of a dental implant based on predetermined success criteria. See: Implant survival, Success rate.

implant-supported prosthesis (ISP): Replacement for missing natural teeth that receives retention, support, and stability from dental implants.

implant surface: External surface of an implant body; the façade of an implant, including its macro and micro surface shape and texture. In the manufacture of an implant, various surface treatments may be used, including, but not limited to, polishing, machining, acid-etching, and grit-blasting, to create the desired surface topography. See: Surface characteristics (implant).

implant surgery: The phase of implant dentistry concerning the selection, planning, and placement of the implant body and abutment.

implant survival: Existence of an implant in the oral cavity under stated criteria. It is generally considered desirable to maximize the bone–implant contact (BIC) (i.e., osseointegration) of a functionally loaded implant. It can be assumed, subjectively, that increased BIC is associated with high implant survival. See: Implant success, Survival rate.

implant system: Group of devices or artificial objects combined for use in a common purpose. Implant systems include all hardware and related instruments/devices used for their application.

implant therapy: See: Implant dentistry.

implant thread: Varied geometric extrusion from the body of a metal implant. Specific design feature of a threaded implant that is manufacturer specific. There are basics in standard screw thread design related to the geometry of a screw. Variations between manufacturers are based on the pitch or slant of the thread and the frequency or number of threads per millimeter along the length of the anchorage component. See: Threaded implant.

implant–tissue-supported prosthesis: An overdenture that derives its support from a combination of intraoral tissues and dental implants. This type of restoration is always removable and may be either partial or complete arch. See: Fixed prosthesis, Removable prosthesis.

implant try-in: See: Trial-fit gauge.

implant type: Classification according to anatomic position, material composition, configuration, shape, surface, and/or implant–tissue interface. Type of implant is determined by the choice of classification system and varies among manufacturers. **Blade i.**: A flat, blade-shaped endosseous implant most commonly made of metal, which gains its support from a horizontal dimension of bone; it may be perforated, smooth, fluted, textured, coated, or wedge shaped, and it may have single or multiple abutments for attachment of the prosthesis. **Endodontic-endosseous i.**: A pin-shaped device that is placed into the root canal space and extends past the tooth's apex into the apical bone. **Endosseous i.**: An implant positioned into the jaw's alveolar and/or basal bone for the purpose of supporting a dental prosthesis. **Fibroosseous (fibroosteal) integrated i.**: A dental implant that has a fibrous connective tissue interface located between the implant and the adjacent bone. **Osseointegrated i.**: A direct physical and functional relationship between organic viable bone and the external surface of a stationary, load-bearing implant as revealed when viewed under a light microscope. **Ramus frame i.**: A complete mandibular arch implant with a tripoidal design that consists a horizontal supragingival connecting bar with terminal left and right posterior ends that pass through the soft tissue and enter the bilateral rami of the mandible. There is also an inferior anterior plate that passes through the soft tissue and enters the bone of the symphyseal area. **Root-form i.**: An endosseous implant that obtains support from the vertical height of alveolar or basal bone. It is frequently made from metal or ceramic and may have a cylinder shape that is tapered, threaded, perforated, solid, and/or hollow. The surface may be coated, smooth, or textured. **Subperiosteal i.**: A dental implant placed on the external surface of the maxillary or mandibular alveolar or basal bone. It is designed to provide support for attachment of a dental prosthesis. The implant is not designed to enter the bone, although there may be retentive screws that do, or, with time, the implant may settle into the supporting bone.

implant uncovering: See: Implant exposure, Stage two surgery.

implantology: A term historically conceived as the study or science of placing and restoring dental implants. See: Implant dentistry, Implant prosthodontics, Implant surgery.

impression: An accurate reproduction, in the negative form, of an individual's dentition and other important anatomical structures contained within the oral cavity.

impression coping: A device that registers the position of a dental implant or dental implant abutment in an impression. It may be retained in the impression (direct) or may require a transfer from intraoral usage to the impression after the attachment of the corresponding analog (indirect).

impression material: Any substance or combination of substances used for making an impression or negative reproduction.

impression taking: Act of recording the negative likeness of anatomic structures in a suitable medium for a positive reproduction in the form of a cast or moulage.

impression tray: Container used to transport impression medium to the mouth and to limit material flow around the structures to be recorded while the material sets to form an impression.

impression wand: Hand-held device used for intraoral digital scanning.

incidence: Rate with which new events or cases occur during a certain period of time. Compare: Prevalence.

incipient: Beginning to exist; coming into existence.

incisal: Cutting surface of incisors or canines.

incisal guidance: 1. The influence of the contacting surfaces of the mandibular and maxillary anterior teeth on mandibular movements. 2. The influences of the contacting surfaces of the guide pin and guide table on articulator movements.

incisal guide: The part of an articulator that maintains the incisal guide angle (GPT-4). See: Anterior guide table.

incisal guide angle: 1. Anatomically, the angle formed by the intersection of the plane of occlusion and a line within the sagittal plane determined by the incisal edges of the maxillary and mandibular central incisors when the teeth are in maximum intercuspation. 2. On an articulator, that angle formed, in the sagittal plane, between the plane of reference and the slope of the anterior guide table, as viewed in the sagittal plane.

incisal guide pin: Adjustable rod attached to one member of an articulator that contacts the guide table on the opposing member to maintain the degree of cast and jaw separation determined in the mouth. See: Articulator.

incision: A cut made in soft tissue. **External bevel i.**: A resective incision angled in an apical-to-coronal direction which is intended to reduce the thickness or amount of mucogingival tissue and allow for healing by secondary intention. Often used during gingivectomy and gingivoplasty. **Internal (inverse, reverse, or inverted) bevel i.**: An acute or oblique surgical incision angled toward the tooth surface in a coronal-to-apical direction which is intended to reduce the thickness or amount of mucogingival tissue. **Releasing i.**: Incision made to increase access to alveolar bone, enhance flap mobility, facilitate lateral or coronal flap advancement, limit the inclusion of nondiseased sites in the surgical field, and/or decrease tension on retracted flaps.

incision and drainage: The surgical procedure of cutting into a lesion to allow the release of exudate.

incisive foramen: An anatomic hole, usually found lingual to the maxillary central incisors, that allows passage of the vascular and neural tissues that supply the anterior maxilla.

incisive foramen: Foramen of the incisive canal containing the nasopalatal nerve and accompanying blood vessels. It is located just palatal to the two maxillary central incisors along the median suture.

incisive papilla: The elevation of soft tissue covering the foramen of the incisive or nasopalatine canal. See: Papilla.

inclined plane: Any of the inclined cuspal surfaces of a tooth.

inclusion criterion: Requirement (such as a diagnostic feature or clinical conditions) that must be met for eligibility to participate in a research project, as specified in the protocol. Compare: Exclusion criteria.

index: Core or mold used to record and/or register relative positions of teeth, anatomic structures, or implants to one another. The recording medium can have reversible or irreversible characteristics. See also: Occlusal index, Remount index, Transfer index.

indirect (closed tray) impression: Impression technique in which a stock or custom-fabricated tray with impression material is used to record the negative likeness of placed copings. Once the impression material is set and the tray is removed from the mouth, the copings are removed from the mouth and seated in the impression with attached laboratory analogs prior to pouring a cast.

indirect fracture: A fracture at a point distant from the primary site of injury due to secondary forces.

indirect retainer: The component of a partial removable dental prosthesis that assists the direct retainer(s) in preventing displacement of the distal extension denture base by functioning through lever action on the opposite side of the fulcrum line when the denture base moves away from the tissues in pure rotation around the fulcrum line.

indirect retention: The effect achieved by one or more indirect retainers of a partial removable denture prosthesis that reduces the tendency for a denture base to move in an occlusal direction or rotate about the fulcrum line.

indirect sinus graft: See: Osteotome technique.

individual suture: See: Interrupted suture.

induction: The act of inducing or causing to occur as referenced in the induction of bone formation.

indurate: To toughen or harden; make hard.

indurated: Hardened; made hard.

infection: Invasion and multiplication of microorganisms in body tissues, which may be clinically inapparent or result in local cellular injury due to competitive metabolism, toxins, intracellular replication, or antigen-antibody response. **Endogenous i.**: Due to activation of organisms previously present in a dormant focus. **Exogenous i.**: Caused by organisms acquired from sources other than the host's own flora.

infectious: Capable of causing infection; caused by or capable of being transmitted by infection; infective.

inferior alveolar artery (arteria alveolaris inferior): Runs with the inferior alveolar nerve and enters the mandibular foramen at the medial aspect of the ramus. It continues through the mandibular canal with the nerve to the mental foramen, where it divides into the mental and incisive branches.

inferior alveolar canal: See: Mandibular canal.

inferior alveolar nerve (IAN): One of the terminal branches of the mandibular nerve, a division of the trigeminal nerve. It enters the mandibular canal branching to the lower teeth, periosteum, and gingiva of the mandible. A branch, the mental nerve, passes through the mental foramen to supply the skin and mucosa of the lower lip and chin.

inferior dental foramen: See: Mandibular foramen.

inflammation: Localized reaction of the body tissues to invasion by pathogenic microorganisms, or to trauma by wounds, burns or chemicals, which serves to destroy, dilute, or wall off both the injurious agent and the injured tissue. It may be acute or chronic and is characterized by some or all five cardinal signs: redness, swelling, pain, a rise in temperature, and loss of function.

informed consent: Principle of biomedical research stating that study participants have the right to know the risks and benefits involved in participating in a research study and that they may not be included in such studies without their explicit written consent.

infrabony: Within the bone. See: Endosseous.

infracture: The controlled fracture of (1) a window prepared in the lateral wall of the maxillary sinus or (2) the floor of the maxillary sinus through an osteotomy prepared in the ridge using an osteotome.

infraorbital artery: A continuation of the internal maxillary artery, but often arises in conjunction with the posterior superior alveolar artery. While in the infraorbital canal, it gives off anterior superior alveolar branches which supply maxillary anterior teeth. It is one of the three primary arterial suppliers to the maxillary sinus.

infrastructure: A metal, ceramic, or resin framework onto which a second framework or prosthesis will be placed or attached using chemical or physical means.

inhalation administration: A technique of administration in which a gaseous or volatile agent is introduced into the lungs and whose primary effect is due to absorption through the gas/blood interface.

initial occlusal contact: The first contact of opposing teeth upon closure of the mandible.

initial stability: (syn): Primary stability. The degree of tightness of a dental implant immediately after placement in its prepared osteotomy. An implant is considered to have initial stability if it is clinically immobile at the time of placement.

injury: See: Trauma, Wound.

innate immunity: Nonspecific immunity present from birth (congenital). Responsible for the initial protection from infectious agents previously unseen by the host. Composed of soluble immune proteins (including complement) and phagocytes.

insertion torque: (syn): Placement torque. The maximum torque recorded at the insertion of a dental implant in an osteotomy, expressed in Newton centimeters (Ncm). It may be used as an indication of the mechanical stability of the implant in the bone.

in situ: In the proper position without invasion of neighboring tissues; in place.

instability: See: Primary stability, Secondary stability.

insulin: A protein secreted from the beta cells of the pancreas responsible for the uptake of glucose into cells, and stimulation of protein synthesis and lipid synthesis in fat cells.

insulin-like growth factor (IGF): Polypeptides structurally similar to insulin. The IGF family consists of two ligands (IGF-I and IGF-II), two cell surface receptors (IGF-1R and IGF-2R) and several IGF binding proteins. They control growth, differentiation, and the maintenance of differentiated function in numerous tissues. In oral tissues, IGFs are involved in tooth growth and development, in the biology of several periodontal structures, and in various aspects of salivary gland homeostasis.

intaglio: In dentistry, the interior surface of a denture.

integration: The action or process of integrating. **Biointegration**: A bonding of living bone to the surface of an implant which is independent of any mechanical interlocking mechanism. **Fibroosseous i.**: The interposition of healthy dense collagenous tissue between implant and bone. Also known as fibroosteal integration. **Osseointegration**: A direct contact, on the light microscopic level, between living bone tissue and an implant.

integrins: Integrins belong to the family of cellular adhesion molecules (CAM) and act as specialized receptors that mediate the interactions between basal epithelial cells and the extracellular matrix.

interalveolar: The area between the alveoli. Situated between the dental alveoli of adjacent teeth.

interalveolar crest: The most coronal portion of the interdental bony septum.

interalveolar septum: Alveolar and trabecular bony partition between adjacent tooth sockets.

interarch distance: The vertical distance between maxillary and mandibular teeth at any given degree of jaw opening.

intercellular: Occurring between cell boundaries.

intercellular adhesion molecules (ICAMs): Molecules with immunoglobulin-like domains found on the surface of endothelial cells whose increased production during inflammation causes leukocytes to adhere to endothelial cells.

interceptive occlusal contact: See: Deflective occlusal contact.

intercondylar: In dentistry, refers to the area between the mandibular condyles.

intercuspal contact: The contact between the cusps of opposing teeth.

intercuspal contact area: The range of tooth contacts in maximum intercuspation.

intercuspation: 1. The cusp-to-fossa relationship of the maxillary and mandibular posterior teeth to each other. 2. The interdigitation of cusps of opposing teeth.

interdental: Between the proximal surfaces of the teeth within the same arch.

interdental alveolar crest: The most coronal portion of the bony septum located between adjacent teeth.

interdental alveolar septum: A component of the alveolar process composed of compact and trabecular bone that extends between the roots of contiguous teeth.

interdental bone height: The distance between the bone crest and the contact point between two teeth.

interdental papilla: Portion of the free gingiva occupying the interproximal space confined by adjacent teeth in contact. See: Papilla.

interdigitation: The interlocking or fitting of opposing parts, as the cusps of the maxillary and mandibular posterior teeth.

interference: A tooth contact that interferes with harmonious mandibular movement.

interferometry: A method used to construct a 3D image of an object scanned using optical scanners.

interferon-gamma (IFN-γ): One of a group of heat-stable soluble basic antiviral glycoproteins of low molecular weight that are produced by T cells in response to either specific antigen or mitogenic stimulation. It regulates the immune response (e.g., by the activation of macrophages and natural killer cells) and is used in a form obtained from recombinant DNA technology in the control of infections and the treatment of neoplasias.

interferons (IFNs): A subset of cytokines classified into two major families, type I and type II, involved in the protection against viral infections and signaling between cells of the immune system.

interfurcation: The area between and at the base of the roots of a multirooted tooth.

interim abutment: See: Temporary abutment.

interim dental implant: A temporary dental implant that allows for the use of a provisional prosthesis. These temporary implants may also be used as stents to guide tissue healing and prevent soft tissue collapse into a healing surgical site. These implants have a smooth machined surface to allow easier removal. Also known as provisional dental implant.

interim denture: See: Interim prosthesis.

interim endosteal dental implant abutment: A type of dental implant abutment used only for a limited time to guide healing or shaping of the adjacent tissues and/or attachment of a transitional prosthesis.

interimplant distance: The horizontal distance between the platforms of two adjacent dental implants.

interimplant papilla: The soft tissue occupying the interproximal space confined by adjacent implant-supported fixed partial dentures in contact.

interim prosthesis: A prosthesis typically used before fabrication of a definitive dental or maxillofacial prosthesis. It can be fixed or removable and is designed to enhance esthetics, stabilize teeth, or improve function for a limited time. Such prostheses often help guide the clinician in designing the appearance and function of the final prosthesis. Also known as a provisional restoration. See: Provisional prosthesis.

interleukins: A family of potent proteins that serve as a link between inducer and effector cells during immune and inflammatory responses; involved in the recruitment of immune and inflammatory precursor cells. Some interleukins have been implicated in the pathogenesis of periodontal diseases. **Interleukin-4** (IL-4): Lymphokine produced by antigen- or mitogen-activated T cells. Its principal role is regulation of IgE- and eosinophil-mediated immune reactions. It stimulates switching of B cells for production of immunoglobulin E (IgE), is a growth and differentiation factor for T cells (particularly helper T cells), is a growth factor for mast cells, and stimulates the expression of some adhesion molecules on endothelial cells. Formerly called B lymphocyte stimulatory factor 1. **Interleukin-6** (IL-6): Lymphokine produced by antigen- or mitogen-activated T cells, fibroblasts, macrophages, and other cells that induce differentiation and maturation of B cells and growth of myeloma cells. It activates and induces proliferation of T cells and stimulates synthesis of immunoglobulin and plasma proteins such as fibrinogen.

interlock: An intracoronal attachment used to segment prosthetic reconstructions.

intermaxillary: Between the maxillary and mandibular jaws.

intermediate abutment: A natural tooth or dental implant located between terminal abutments that provides added stability and retention for the fixed or removable prosthesis.

internal bevel incision: (syn): Inverse bevel incision, inverted bevel incision, reverse bevel incision. Blade cut made in a coronal to apical direction, designed to reduce the thickness of gingiva or periimplant mucosa from its internal surface (i.e., sulcular side). See: External bevel incision.

internal connection: A prosthetic connection interface internal to a dental implant platform. Examples include internal hexagon and Morse taper. See: External connection.

internal connector: A device of varying geometric designs used to unite parts of a fixed partial denture.

internal derangement: Abnormal positioning of the articular disk in relation to the condyle, fossa, or articular eminence; a deviation in form or function of the joint capsule.

internal hexagon (hex): A hexagonal connection interface of the platform of an implant within its coronal aspect. It prevents gross rotation of attached components. See: External hexagon.

internal irrigation: Method of irrigation during the drilling of osteotomies for the placement of root-form dental implants, whereby the cooling solution passes inside the shaft of the drilling bur and is delivered through an exit at the working end. This method delivers the cooling solution inside the osteotomy. **internally threaded**: Having a thread pattern within the body of a dental implant.

internal sinus graft: See: Osteotome technique, Sinus graft.

interocclusal: Between the occlusal surfaces of opposing teeth.

interocclusal clearance (freeway space): The space between the maxillary and mandibular opposing teeth when the mandible is suspended in postural (rest) position.

interocclusal record: A record or registration of the positional relationship of the teeth or jaw position.

interocclusal rest space: The measured difference in tooth position between the vertical dimension of occlusion.

Interpore: Proprietary product name for porous coralline hydroxyapatite.

interpositional graft: Placement of graft material within a three-four, or five-walled bone compartment. Examples include the sinus graft, socket graft, and ridge expansion.

interproximal space: Intervening distance between adjacent teeth in the dental arch.

interpupillary line: Imaginary line connecting the pupils of the eyes. It is useful for evaluating frontal facial symmetry and orientation of the occlusal plane when arranging artificial teeth.

interquartile range (IQR): Range of values containing the central half of the observations, i.e., the range between the 25th and 75th percentiles. It is used with the median value to report data that are markedly non-normally distributed. See: Median.

interradicular: Between the roots of teeth.

interradicular septum: Part of the alveolar process that separates individual roots of the same tooth. See: Interalveolar septum.

interrupted suture: Suture made from a single tissue penetration of the flap(s).

interstitial: Positioned between parts or spaces of a tissue envelope.

interstitial collagenase: See: Mammalian collagenase.

intrabony: Within a bone. Used for description of bony defects or periodontal pockets with their base apical to adjacent bone crest. Called also infrabony.

intracoronal attachment: **1.** A retainer consisting of a metal receptacle (matrix) and a closely fitting part (patrix); the matrix is usually contained within the normal or expanded contours of the crown on the abutment tooth/dental implant and the patrix is attached to a pontic or the removable dental prosthesis framework. 2. An interlocking device, one component of which is fixed to an abutment or abutments, and the other is integrated into a removable dental prosthesis in order to stabilize and/or retain it.

intramembranous ossification: Bone formation in which connective tissue serving as a membrane becomes a template for bone deposition without any intermediate formation of cartilage. Flat bones are embryonically formed in this way. When sufficient vascularity is present adjacent to the condensed mesenchyme, the osteoblasts begin to produce osteoid. A similar process takes place in healing of bone defects.

intramobile connector: Implant-abutment connection incorporating a movable or flexible interpositional component intended to modify or reduce the load transferred from the prosthesis to the underlying implant and its surrounding bone. A connector intended to simulate mobility of the periodontal ligament.

intramobile element (IME): See: Intramobile connector.

intramucosal: Found within the confines of mucosa; for example, submucosal inserts attached to removable appliances to add retention.

intramucosal implant: See: Mucosal insert.

intramucosal insert: See: Mucosal insert.

intraoral (internal) distraction: A distraction procedure in which the distraction device is located completely within the oral cavity.

intraoral distractor: Distraction device designed to be placed within the oral cavity for alveolar distraction osteogenesis. Called also internal distractor. See: Distraction osteogenesis (DO).

intraoral scanning: The process of scanning and capturing the intraoral cavity for translation into a digital file format, such as STL.

intraosseous: syn. Endosseous. Within the bone.

intraosseous distractor: See: Endosseous distractor.

intrasulcular incision: Incision approach made along the sulcus of a tooth.

intrinsic coloring: Shading or actual coloring found within the material of a restoration.

intrusion: A translational form of tooth movement directed apically and parallel to the long axis of a tooth.

inverted basket: See: Implant basket.

investing: The process of covering or enveloping, wholly or in part, an object such as a denture, tooth, wax form, crown, etc. with a suitable investment material before processing, soldering, or casting.

investment casting: See: Casting wax.

in vitro: Outside the living organism or natural system. Usually refers to artificial experimental systems such as cultures or cell-free extracts.

in vivo: Within a living body.

iontophoresis: The act or process of introducing therapeutic agents into tissues using an electrical current or electrochemical gradient.

ipsilateral: Belonging to or occurring on the same side of the body.

IQR (abbrev.): Interquartile range.

irradiation: Process by which an organ or tissue is exposed to radiation. See: Radiation.

irrigation: 1. Technique of using a solution, usually physiologic saline, to cool the surgical bur and flush away the surgical debris. 2. Act of flushing an area with a solution. See: External irrigation, Internal irrigation.

irritant: An agent capable of inducing functional derangements or organic lesions in tissues.

ischemia: Deficiency of blood in an area due to a functional constriction or actual obstruction of a blood vessel(s); blockage or inadequate supply of oxygenated blood to tissues or organs; may be caused by overzealous tight suturing.

isoforms: Approximately 20 BMP family members (isoforms) have been identified and characterized. Each isoform is involved in some developmental process, and BMP-2 has been the most studied isoform for therapeutic purposes in bone regeneration.

isogeneic graft: See: Isograft.

isograft: (syn): Isogeneic graft, isologous graft, syngeneic graft. A tissue graft transplanted from one genetically identical individual to another, as in monozygotic twins.

isotonic: See: Contraction, isotonic.

isotonic solution: One having osmotic pressure equal to that of blood.

isotropic: Quality of having the same properties in all dimensions, irrespective of direction.

isotropic surface: Surface textures that are randomly distributed so the surface is identical in all directions. See: Anisotropic surface.

ISP (abbrev.): Implant-supported prosthesis.

ISQ (abbrev.): Implant stability quotient.

J

jaw: Either of two bony structures (maxilla or mandible) that are intended to bear natural teeth or support prosthetic teeth.

jaw malposition: Abnormal or anomalous position of the mandible.

jaw relation: Any relation of the mandible to the maxilla. See: Centric relation, Centric occlusion. **Eccentric j.r.**: Any jaw relation other than centric relation. **Median j.r.**: Any jaw relation when the mandible is in the median sagittal plane. **Protrusive j.r.**: A jaw relation resulting from an anterior positioning of the mandible. **Rest j.r.**: The habitual postural jaw relation when the head is in an upright position and the condyles are in neutral, unstrained positions in the glenoid fossae. **Retrusive j.r.**: A jaw position resulting from a posterior positioning of the mandible.

jig: A device used to maintain mechanically the correct positional relationship between a piece of work and a tool or between components during assembly or alteration.

joint: Where two or more skeletal bones meet (intersect); functions to allow the movement of the individual bones. See: Prosthetic joint, Temporomandibular joint.

joint replacement: See: Prosthetic joint.

joint-separating force: Tensile force applied to separate two or more contacting components. Generally applied to bolted or friction fit joints.

JPEG 2000: Image compression standard and coding system. It was created by the Joint Photographic Experts Group committee in 2000 with the intention of superseding their original discrete cosine transform-based JPEG standard (created in 1992) with a newly designed, wavelet-based method.

jumping distance: See: Gap distance.

junction: The process of joining together, as in two different structures. **Cementodentinal j.**: The zone where the dentin and cementum meet. **Cementoenamel j.**: The zone where the cementum and enamel meet at the cervical section of the tooth. **Dentinoenamel j.**: The zone where the dentin and enamel meet. **Mucogingival j.**: The zone where the gingiva and alveolar mucosa meet.

junctional epithelium: The epithelium adhering to the surface of a dental implant or tooth surface at the base of the sulcus. It constitutes the coronal part of the biologic width. It is formed by single or multiple layers of nonkeratinizing cells. The junctional epithelial cells have a basal membrane and hemidesmosomal attachments to the implant or tooth surface. See: Epithelial attachment.

juvenile periodontitis: A deteriorating periodontal disease found in adolescents in which the periodontal damage is greater than what would normally be expected when considering the localized irritating factors found on adjacent teeth. Inflammatory changes become excessive, leading to observed bone loss, tooth migration, and/or extrusion. Juvenile periodontitis is now called aggressive periodontitis.

juxtaposition: Two things placed side by side or in close proximity; in apposition, contiguous.

Glossary of Dental Implantology, First Edition. Khalid Almas, Fawad Javed and Steph Smith.
© 2018 John Wiley & Sons, Inc. Published 2018 by John Wiley & Sons, Inc.

K

Kaplan–Meier analysis: A statistical method used to estimate a population (e.g., dental implants) survival curve from a sample. Survival over time can be estimated, even when patients drop out or are studied for different lengths of time. Statistical method used in survival (time-to-event) analysis to estimate the probability of an event, such as implant loss, at different times in the study.

Kaposi's sarcoma: An infectious granuloma or a reticuloendothelial hyperplasia that may be neoplastic in nature. Clinically, multiple reddish or brownish-red nodules can involve the skin, oral mucosa, visceral organs, and lymph nodes.

keeper: A device used for holding something in a desired position. In dentistry, this is typically understood to mean a magnetized alloy fixed to one component of a restoration to which a magnet may adhere.

Kennedy classification of removable partial dentures: The most widely accepted and used classification system for removable partial dentures. The Kennedy classification is based on the location of the missing teeth.

- **Class I**: Characterized by bilateral edentulism located distal to the remaining natural teeth.
- **Class II**: Characterized by unilateral edentulism distal to the remaining natural teeth.
- **Class III**: Characterized by unilateral edentulism when natural teeth are located both mesially and distally to the edentulous area.

- **Class IV**: Observed when the edentulism is located mesially to the natural teeth.

keratinized gingiva: The portion of the gingiva extending from the mucogingival junction to the gingival margin.

keratins: A multigene family of approximately 30 proteins that form the intermediate filaments of the epithelial cell cytoskeleton.

keratocyst: A cutaneous cyst that is similar to epidermoid cysts but is not limited to a specified location on the body. They are frequently reported in persons with nevoid basal cell carcinoma syndrome.

keratosis: A horny, keratinous growth, particularly on the skin. Also known as a wart or callus.

keyway: An interlock connection that uses a matrix and patrix between the units of a fixed dental prosthesis. Once it is soldered in place, it holds the pontic in its proper relationship to the edentulous ridge and the opposing teeth and reinforces the connector.

knife-edge: Term used to describe a sharp or narrow morphology of a residual ridge.

knife-edge ridge: Severely atrophic edentulous maxillary or mandibular alveolar ridge with a sharp crest resulting from progressive resorption, especially after long periods of denture wearing. Cawood and Howell class 4 for the anterior maxilla and mandible. See: Alveolar ridge.

Glossary of Dental Implantology, First Edition. Khalid Almas, Fawad Javed and Steph Smith.
© 2018 John Wiley & Sons, Inc. Published 2018 by John Wiley & Sons, Inc.

L

labial: Of or relating to the lip; toward the lip.

labial flange: The ridge, edge, or projection of a denture that is positioned toward the vestibule located on the lip side of the mouth.

labial plate: See: Buccal plate.

labial vestibule: The segment of the oral cavity that is anterior to the bicuspids and lies between the lips and the adjacent teeth or the corresponding edentulous residual ridge.

labioversion: Any deviation from the normal arrangement of the dental arch toward the lip.

laboratory analog: Copy of a prosthetic or implant element used in laboratory fabrication procedures. See: Analog/analogue.

laboratory screw: Threaded component matching the abutment screw, used by the laboratory technician in the fabrication of the prosthetic reconstruction. Its use avoids damage to the prosthetic screw which is reserved for the intraoral fixation of the prosthesis.

lacerate: To mangle; to tear; to cut so that the margin is irregular.

Lactobacillus spp: Gram-positive bacteria that contribute to caries progression. The bacteria are rod-shaped and motile, and can exist under anaerobic conditions.

lacuna: A depression; a hollow space.

lamella: A thin layer, membrane, plate, or scale, as of bone, tissue, or cell walls.

lamellar bone: Adult, mature bone consisting of 3–5 μm-wide layers of mineralized collagen fibrils. The orientation of fibrils changes from layer to layer; this construction is often compared with that of plywood. It appears birefringent in polarized light and is found in mature cortical as well as trabecular bone.

lamina: One of the thin layers or flat plates of a larger composite structure, such as bone or tissue.

lamina dura: The sheet of compact bone that forms the tooth alveolar wall or tooth alveolus.

- **Crestal lamina dura:** The layer of compact bone at the alveolar crest.

lamina propria: Connective tissue that is highly vascularized and lies beneath the basement membranelining the epithelium; vascularized connective tissue layer of mucous membranes.

laminate: Layered material. In dentistry, a thin layer or veneer of restorative material applied to the surface of a tooth, usually for cosmetic purposes.

laminin: A high molecular weight glycoprotein composed of three polypeptide chains that are organized in a cross-like manner; functional domains of this molecule have affinity for cell surface receptors and extracellular matrix components.

lancinating pain: A sharp, piercing, cutting, knife-like pain that is usually intermittent.

land area: The area of a dental cast that denotes the end of the replicated anatomic surface of the mouth and the beginning of a border of the cast.

lap: To cover, fold over, or lie on top of, as in the ridge lap of an artificial tooth that covers the residual ridge.

Glossary of Dental Implantology, First Edition. Khalid Almas, Fawad Javed and Steph Smith.
© 2018 John Wiley & Sons, Inc. Published 2018 by John Wiley & Sons, Inc.

lapping tool: Instrument used with or without abrasives to improve the adaptation of two opposing surfaces. In the laboratory, an instrument, often rotating, used to remove casting irregularities by means of grinding or polishing.

laser: Acronym for light amplification by stimulated emission of radiation. A technique that converts light from several frequencies into an intense, visible, small, nondivergent, monochromatic radiation beam that is capable of creating immense localized heat and power when concentrated and directed at a short distance.

laser etching: Application of a laser beam to selectively ablate a material from a surface (e.g., dental implant).

laser phototherapy (LPT): The clinical use of nonionizing laser sources for nonsurgical applications.

laser scanner: A machine that uses a laser beam or plane to scan an object in 3D.

laser scanning: Creates a 3D image through a triangulation mechanism. A laser dot or line is projected onto an object from a handheld device, and a sensor (typically a charge-coupled device, CCD, or position-sensitive device) measures the distance to the surface. Data are collected in relation to an internal coordinate system, and therefore to collect data where the scanner is in motion, the position of the scanner must be determined. The position can be determined by the scanner using reference features on the surface being scanned or by using an external tracking method.

laser therapy: The use of concentrated light beams to specifically cut, burn, remove, or destroy soft tissue.

laser welding: Technique of joining pieces of metal (e.g., a bar) through the use of a laser beam. The beam provides a concentrated heat source, allowing for high-strength, narrow, and deep welds.

late closing click: A sound made in the temporomandibular joint just before jaw closure as the disk slips from anterior displacement to its original position between the glenoid fossa and the head of the condyle.

late implant failure: (syn): Secondary implant failure. The failure of a dental implant after osseointegration has been established. This type of failure may be due to or accompanied by periimplantitis or overload.

late implant loss: Outcome related to the loss of an implant that occurred after implant osseointegration. Compare: Early implant loss.

late implant placement: Implant placement at least 6 months following tooth extraction. The chosen time period should allow for sufficient bone regeneration of the extraction socket, and consequently, implant placement without bone augmentation procedure. Late implant placement bears the risk of bone atrophy in the orofacial direction, particularly in the anterior maxilla.

late opening click: A sound made in the temporomandibular joint just before maximum jaw opening as the disk slips from anterior displacement to its original position between the glenoid fossa and the head of the condyle.

latency period: See: Consolidation period, Distraction osteogenesis.

lateral: Any position that is right or left of the midline.

lateral antrostomy: See: Lateral window technique, Sinus graft.

lateral Bennett shift: See: Bennett angle.

lateral cephalograph: Extraoral radiograph showing the region of the skull that comprises the bones of the face (i.e., the viscerocranium). It requires a 18×24 cm or 20×25 cm image receptor and is intended for diagnosis in orthodontics. It also has been used in preoperative implant examination to determine the size and length of implants to be placed in the interforaminal region.

lateral condylar inclination: The angle made by the moving condyle within the horizontal plane (superior-inferior movement) and the median plane (anterior-posterior movement) as the jaw moves laterally. The condylar deviation or the degree of deviation (slant) from its original horizontal and vertical orientation when it is moved to one side.

lateral interocclusal record: Bite registrations of the teeth in right and then left lateral working positions, used to estimate the opposite side lateral condylar path and inclination.

lateral relation: An obsolete term for the positional relationship between the mandible and the maxillae when the lower jaw is to the left or the right side of the centric relation.

lateral window technique: Surgical technique using a window into the lateral wall of the maxillary sinus to gain access to the maxillary sinus membrane. Following mobilization and elevation of the sinus membrane, bone augmentation materials (i.e., autografts, allografts, alloplasts, xenografts, or combination mixtures) are used to elevate the sinus floor and allow the placement of dental implants. If the original bone height permits sufficient primary implant stability, then a simultaneous procedure can be used. Otherwise, a staged approach is recommended. Compare: Osteotome technique. See: Maxillary sinus floor elevation.

laterotrusion: The movement of the mandibular condyle on the working side in the horizontal plane. This description of mandibular condyle movement is used in conjunction with other types of condylar movement in other planes, such as laterodetrusion, lateroprotrusion, lateroretrusion, and laterosurtrusion.

layered manufacturing: See: Solid freeform fabrication (SFF).

Le Fort fracture (Leon Clement Le Fort, French surgeon, 1829–1893): Eponym for a midfacial fracture, classified into three categories (I, II, III).

- **Le Fort I fracture**: horizontal segmented fracture of the alveolar process of the maxilla, in which the teeth are usually contained within the detached portion.
- **Le Fort II fracture**: pyramidal fracture of the midfacial skeleton with the principal fracture lines meeting at an apex at or near the superior aspect of the nasal bones.
- **Le Fort III fracture**: craniofacial dysjunction fracture in which the entire maxilla and one or more facial bones are completely separated from the craniofacial skeleton.

Le Fort osteotomy: Surgical sectioning of the maxilla from the rest of the skull. Le Fort I osteotomy sections the midface through the walls of the maxillary sinuses, the lateral nasal walls, and the nasal septum, just superior to the apices of the maxillary teeth. Le Fort II osteotomy is similar to Le Fort I, except that instead of continuing anteriorly across the pyriform aperture, the osteotomy continues superiorly towards the orbit. Le Fort III osteotomy is designed to separate the entire facial mass from the cranial base along the interfrontofacial and interpterygomaxillary planes.

leaf gauge: A device consisting of a set of blades or leaves of graduated thicknesses that is placed in the oral cavity to make accurate measurements between two points or to provide a metered separation.

lengthening of the clinical crown: A surgical procedure performed to increase the extent of supragingival tooth structure by apically repositioning the gingival tissue around the tooth; often includes removing a portion of the surrounding alveolar bone. This procedure is typically performed for restorative or esthetic purposes.

Leptotrichia ssp.: Gram-negative, nonmotile, anaerobic, rod-shaped bacteria found in marginal and subgingival plaque.

lesion: Any pathological change to a tissue or organ, local in nature, caused by injury, surgical procedures, chemicals, or infection that may result in a loss of normal function. **Chemically induced l.:** A lesion resulting from local contact with chemically irritating substances such as aspirin, cocaine, pyrophosphates, detergents (e.g., sodium lauryl sulfate), smokeless tobacco, betel nut, and tooth- whitening agents. **Traumatic l.:** A self-inflicted (factitious), accidental, or iatrogenic injury which may manifest as recession, abrasions, ulcerations, lacerations, erythematous or white lesions, or combinations of several of these features.

leukemia: A generalized neoplastic disorder of the blood-forming tissues, primarily those of the leukocyte series.

leukocidin: See: Leukotoxin.

leukocyte: Blood cell that is colorless, lacks hemoglobin, and contains a nucleus. Leukocytes are involved with host defense and are classified in two large groups: granular leukocytes (basophils, eosinophils, and neutrophils) and nongranular leukocytes (lymphocytes and monocytes). Called also white blood cell.

leukopenia: Reduction in the number of leukocytes in the blood below 5000 per cubic mm. See: Agranulocytosis, Neutropenia.

leukoplakia: A nonspecific white patch in the oral cavity which will not rub off.

leukotoxin: A toxin produced by certain bacteria, including *Aggregatibacter actinomycetemcomitans*, which is toxic to leukocytes, particularly polymorphonuclear leukocytes. Also known as leukocidin.

leukotrienes: A group of potent biologic mediators of inflammation consisting of 20 carboxylic acids with at least two oxygen substitutes and three double bonds; derived from arachidonic acid by the lipoxygenase pathway; mediator of inflammatory reactions.

levofloxacin: Fluoroquinolone antibiotic with a broad spectrum of action, which may be used orally or parenterally. It is used in implant dentistry for severe infections, especially in the maxillary sinus.

L-forms: A phase of bacteria that have lost the cell wall. Bacteria in this phase retain the ability to reproduce and divide and often have pleiomorphic cell morphologies. The role of L-forms in nature is unclear, but may be associated with disease when found in humans.

lichen planus: An inflammatory mucocutaneous disorder characterized by discrete skin papules with a keratinized covering which often appears in the form of adherent scales. Oral lesions with characteristic radiating white striae are common.

life table analysis: Statistical method to describe the survival (e.g., dental implants) in a sample. The distribution of survival times is divided into intervals. For each interval, one can compute the number and proportion of cases that entered the respective interval "alive," the number and proportion of cases that failed in the respective interval (i.e., number of cases that "died"), and the number of cases that were lost to follow-up or censored in the respective interval.

ligament: A band of fibrous tissue that connects bones and cartilages, serving to support and strengthen joints.

ligate: To tie or bind, usually in the therapeutic sense, for the purpose of stopping bleeding or immobilizing a structure.

ligation, teeth: The binding together of teeth with ligatures for stabilization and immobilization. See: Splint.

ligature: 1. Any substance, such as gut, nylon, silk, or wire, used to tie an object or strangulate a part. 2. A wire or other material used to secure an orthodontic attachment. **Orthodontic l.:** A wire or other material used to secure an orthodontic attachment or tooth to an archwire.

lightness: The perception by which objects are distinguished as white or gray and light or dark; equivalent to shading in grays, in the Munsell color order system. Lightness (also called brightness) is one dimension of the three achromatic dimensions (the others being hue and saturation) describing the three-dimensional nature of color.

line angle: The point of convergence of two planes in a cavity preparation.

line of occlusion: A line passing through the cusp tips of adjacent teeth on one side of the arch forming a plane when viewed horizontally. See: Occlusal plane.

linear gingival erythema: A distinct erythematous linear band limited to the free gingiva; commonly a manifestation of immunosuppression that does not predictably respond to plaque removal.

linear occlusion: An occlusal arrangement of artificial teeth developed to enhance stability for complete denture prosthetics. This arrangement is described as a mandibular flat plane or monoplane arrangement, opposed by a line or bladed arrangement of the maxillary teeth with no anterior interferences in protrusive or lateral movements.

lingual: Related to the tongue; adjacent to or toward the tongue.

lingual artery: Branch of the carotid artery, with a distribution to the undersurface of the tongue, terminating as the deep artery of the tongue, and with subdivisions to the suprahyoid and dorsal lingual branches and the sublingual artery.

lingual bar connector: A major connector of a partial removable dental prosthesis located lingual to the dental arch.

lingual flange: The portion of a mandibular denture that occupies the space between the tongue and residual alveolar ridge.

lingual inclination: Deviation of the coronal portion of a tooth from the vertical plane toward the tongue.

lingual nerve: Branch of the mandibular division of the trigeminal nerve. It lies inferior to the lateral pterygoid and medial and anterior to the inferior alveolar nerve. It supplies sensory innervations to the mucous membrane of the anterior two-thirds of the tongue and the gingiva on the lingual side of the mandibular teeth.

lingual plate: 1. Bony wall at the lingual aspect of an alveolus consisting of alveolar bone proper, cortical bone, with or without intervening cancellous bone. 2. The portion of the major connector of a partial removable dental prosthesis contacting the lingual surfaces of the natural teeth. Also spelled linguoplate.

lingual rest: A metallic extension of a partial removable dental prosthesis framework that fits into a prepared depression within an abutment tooth's lingual surface.

lingual splint: A dental splint conforming to the inner aspect of the dental arch.

lingualized occlusion: An occlusal relationship commonly used in full denture prostheses characterized by maxillary palatal cusp contact against the central fossa of the mandibular teeth, where the buccal cusps of the mandibular teeth do not contact the opposing maxillary teeth and the position of the mandibular teeth is lingual to the alveolar ridge.

linguocclusion: An occlusal relationship where the teeth are located in a lingual position to their normal location.

linguoversion: Deviation of a tooth lingual in direction to the regular arch alignment.

lining cells: Old osteoblasts occupying the surface of mineralized bone with the primary function of nutritional transfer from the surface to osteocytes via cellular extensions. They participate in the normal physiologic remodeling of bone by digesting the osteoclast-resistant surface layer, whereby the bone matrix is opened and osteocalcin is released from the bone matrix. The osteocalcin is osteoclast-chemotactic.

lining mucosa: See: Alveolar mucosa, Oral mucosa.

lip line: Contour of the inferior border of the upper lip at rest or during maximum muscular retraction; reference for position of the residual ridge crest and for orientation of the occlusal plane when planning for esthetics and function during restorative treatment. The lower lip line is the relative position of the lower lip at rest or during voluntary retraction.

lip switch operation: A procedure in which tissue obtained from one lip is transferred to the other lip of the same patient. Also used to describe a modified vestibuloplasty procedure.

lipopolysaccharide (LPS): A large molecule consisting of lipids and sugars joined by chemical bonds. It is a major component of the cell wall of gram-negative bacteria, a type of endotoxin, and an important group-specific antigen. See: Endotoxin.

litigation: See: Malpractice litigation, Product liability litigation.

LLLT (abbrev.): Low-level laser therapy.

load: Any external mechanical force applied to a prosthesis, dental implant, abutment, tooth, skeletal organ, or tissue. In implant dentistry, generally meant to be the placement of a superstructure on an implant to bring it into contact with the opposing teeth during function. See: Occlusal force.

loading: Application of a force directly or indirectly onto a dental implant, tooth, or prosthesis. See: Immediate loading, Progressive loading. **Effects of l. on bone–implant contact:** It is generally assumed that loading within a range of physiologic tolerance stimulates increased bone–implant contact, while loading in a magnitude greater than the range of physiologic tolerance may cause loss of bone–implant contact. See: Bone–implant contact (BIC). **Effects of l. on framework:** Load distribution to supporting implants is affected by the relative stiffness of the prosthesis connecting the implants. With a rigid prosthesis, load is transferred relatively equally to all underlying implants. With a more resilient prosthesis, loading tends to be greatest at the implant closest to the point of load application. **Screw joint effects on l.:** Mechanical effect of loading, usually cyclic in nature, on the stability of bolted or screw-retained joints. Micromotion and fatigue are potential negative occurrences that may result from such loading.

loading dose: The larger dose given at the initiation of treatment in order to quickly achieve the desired blood or tissue final concentration.

lobe: A curved or rounded projection or division, especially of a body organ or part.

local contributing factor: An event occurring locally that can influence the manner in which a disease or condition is manifested.

localized ridge augmentation: See: Alveolar reconstruction, Alveolar ridge augmentation, Guided bone regeneration (GBR).

logistic regression analysis: Statistical approach to predict or estimate the value of a response variable from the known values of one (termed simple regression) or more (termed multiple regression) explanatory variables. Logistic regression is when the response variable is a binary categorical variable (such as diseased or not diseased) and it can be simple or multiple.

long axis: An imaginary line passing longitudinally through the center of a body.

long buccal nerve: Branch of the mandibular division of the trigeminal nerve. It passes anteriorly between the heads of the lateral pterygoid muscle and descends inferiorly to the anterior border of the masseter muscle. It supplies the skin over the buccinator muscle as well as the mucous membrane lining its inner portion and the buccal gingiva of the mandibular molars.

longitudinal study: A study in which observations on subjects are made at two or more points in time.

low-energy laser therapy: See: Low-level laser therapy.

low-intensity laser: See: Low-level laser therapy.

low-level laser therapy: Type of laser therapy applied for the stimulation of cell function. Unlike high-power surgical lasers used to cut, coagulate, and evaporate tissues for surgical procedures, their biologic effect is not thermal. Called also biostimulating lasers or low-intensity lasers.

low lip line: 1. The lowest position of the inferior border of the resting upper lip. 2. When the patient voluntarily smiles or retracts the lips, the lowest position of the superior border of the lower lip.

low-power laser therapy: See: Low-level laser therapy.

LPS (abbrev.): Lipopolysaccharide.

LPT (abbrev.): Laser phototherapy.

Lucia jig: Eponym (Victor O. Lucia) for an anterior muscle programming device used to obtain an accurate dental arch centric relationship by allowing the condyles to seat in their most superior position.

luminance: The intensity of light emitted from a surface per unit area.

lute: To attach two surfaces by means of a cement or other adhesive material.

luting agent: Any material used to attach or cement indirect restorations to prepared teeth.

luting of crowns: See: Cementation.

luxation: 1. Dislocation or displacement. 2. Partial or complete dislocation of a tooth from its alveolus.

lymphocyte: Mononuclear, nonphagocytic leukocyte that originates from stem cells and differentiates in lymphoid tissue (as of the thymus or bone marrow). It is the typical cellular elementsof lymph and constitutes 20–30% of the white blood cells of normal human blood. Divided on the basis of ontogeny and function into two classes: B, T lymphocytes, responsible for humeral and cellular immunity, respectively.

lymphokine: Soluble factors released from lymphocytes that transmit signals for growth and differentiation of various cell types.

lymphotoxin: A lymphokine that results in direct cytolysis following its release from stimulated lymphocytes; also termed tumor necrosis factor beta.

lyophilization: Creation of a stable preparation of a biologic substance (e.g., blood plasma, serum) by rapid freezing followed by dehydration under high vacuum. See: Freeze-drying.

lysis: The process of cell dissolution; the action of a lysin.

lysosomes: Intracellular cytoplasmic vesicles filled with hydrolytic enzymes; especially prominent in phagocytic cells such as polymorphonuclear leukocytes and macrophages.

lysozyme: The cationic low molecular weight enzyme present in tears, saliva, and nasal secretion that functions as an antibacterial hydrolase by catalyzing the hydrolysis of specific glycosidic linkages in the cell wall of susceptible bacteria.

M

machined implant surface: See: Turned implant surface.

machined surface: (syn): Turned surface. A dental implant surface that results from the milling process of a metallic rod. The scratches of the tooling on the implant form a machined pattern of lines and grooves.

macroglossia: Excessive size of the tongue.

macro-interlock: Fixation by mechanical interlocking between bone and dental implant macro-irregularities such as threads, holes, pores, grooves, etc., which have dimensions in the range of 50 microns or greater.

macromotion: Motion that is substantial in nature. It is generally applied to the implant body in situations where implant stability is lacking at the time of placement or as a result of loss of osseointegration.

macrophage: A large phagocytic cell of the monocyte series. Important as an antigen-presenting cell and as a producer of certain cytokines, i.e., interleukin-1 and gamma-interferon, and growth factors.

macrophage-derived angiogenic factor (MDAF): Macrophage-derived factor that promotes proliferation of new blood vessels. It is released by hypoxic macrophages at the edges or outer surfaces of wounds and initiates revascularization in wound healing.

macula: A small spot, perceptibly different in color from the surrounding tissue. It is neither elevated nor depressed from the surface.

macule: A completely flat circumscribed change in the color of skin that can only be appreciated by visual inspection and not by touch.

magnet: Certain metals or ferromagnetic alloys that demonstrate an attractive or repulsive force between these materials.

magnet attachment system: Retentive mechanism that is nonmechanical but dependent on the attraction properties of rare earth composition, such as samarium-cobalt, and a ferromagnetic alloy. Elements consist of a magnet and a keeper, which is made of a ferromagnetic alloy. See: Magnetic attachment.

magnetic attachment: Retentive device mainly used for retention of overdentures.

magnetic resonance imaging (MRI): Imaging that uses magnetic fields and radio waves to produce high-quality two- or three-dimensional images without use of ionizing radiation (X-rays) or radioactive tracers. During an MRI scan, a large cylindrical magnet creates a magnetic field around the patient through which radio waves are sent. Medical MRI most frequently relies on the relaxation properties of excited hydrogen nuclei in water. The vast quantity of nuclei in a small volume sum to produce a detectable change in a magnetic field, which can be measured from outside the body. When the magnetic field is imposed, each point in space has a unique radiofrequency at which the signal is received and transmitted. Sensors read the frequencies and a computer uses the information to construct an image.

maintenance: Procedures performed at selected time intervals to assist in the

Glossary of Dental Implantology, First Edition. Khalid Almas, Fawad Javed and Steph Smith.
© 2018 John Wiley & Sons, Inc. Published 2018 by John Wiley & Sons, Inc.

maintenance of the prosthetic reconstruction, periodontal and periimplant tissue health.

major aphtha: A type of recurrent aphthous stomatitis that occurs in 10–15% of patients with the condition; usually manifested by the appearance of one or two large, painful ulcerations on movable, nonkeratinized oral mucosa, lasting for up to 6 weeks.

major connector: The part of a partial removable dental prosthesis that joins the components on one side of the arch to those on the opposite side.

major (thread) diameter: The largest diameter of a screw thread. It corresponds to the diameter by which the screw is designated.

malalignment, dental: The displacement of a tooth from its normal position in the dental arch.

malignant: In the case of a neoplasm, having the properties of anaplasia, invasion, and metastasis.

malleable: Capable of being extended or shaped with a hammer or with the pressure of rollers.

malocclusion: 1. Any deviation from a physiologically acceptable contact between the opposing dental arches. 2. Any deviation from a normal occlusion. See: Angle's classification of occlusion.

- **Angle's classification of malocclusion class I (neutrocclusion)**: The normal mesiodistal relation of the maxillary and mandibular teeth with the mesiobuccal cusp of the maxillary first permanent molar occluding in the buccal groove of the mandibular first molar.
- **Angle's classification of malocclusion class II (distocclusion)**: The dental relationship wherein the mandibular dental arch is posterior to the maxillary arch; the mandibular first molar is located distal to that seen in neutrocclusion.
- **Angle's classification of malocclusion class II (retrognathism)**: The dental relationship wherein the mandibular dental arch is posterior to the maxillary arch; the mandibular first molar is located distal to that seen in neutrocclusion.

- **Angle's classification of malocclusion class II (distocclusion) division 1**: Angle's Class II in combination with excessive proclination of the maxillary incisors. The term 'subdivision' indicates a unilateral condition.
- **Angle's classification of malocclusion class II (distocclusion) division 2**: Angle's Class II in combination with excessive retroinclination of the maxillary incisors. The term 'subdivision' indicates a unilateral condition.
- **Angle's classification of malocclusion class III (prognathism)**: The dental relationship wherein the mandibular dental arch is anterior to the maxillary arch; the mesiobuccal groove of the mandibular first molar lies anterior to the cusp of the maxillary first molar.

malpositioned implant: A dental implant placed in a position creating restorative, biomechanical, and esthetic challenges for an optimal result.

malpractice litigation: Legal proceeding in a court or a judicial contest to determine a dereliction from professional duty or a failure to exercise an accepted degree of professional skill or learning by one rendering professional services that results in injury, loss, or damage.

mammalian collagenase: Proteolytic enzyme that degrades native collagen. After initial cleavage, less specific proteases will complete the degradation. Collagenases from mammalian cells are metalloenzymes and are collagen-type specific (collagenase 1, collagenase 2, and collagenase 3). They may be released in latent form (proenzyme) into tissues and require activation by other proteases before they will degrade fibrillar matrix. They are involved in the degradation of collagen during tissue repair or during embryonic and fetal development. Called also interstitial collagenase.

mandible: Lower jaw consisting of the horizontal body and two perpendicular rami that end in the coronoid and condylar processes. The condyle articulates in the temporal fossae with the temporomandibular joint.

mandibular: concerning the lower jaw (mandible).

mandibular anteroposterior ridge slope: Usually produced in an edentulous patient by resorption of alveolar bone of the lower jaw (mandible). This slope of the crest of the ridge from the third molar region to the greatest anterior aspect relative to the inferior border of the mandible as observed in profile is of particular significance for the design and fabrication of a lower prosthesis as it can affect movement of the denture in an anterior direction during normal occlusion and function.

mandibular block graft: Intraoral source of autogenous block graft taken from the patient and fixed to a defect site. The block may be harvested either from the ramus buccal shelf or the mandibular symphysis.

mandibular block graft: **M.b.g from the ramus**: Ramus block graft taken from the buccal shelf area. Advantages include less donor site morbidity; disadvantages include limited block dimension and a low cancellous component. **M.b.g. from the symphysis**: Block graft taken from the symphysis region apical to the incisors. Advantages include greater block dimensions, a greater cancellous portion, and easier surgical access. Disadvantages include the potential of sensory disturbances following surgery.

mandibular canal: (syn): Inferior alveolar canal. The canal within the mandible that houses the inferior alveolar nerve and vessels. Its posterior opening is the mandibular foramen. Its anterior opening is the mental foramen.

mandibular dislocation: A unilateral or bilateral displacement of the mandibular condyle(s) out of the glenoid fossa(e) that precludes normal occlusion of the teeth.

mandibular dysplasia: A condition in which the two halves of the mandible lack symmetry in size or form.

mandibular equilibration: Adjustments to the occlusal surfaces of the natural teeth or prosthetic teeth in the lower arch (mandible) that place the mandible in a condition whereby forces placed on it by the opposing dentition are neutralized and a state of equilibrium is created.

mandibular flexure: The medial deformation in the body of the mandible due to the contraction of the pterygoid muscles during opening and protrusion.

mandibular foramen: The opening into the mandibular canal on the medial surface of the ramus of the mandible giving passage to the inferior alveolar nerve, artery, and vein.

mandibular glide: The side-to-side, protrusive, and intermediate movements of the mandible occurring when the teeth or other occluding surfaces are in contact.

mandibular hinge position: An obsolete term referring to the mandibular position that allows for hinge axis-type movements upon opening and closing relative to the maxilla.

mandibular micrognathia: A mandible that is atypically small and characteristically associated with a diminished chin form.

mandibular movement: Movement of the mandible as it changes position relative to the maxilla or other structures.

mandibular nerve: A part of the trigeminal nerve referred to as the third division. The trigeminal nerve exits the skull via the foramen ovale. The mandibular nerve feeds motor innervation to the muscles of mastication, tensor veli palatini muscle, tensor tympani muscle, anterior belly of the digastric muscle, and mylohyoid muscle. Sensory innervation is provided to the mandibular gingiva and teeth, epithelium of the anterior two-thirds of the tongue, skin of the lower face, and floor of the mouth.

mandibular overdenture: See: Overdenture.

mandibular plane: In cephalometrics, a plane that passes through the inferior border of the mandible.

mandibular ramus: A quadrilateral process projecting upward and backward from the posterior part of the body of the mandible, and ending on the other end at the temporomandibular joint in a saddle-like indentation (sigmoid notch) between the coronoid and condylar processes. It may serve as a source for bone grafting.

mandibular ramus graft: See: Ramus graft.

mandibular relationship record: A record or registration of the correlation of the mandible to maxilla.

mandibular repositioning: Guidance of the mandible to cause closure in a predetermined, altered position.

mandibular retraction: Movement of the mandible posteriorly by surgical or orthopedic/orthodontic means.

mandibular rest position: See: Physiologic rest position.

mandibular staple: A dental implant that is placed transosteally from the inferior border of the mandible with threaded rods that pass through the anterior body of the mandible and emerge through the oral mucosa between the mental foramen.

mandibular staple implant: (syn): Transmandibular implant. Form of transosseous dental implant whereby a plate is fixed at the inferior border of the mandible. Retentive pins are placed partially into the inferior border with two continuous screws going transcortically and penetrating into the mouth in the canine areas and used as abutments.

mandibular symphysis: The line of fusion of the lateral halves of the body of the mandible, which splits inferiorly to form the mental protuberance. It may serve as a source for bone grafting.

mandibular symphysis graft: See: Chin graft.

mandibular torus: See: Torus.

mandibular translation: Anterior movement of the mandible on opening.

mandibular trismus: Tonic contraction of the muscles of mastication that leads to limited opening of the mandibular jaw.

mandrel: 1. Usually a tapered or cylindrical axle, spindle, or arbor placed in a hole to support it during machining. 2. A metal bar which serves as a core about which material may be cast, molded, compressed, forged, bent, or shaped. 3. The shaft and bearings on which a tool is mounted.

marginal: Pertaining to or connected with a margin or border.

marginal gingiva: The terminal edge (most coronal aspect) of the gingiva surrounding the teeth, forming the wall of the gingival sulcus.

marginal periimplant area: The mucosal periimplant tissues and crestal bone.

marginal ridge: The rounded enamel border at the junction of the occlusal and mesial/distal tooth surfaces.

marginal tissue recession: See: Gingival recession.

marking bur: Rotary cutting tool used to score the bone at the site of an osteotomy.

marrow: The soft material rich in fat, connective tissue fibers, and cells that fills the cavities of bones.

marrow cavity: Central portion of bone between the cortices where marrow is formed.

Maryland bridge: See: Resin-bonded splint.

masking: The process of applying an opaque covering to camouflage the metal component of a prosthesis.

massage: The act of manipulating soft tissue in the hope of increasing circulation and keratinization, and enhancing tissue tone. Data documenting the treatment efficacy of this procedure is not currently available.

mast cell: A tissue cell, often found around blood vessels, which produces histamine, heparin, leukotrienes, and platelet activation factor. Important in immediate hypersensitivity reactions.

master (definitive) cast: Final cast used for the fabrication of a prosthesis.

master impression: The negative likeness reproduction of the dental arch characterized by high dimensional accuracy and surface detail made for the construction of a master cast on which the prosthesis will be fabricated.

mastication: Act of grinding or crushing food (chewing) preparatory to deglutition and digestion. The masticatory cycle involves three-dimensional movements of the mandible observed in the frontal, horizontal, and sagittal planes. See: Mandibular movement.

masticatory mucosa: Keratinized and attached oral mucosa of the gingiva and hard palate.

masticatory system: The organs and structures functioning in mastication, including the jaws, teeth with their supporting structures, temporomandibular articulation, mandibular musculature, tongue, lips, cheeks, oral mucosa, and associated nervous system.

materia alba: Loosely adherent, white curds of matter composed of dead cells, food debris, bacteria, and other components of the dental plaque that lack the organized structure of a biofilm and are found on tooth or oral implant prosthesis surfaces.

matrix: 1. An intricate network of natural or synthetic fibers that aids in the reinforcement and development of tissues by supplying a scaffold on which cells may grow, migrate, and proliferate. 2. The female part of an attachment.

matrix component: The part of an attachment designed specifically as a receptacle for the matching or mate component (patrix), such that when engaged it provides mechanical retention. Attachment systems that use mechanical retention are available in various designs.

matrix metalloproteinase(s) (MMPs): A group of zinc- and calcium-dependent proteinases that degrade components of the extracellular matrix, such as collagen. These proteinases play a central role in many biological processes.

mattress suture: Suture made by a double penetration of the flap(s), not crossing over the incision line. Its purpose is to hold together the deeper tissues in order to reduce the tension of a flap upon approximation. It may be done in a horizontal or vertical direction.

maxilla: Paired bone making up a large part of the facial skeleton, including the body of the maxilla and the frontal, palatine, alveolar, and nasal processes.

maxillary antroplasty: See: Sinus graft.

maxillary antrum: See: Maxillary sinus.

maxillary artery: A branch of the external carotid artery that arises behind the neck of the mandible. It passes forward between the mandibular ramus and the sphenomandibular ligament, towards the pterygopalatine fossa. It supplies the deep structures of the face, and may be divided into mandibular, pterygoid, and pterygopalatine portions.

maxillary cross-arch splint: See: Cross-arch stabilization.

maxillary micrognathia: A condition in which the volume of maxillae bone is less than normal and usually visible as smaller bone structures found in the middle third of the face. This smaller middle third of the face occludes with a normal-sized mandible (lower third of the face).

maxillary overdenture: See: Overdenture.

maxillary protraction: A condition in which the upper jaw bone (maxillae) volume of bone and its supporting tissue structures are less than normal for the size of the mandibular bone and its supporting tissue structures.

maxillary pseudocyst: A nonsecreting cyst within the maxillary sinus that is usually present on the sinus floor and is caused by accumulation of fluid between the sinus membrane and the sinus floor. It is not a true cyst because it lacks an epithelial lining.

maxillary retention cyst: A secretion cyst, not usually seen radiographically, that is caused by blockage of the seromucinous gland duct. As secretions collect, they expand the duct, producing a cyst that is encompassed by respiratory or cuboidal epithelium. It may be located on the sinus floor, near the ostium, or within antral polyps. It may be caused by sinus infections, allergies, or odontogenic infections.

maxillary rhinosinusitis: A bacterial infection within the maxillary sinus with radiographic signs of an air–fluid level at its acute stage. Symptoms include purulent nasal discharge, nasal congestion, and facial pain. As the condition progresses from acute to chronic, anaerobic bacteria become the predominant pathogens. It is considered chronic if it does not resolve in 6 weeks and/or becomes recurrent.

maxillary sinus: (syn): Antrum of Highmore, maxillary antrum. Air cavity in the body of the maxilla that is lined by the Schneiderian membrane consisting of a pseudostratified ciliated columnar epithelium. It normally lies superior to the roots of the maxillary premolars and molars and generally extends anteroposteriorly from the canine or premolar region to the molar or tuberosity region. Anatomically, it is a pyramidal cavity, with thin bony walls corresponding to the orbital, alveolar (floor), facial, and infratemporal aspects of the maxilla. Its apex extends into the zygomatic process. Its base is medial, forming the lateral wall of the nasal cavity. It communicates with the nasal cavity through an opening in the middle meatus called the ostium. The floor is formed by the maxillary alveolar process and partly by the hard palate. The floor exhibits recesses and depressions in the premolar and molar regions. Each sinus usually has a volume of about 5 mL.

maxillary sinus aplasia: Developmental pathology characterized by the failure of the maxillary sinus to develop. It is diagnosed radiologically by an opaque maxillary antrum. It may be misdiagnosed as a sinusitis or a neoplasm.

maxillary sinus augmentation: See: Sinus graft.

maxillary sinus floor: (syn): Antral floor. Inferior wall of the maxillary sinus, in relation with the maxillary roots of the molars and premolars, or the edentulous ridge.

maxillary sinus floor elevation: Augmentation procedure for the placement of implants in the posterior maxilla where pneumatization of the maxillary sinus and/or vertical loss of alveolar bone have occurred. Autografts are often mixed with bone substitutes to increase the volume of the augmentation material or prevent graft resorption during remodeling. Two surgical techniques are well known and routinely used in daily practice: the lateral window technique, first described by Boyne and James in 1980, and the transalveolar osteotome technique, first described by Summers in 1994. See: Sinus graft.

maxillary sinus floor graft: Graft used to augment the vertical height in the maxillary sinus for implant placement. A particulate mixture of autogenous bone and a bone substitute is often used. See: Maxillary sinus floor elevation.

maxillary sinus hypoplasia (MSH): Developmental pathology characterized by the underdevelopment of the maxillary sinus. It is diagnosed radiologically by a centripetal opacification of the maxillary antrum. It may be congenital or a direct result from trauma, infection, surgical intervention, or irradiation of the maxilla during the development of the maxillary bone.

maxillary sinus membrane: Thin mucous membrane lining the sinus cavity and characterized by respiratory epithelium. Formerly called Schneiderian membrane. **Perforation of the m.s.m.**: Iatrogenic perforation or tear of the maxillary sinus membrane during sinus floor elevation; the most common complication of this procedure. Small perforations may not need treatment if the elevation can continue uneventfully; larger perforations may be covered by collagen membranes and/or by a fibrin sealant. Incidence of maxillary sinus membrane perforation does not appear to affect the outcome of implant success. See: Valsalva maneuver.

maxillary sinus pneumatization: The maxillary sinuses are usually fluid-filled at birth. Pneumatization, or filling of the sinus cavity with air, takes place during the later phase of growth as the permanent teeth develop and erupt. Pneumatization can be so extensive as to expose tooth roots with only a thin layer of soft tissue covering them. Later with tooth loss, further pneumatization can take place, leading to a reduced vertical height in the alveolar bone. This often requires sinus floor elevation procedures to allow the placement of dental implants.

maxillary sinus septum: (syn): Underwood cleft. Anatomic spine-like bony structure or web formation present in some maxillary sinuses. It may divide the inferior portion of the sinus into sections or loculi.

maxillary sinusitis: Infection in the maxillary sinus, either acute or chronic in nature, which can be caused by dental pathology, such as root tips, periapical lesions, over-filled endodontic material, and oroantral fistulae or openings, among others. Acute sinusitis is an absolute contraindication for surgery, whereas chronic sinusitis is a relative contraindication where implant and/or sinus floor elevation procedures may still be performed. See: Sinusitis (maxillary).

maxillary torus: See: Torus.

maxillary tuberosity: The most distal aspect of the maxillary ridge, bilaterally. It may be used as a source of autogenous bone or for support of a prosthesis.

maxillectomy: Removal of part or all of the maxillary (upper) jaw bone structure. Also known as a maxillary resection.

maxillofacial: Concerning or relating to the teeth, jaws, face, head, and neck.

maxillofacial prosthesis: Restoration replacing oral, stomatognathic, or craniofacial structures with a fixed or removable prosthesis. Support and/or retention is provided by natural teeth and supporting tissues, endosseous implants, or adhesives.

maxillofacial prosthetic adhesive: A material used to hold or adhere an external facial appliance or device to the skin and its accompanying structures adjacent to the margins of an anatomic defect for the purpose of preventing its dislodgement during normal function.

maxillofacial prosthetics: The subspecialty of dental prosthodontics concerned with the prosthetic replacement or reconstruction of lost stomatognathic and/or craniofacial structures with fixed or removable prostheses.

maxillomandibular dysplasia: Disharmony between the right and left portions of the mandible and the maxillary jaw.

maxillomandibular fixation: A temporary fixed connection of the maxillary and mandibular teeth, typically with wire, for use in treating a mandible fracture.

maxillomandibular relationship: Any spatial relationship of the mandible to the maxilla.

maxillomandibular relationship record: A registration of any position of the mandible with respect to the maxillae. These records often capture the vertical, horizontal, and oblique planes of relationship.

maximal intercuspal contacts: Position that results in maximal tooth contact between the mandibular and maxillary dental arches when the jaws are in a closed position.

maximal intercuspal position: Sometimes referred to as centric occlusion, this is the best fit of the upper teeth to the lower teeth regardless of the position of the mandibular condyle. Called also maximal intercuspation. Compare: Centric occlusion.

maximum bite force: The greatest load a patient can generate by intentionally biting down on an indicating device. This measurement may influence prosthetic design, especially if the patient can develop extreme loads.

MBC (abbrev.): Minimum bactericidal concentration.

McGill Consensus Statement: Conclusion from a 2002 meeting of experts held at McGill University in Montreal, Canada, discussing implant overdenture therapy. Consensus on the use of overdentures was that a two-implant supported overdenture was the first choice for restoration of the edentulous mandible and not a conventional denture.

MDAF (abbrev.): Macrophage-derived angiogenic factor.

mean: Arithmetic average of a group of values. The mean is a common descriptive statistic best used to summarize the central tendency of normally distributed data. In this use, it is usually accompanied by the standard deviation.

mechanical failure: Failure of a component caused by mechanical forces. It may be catastrophic in nature or the result of wear, fatigue, or plastic deformation.

mechanicoreceptor: Nerve ending (receptor) that is excited by mechanical pressure. The mechanical pressure may result from muscle contraction, external pressure (including sound), or touch.

median: Value that separates the highest 50% of the scores from the lowest 50%.

Useful in describing the central tendency of abnormally distributed data, because it is less influenced by the outlier data (i.e., extreme values) that skew the distribution and can have a disproportionate effect on the mean.

median jaw relation: Any jaw relation when the mandible is in the median sagittal plane.

median line: A hypothetical line that divides the body into left and right halves.

median mandibular point: An obsolete term referring to a point in the median sagittal plane that is in the center (measuring anterior to posterior) of the mandibular ridge.

median plane: A hypothetical plane passing from anterior to posterior that divides a body into right and left halves.

medical device: Instrument, apparatus, machine, or other related article, including any components (part or accessory), intended for use in the diagnosis of disease or other conditions, for the cure, mitigation, treatment, or prevention of disease in humans.

medical-grade calcium sulfate (MGCS): Bioengineered form of calcium sulfate, a bone substitute used for intraoral grafting procedures. The shape and size of the hemihydrate crystals are modified to ensure a controlled and slower resorption profile.

medical image registration: Data of the same patient taken at different points in time, such as change detection or tumor monitoring.

mediotrusion: Movement of the nonworking condyle toward the midfacial sagittal plane.

medullary: Pertaining to the bone marrow.

medullary bone: 1. Any substance resembling marrow in structure. 2. Bone formed as an outgrowth from the endosteal lining of the shaft of long bones in birds. The main purpose is accumulation of calcium to be used in the formation of an egg shell. When the shell is being calcified, the medullary bone is destroyed and the calcium is released.

megapascal (MPa): A unit of pressure or stress equal to 1 million pascals. It is equivalent to 145 psi(lb/in^2) or 9.87 kg/cm^2.

melanin: The dark, amorphous pigment of the skin, hair, various tumors, the choroid coat of the eye, and substantia nigra of the brain.

melanoma: A neoplasm made up of melanin-pigmented cells. When used alone, the term refers to malignant melanoma.

melanoplakia: Patches of pigmentation on the oral mucosa.

membrane: 1. A thin, soft, pliable sheet or layer, especially of plant or animal origin. 2. A thin layer of tissue that lines a cavity, envelops a vessel or part, or separates a space or organ. See: Barrier membrane, Collagen membrane, Expanded polytetrafluoroethylene (e-PTFE) membrane, Nonresorbable membrane, Resorbable membrane.

membrane exposure: See: Exposure.

membrane tack: A metal device used to stabilize a membrane by fixing it to the alveolar bone, providing for stability.

membranous bone: See: Intramembranous ossification.

meniscal displacement: See: Temporomandibular disorders, Internal derangement.

meniscectomy: Surgical removal of the intraarticular disk. See: Discectomy.

meniscus: The fibrocartilaginous articular disk of the temporomandibular joint.

mental foramen: The anterior opening of the mandibular canal on the lateral aspect of the body of the mandible in the region of the first premolar, giving passage to the mental neurovascular bundle.

mental nerve: Terminal branch of the inferior alveolar nerve, arising in the mandibular canal and passing through the mental foramen providing sensation to the chin and lower lip.

merging: The process of combining all individual elements (meshes, copings, connectors, etc.) into one or more meshes suitable for additive or subtractive manufacturing.

MES (abbrev.): Minimum effective strain.

mesenchymal cell: Type of pluripotential cell that constitutes the mesenchyme.

mesenchymal progenitor cell (MPC): See: Mesenchymal stem cell (MSC).

mesenchymal stem cell (MSC): Contributes to the regeneration of mesenchymal tissues (e.g., bone, cartilage, muscle, ligament, tendon, adipose, and stroma) and is essential in providing support for the growth and differentiation of primitive hemopoietic cells within the bone marrow microenvironment for the repair of bony defects. The most accessible source of mesenchymal stem cells is bone marrow, although they have been isolated from a number of tissues, including the liver, fetal blood, cord blood, and amniotic fluid.

mesenchyme: Mass of tissue that develops primarily from the mesoderm (i.e., the middle layer of the trilaminar germ disk) of an embryo. Viscous in consistency, mesenchyme contains collagen bundles and fibroblasts and later differentiates into blood vessels, blood-related organs, and connective tissues.

mesh: A general term used to describe the surface referencing of a scanned point cloud resulting in a 3D object typically composed of triangular faces. A mesh object has no true curvature. The appearance of curvature is achieved by increasing the number of faces (level of detail).

mesial: Near or toward the centerline of the dental arch; toward the median sagittal plane of the face, following the curvature of the dental arch.

mesioversion: The location of a tooth nearer than normal to the median line of the face along the dental arch.

mesostructure: The part of a reconstruction that couples the dental implant complex (infrastructure) to the superstructure.

metaanalysis: A quantitative method of combining the results of independent studies meeting specified protocol criteria (usually drawn from the published literature) and synthesizing summaries and conclusions that may be used to evaluate therapeutic effectiveness and plan new studies.

metabolic syndrome: A combination of medical disorders that, when occurring together, increase the risk of developing cardiovascular disease and diabetes.

metal artifact: Metal objects in the scan field can lead to severe streaking artifacts. This presents a loss of detail, transferring as a loss of information in the reconstruction of a 3D model.

metal ceramic restoration: A tooth- and/or implant-retained fixed dental prosthesis that uses a metal substructure upon which a ceramic veneer is fused.

metal collar: A narrow band of highly polished metal immediately adjacent to the facial/buccal margin on a metal-ceramic restoration.

metal encapsulator: See: Metal housing.

metal housing: (syn): Metal encapsulator. 1. Part of an attachment mechanism incorporated in a removable prosthesis. The interchangeable retentive component is inserted in the metal housing and replaced when necessary. 2. Metallic enclosure in a removable prosthesis into which replaceable plastic retentive elements are placed to stabilize the restoration.

metal tap: See: Tap.

metamer: One of two objects whose colors appear to match when viewed under certain conditions but under alternative viewing conditions may appear different.

metameric pair: Two objects matching in apparent color under some lighting conditions but not others.

metamerism: Pairs of objects that match in a given hue of light but not in others.

metaphysis: Growing part of a long bone, consisting of the epiphysial cartilage plate united with the diaphysis by columns of trabecular bone.

metaplasia: A change from one adult cell type to another form which is not normal to that tissue.

metastasis: Transfer of disease from one body part or organ to another not directly connected to it. Classically, the transfer of cells, as in malignant tumors, or the transfer of pathogenic microorganisms.

methyl methacrylate resin: A transparent, thermoplastic acrylic resin used in dentistry by mixing liquid methyl methacrylate monomer with the polymer powder. The resultant mixture forms a pliable plastic termed dough, which is packed into a mold prior to initiation of polymerization.

methylprednisolone: An intramuscular, intravenous, and oral glucocorticoid with an intermediate half-life. See: Glucocorticoid.

metronidazole: Antiprotozoal and antibacterial drug ($C_6H_9N_3O_3$) with a spectrum confined to obligate anaerobes, some microaerophilic organisms, and some anaerobic protozoa that act to damage or inhibit DNA synthesis; may induce a disulfiram-like reaction. This antibiotic is commonly used to treat periodontitis and periimplantitis infections caused by gram-negative anaerobic pathogens.

MGCS (abbrev.): Medical-grade calcium sulfate.

MIC (abbrev.): Minimum inhibitory concentration.

microaerophilic: Refers to bacteria that grow under conditions of reduced oxygen concentration. Used to describe conditions in which the oxygen concentration is lower than atmospheric levels.

microbial resistance: The ability of microorganisms to resist the effects of antibiotics; usually due to chromosomal mutation or the transfer of resistant genes from already resistant organisms; mechanisms include antibiotic enzymatic destruction.

microbiota: The microscopic living organisms of a region.

microcrack: In porcelain, one of the numerous surface flaws that contribute to stress concentrations and results in strengths below those theoretically possible.

microgap: Microscopic space between two components, specifically between an implant and an abutment. It is usually considered to be a source of chronic irritation or contamination creating an inflammatory response. See: Implant-abutment junction (IAJ).

microglossia: Having an abnormally small tongue.

micrognathia: Abnormal smallness of the jaw, particularly the mandible, that can be congenital or acquired. See: Mandibular micrognathia, Maxillary micrognathia.

micro-interlock: Fixation by mechanical interlocking of bone to micro-irregularities at textured dental implant surfaces, including those created by grit blasting, coating, or ion bombardment, which have dimensions in the range of less than 10 microns.

microleakage: Microscopic movement of fluids or contaminants across a barrier or between chambers that cannot be observed without magnification.

micromotion: Relative motion on a microscopic scale. It generally describes the relative motion between an implant and its osteotomy site during the initial healing period or relative motion between mechanical components of the implant stack.

microorganism: A microscopic organism; those of medical interest include bacteria, viruses, fungi, yeasts, and protozoa.

microradiography: Radiographic recording of the details within the structure of thin specimens at a high magnification. Also known as X-ray micrography. "The technique of passing X-rays through a thin metal section in contact with a fine-grained photograph to obtain a radiograph which can be viewed at 50× to l00× to observe constituents and voids."

microstomia: Having an abnormally small oral orifice.

microtextured surface treatment: Treatment providing a microscopically roughened surface.

midcrestal incision: An incision made in the middle of the crest of an edentulous ridge.

middle superior alveolar nerve: Branch of the infraorbital nerve arising at the infraorbital groove. It runs downwards and forward in the lateral wall of the sinus to supply the maxillary premolars.

midfacial fracture: Fracture of the middle third of the face, including zygomatic, maxillary, nasal, and other associated bones of the midface.

midpalatal implant: See: Palatal implant.

migration, pathologic dental: The movement of a tooth out of its former position when the etiology or etiologies responsible for such movement are associated with a disease process.

mill: 1. To subject to an operation or process in a mill; to grind. 2. To shape or dress by means of instruments.

milling: The machining process of using rotary cutters (burs) to remove material from a workpiece by advancing it (or feeding) at an angle with the axis of the tool. It covers a wide variety of different operations and machines, on scales from small individual parts to large, heavy-duty milling operations. It is one of the most commonly used processes to fabricate dental restorations with high precision. Mills have multiple axes (e.g., 3-axis, 4-axis, 5-axis) that determine their ability to create final detail and complex geometries with undercuts, concave contours, and holes.

millipore filter: One of the first barrier membranes used as proof of principle for the regeneration of membrane-protected defects. Millipore filters have been used in initial studies for guided tissue regeneration for periodontal defects.

mineral corticoid: A group of C2l steroid hormones (aldosterone, etc.) that regulates electrolyte and water balance in the kidney; secreted from the adrenal cortex; a corticosteroid.

mineralization front: Transitional area of bone mineralization; a seam that separates the osteoid zone from the mineralized part of the bone. See: Tetracycline bone labeling.

mineralize: The precipitation of calcium and other salts into an organic matrix to form a hard deposit, such as dental calculus.

mini-implant: A narrow diameter root-form dental implant which may be in one piece or two pieces. It is used for the support and/or retention of a provisional or definitive prosthesis. See: Transitional implant.

minimal sedation: A minimally depressed level of consciousness, produced by a pharmacological method, that retains the patient's ability to independently and continuously maintain an airway and respond normally to tactile stimulation and verbal command.

minimum bactericidal concentration (MBC): The minimum concentration of an antimicrobial agent required to kill a pure population of bacteria *in vitro*.

minimum effective strain (MES): Derived from Frost's mechanostat theory for bone adaptation, the MES is essentially a minimum value of strain that must be exceeded to provoke an adaptive response in bone; stimulus for bone remodeling. Called also minimum effective strain for remodeling (MESr).

minimum inhibitory concentration (MIC): The minimum concentration of an antimicrobial agent required to inhibit the growth and/or reproduction of a pure population of bacteria *in vitro*.

miniscrew: Small titanium threaded implant used for temporary orthodontic anchorage via mechanical monocortical bone retention. See: Orthodontic implant, Temporary anchorage device.

minor aphtha: The most common form of recurrent aphthae. Also known as a canker sore. Shallow, painful, nonscarring ulcers surrounded by an erythematous halo that are usually found on movable, nonkeratinized oral mucosa.

minor connector: The connecting link between the major connector or base of a partial removable dental prosthesis and the other units of the prosthesis, such as the clasp assembly, indirect retainers, occlusal rests, or cingulum rests.

minor (thread) diameter: The smallest diameter of a screw thread.

mirroring: The process of symmetrically copying and transferring one dental design feature (e.g., crown) to the contralateral side. For example, mirroring a maxillary central incisor so that its pair is an exact, mirrored duplicate.

misfit: Lack of precise adaptation of one component to another, particularly the lack of ideal passive fit of a multiple-unit prosthesis to two or more implants. Misfit is considered to be detrimental in that it may lead to increased occurrence of component loosening or fracture and may contribute to attachment loss adjacent to an implant.

mitogen: A substance that causes DNA synthesis, blast transformation, and mitosis in lymphocytes.

MMP (abbrev.): Matrix metalloproteinase.

mobility (implant): See: Implant mobility.

mobility, tooth: The movement of a tooth in its socket resulting from an applied force.

mode: Value with the largest number of observations, namely the most frequent value or values.

model: A facsimile representation of something; an analog or emulation used for display purposes. See: Cast.

model scanning: The process of acquiring the 3D image of a dental model for translation into a digital file format, such as STL. The digital file can be stored for future reference or used in a CAD software program for the design and fabrication of a dental prosthesis.

modeling (bone): Independent sites of formation and resorption that result in a change of the shape or size of bone. It occurs during growth and during healing.

moderate sedation: A drug-induced depression of consciousness during which patients respond purposefully to verbal commands, either alone or accompanied by light tactile stimulation. No interventions are required to maintain a patent airway and spontaneous ventilation.

modified occlusal anatomy: Application of nonanatomic occlusal surfaces of artificial teeth in an attempt to control or modify the direction and/or magnitude of forces generated during function or parafunction.

modified ridge lap: A ridge lap surface of a pontic that is reduced, shaped, and adapted to only the facial or buccal aspect of the residual alveolar ridge.

modifier: Any substance that changes the color or properties of a given substance.

modulus of elasticity: (syn): Elastic modulus. Ratio of stress over strain, when the deformation is elastic. It is a measure of stiffness or flexibility of a material. A stiff material has a high modulus of elasticity and a flexible material has a low modulus of elasticity. Also called Young's modulus.

mold: A matrix used to fabricate or duplicate a prosthetic device.

mold chart: Representation of the different dimensions of a denture tooth's (or teeth's) shape and size.

mold guide: A selection of artificial teeth demonstrating the dimensions and shape of commercially available artificial teeth.

moment: The magnitude of force applied to a rotational system at a distance from the axis of rotation.

moment of inertia: Resistance to rotation of a body; used to explain the relative change if bending moments are based upon the cross-sectional radius of a structure.

monocyte: Mononuclear phagocytic leukocyte, 13–25 µm in diameter, with an ovoid or kidney-shaped nucleus. Precursor to a macrophage, it is formed in the bone marrow from a promonocyte and is transported to tissues such as the lung and liver, where it develops into a macrophage.

monomer: The chemical initiator of a polymerization process.

monoplane: The occlusal surface of teeth where all cusp heights are within the same plane.

monoplane articulation: The arrangement of teeth in a single plane of occlusion.

monoplane occlusion: The arrangement of teeth where tooth contact in all excursions occurs in a single plane of occlusion.

mora device: Acronym for mandibular orthopedic repositioning appliance; an appliance designed to optimize jaw relationships and neuromuscular balance.

morbidity: The condition of being in a diseased state.

Morgan and James model of prosthesis loading: Model of implant prosthesis loading with rigid implant-to-prosthesis connections.

morphogen: Morphogenetic proteins guiding cellular morphodifferentiation.

morphological tooth adaptation: A digital technique to improve the performance and/or esthetics of a tooth among its neighbors. A simple version of adaptation is scaling, where the mere size of the tooth is altered (smaller or larger) to achieve better occlusion or improved arch length, or to close interproximal diastemata.

Morse taper connection: An internal connection interface consisting of a converging circular surface, which forms a mechanical locking friction-fit. Also known as a cold weld and morse taper connection: taper of 3°

(6° total convergence) or a reduction of 5/8 inch per linear foot of cylinder length. It describes one method of internal abutment connection, although the Straumann implant- abutment connection to which the term is applied is not technically a morse taper but rather an 8° (16° total convergence) cylindrical taper.

motion artifact: A feature that appears in an image but which was not present in the original, caused by movement of the patient, usually appearing as shading or streaking in a reconstructed image.

motion-sensing device (implant): Tool evaluating the relative mobility of a dental implant in relation to its surrounding bone.

motion tracking: Tracing the spatial position of moving objects relative to a reference coordinate system. See: Handpiece motion tracker, Patient motion tracker.

mount: See: Implant mount.

mounting: When maxillary and mandibular dental casts are attached to an instrument (articulator) that maintains the occluded relationship of dental casts to each other, yet the casts may be separated as the instrument facilitates the opening and return of the casts to the intended occluded relationship.

mounting plate: Removable flat, round components made of metal or resin that facilitate the attachment of dental casts to the upper and lower members of an articulator.

mouth breathing: The process of breathing primarily through the oral cavity rather than the nasal passages. May be associated with gingival enlargement and inflammation.

mouth guard: A removable dental appliance made of resilient or hard materials used to protect the teeth and surrounding tissues from injury. See: Occlusal guard.

mouth rehabilitation: Restoration of the form and function of the masticatory apparatus to as near normal as possible.

mouth stick: A prosthesis that is held in position by the teeth and used by a disabled person to perform certain functions (e.g., as a rod for the purposes of pointing).

MPa (abbrev.): Megapascal.

MPC (abbrev.): Mesenchymal progenitor cell.

MPD (abbrev.): Myofascial pain dysfunction syndrome.

MRI (abbrev.): Magnetic resonance imaging.

MSC (abbrev.): Mesenchymal stem cell.

MSH (abbrev.): Maxillary sinus hypoplasia.

mucobuccal fold: The cul-de-sac formed where the mucous membrane is reflected from the mandible or maxilla to form the cheek.

mucobuccal fold incision: (syn): Vestibular incision. An incision made in the mucobuccal fold. See: Crestal incision, Midcrestal incision

mucocele: "Epithelium-lined sac containing mucus. Mucous cysts in the sinus may appear as spherical, radiopaque areas."

mucocutaneous disorders: Mucosal changes characterized by epithelial desquamation, erythema, ulceration, and/or the presence of vesiculobullous lesions of the gingiva or other oral tissues; often triggered by autoimmunity, sensitivity reactions, or medications.

mucogingival: The portion of the oral mucosa that covers the alveolar process including the gingiva (keratinized tissue) and the adjacent alveolar mucosa.

mucogingival deformity: A departure from the normal dimension and morphology of and/or interrelationship between gingiva and alveolar mucosa; the abnormality may be associated with a deformity of the underlying alveolar bone.

mucogingival junction: The junction or area of union of the gingiva and the alveolar mucosa.

mucogingival surgery: Group of surgical procedures used in periodontics to augment the band of keratinized mucosa around teeth, to cover recession-type defects, or to augment other types of soft tissue defects. Techniques include the use of free gingiva grafts, subepithelial connective tissue grafts, pedicle flaps, and use of barrier membranes, among others. Similar techniques have been adopted for implant patients.

mucogingival therapy: Nonsurgical and surgical treatment procedures for correction of defects in morphology, position, and/or amount of soft tissue and underlying bone support at teeth and implants.

mucolabial fold: The line, bend, crease, or area of change as the oral mucous membrane passes from its role as the mucosal tissue of the mandible or maxilla to form the lip.

mucoperiosteal flap: Full-thickness mucosal flap, generally including gingiva, alveolar mucosa, and periosteum.

mucoperiosteum: Layer of periosteum, connective tissue and epithelium that covers bone of the maxilla and mandible.

mucopolysaccharide: See: Glycosaminoglycan.

mucosa: Mucous membrane that forms the soft tissue barrier to the environment, particularly in the oral cavity. It is loosely attached to the periosteum, is movable, and consists of epithelium, basement membrane, and lamina propria. **Alveolar mucosa**: Mucosa covering the basal part of the alveolar process and continuing without demarcation into the vestibular fornix and the floor of the mouth. **Masticatory mucosa**: The gingiva and the mucosal covering of the hard palate. **Oral mucosa**: The tissue lining the oral cavity.

mucosal cell: Cells that secrete mucus, such as those found in the oral cavity.

mucosal implant: See: Mucosal insert.

mucosal insert: (syn): Button implant, epithelial implant, intramucosal insert, mucosal implant. Mushroom-shaped device fastened to the tissue surface of a removable denture that fits within a prepared gingival receptor site. The use of multiple mucosal inserts enhances a denture's retention and stability.

mucosal periimplant tissue: Mucosal tissue around dental implants, which forms a tightly adherent band consisting of a dense collagenous lamina propria covered by stratified squamous keratinizing epithelium. The sulcular and junctional epithelium are similar to a natural tooth. The difference is noticed in the connective tissue which is not attached to the implant like in the tooth.

mucositis: A painful inflammatory response of the oral mucous membrane. May be caused by local irritants, including prostheses, or may be systemically induced.

mucostatic: 1. Refers to oral mucosa at a state of rest, without displacement. 2. Prohibiting the flow of mucus.

mucous membrane: See: Mucosa.

mucus: The clear, viscous secretion of the mucous membranes, composed of secretions of the glands, along with various inorganic salts, desquamated cells, and leukocytes.

multicenter study: A clinical trial conducted according to a single protocol but at more than one research center, and therefore carried out by a group of investigators.

multidisciplinary treatment: Team approach to provision of patient treatment, encompassing the services of clinicians from various disciplines and adjunct laboratory personnel.

multiple regression: "To predict the value of a single response variable from a combination of explanatory variables."

Munsell chroma: One of the three main components of the Munsell color order system. It indicates the purity or saturation of any particular color, from vivid to washed out.

Munsell color order system: A color classification system that uses numeric nomenclature to characterize any color using hue, value, and chroma. This is the basis for most shade matching systems in dentistry.

Munsell hue: One of the three main components of the Munsell color order system. It is divided into five principal color families: red, yellow, green, blue, and purple.

Munsell value: One of the three main components of the Munsell color order system. It indicates the relative lightness or darkness of a particular color, from white to neutral gray to black.

muscle contracture: A pathologic condition in which there is permanent shortening and loss of strength and flexibility in a muscle.

muscle fiber: See: Fiber.

muscle hyperalgesia: Increased awareness of pain in a muscle out of proportion to physical findings.

muscle hypertonicity: Hyperactivity of a muscle related to increased involuntary contractions.

muscle relaxant: A medication used for treating muscle tension or spasm.

muscle spasm: An abrupt involuntary contraction of a muscle that is associated with pain and can occur even when the muscle is at rest.

muscle spasticity: A clinical situation when opposing muscles have increased contractibility and tension, impeding movements of the agonistic muscles.

muscle splinting: Slang for a muscle contraction initiated to avoid the pain associated by passively stretching the muscle.

muscular splinting: Muscular contraction at a nonrest state that impairs function. It is associated with involuntary movements.

musculoskeletal pain: Deep, somatic pain that originates in skeletal muscles, facial sheaths, and tendons (myogenous pain), bone and periosteum (osseous pain), joint, joint capsules, and ligaments (arthralgic pain), and in soft connective tissues.

mush bite: An obsolete slang term for a record of the mandible in relation to the maxilla without using baseplates but instead by using a nonrigid material alone (i.e., wax).

mutually protected articulation: An occlusal scheme where all the posterior teeth disocclude during mandibular movements while the occlusion is supported by the anterior teeth. At maximum intercuspation, the posterior teeth reduce the occlusal forces applied on the anterior teeth so the forces applied on the anterior teeth are not excessive.

mutually protected occlusion: See: Mutually protected articulation.

myalgia: Pain in a muscle or muscles.

Mycoplasma spp.: Small cell intermediate in physiologic properties between bacteria and viruses, lacking a cell wall but able to grow and multiply. Able to agglutinate red blood cells and sometimes found in association with human periodontal disease.

mycotic: A clinical situation where fungus has been attributed to an established infection or lesion.

mylohyoid concavity: A fossa found in the molar region of the mandible that is inferior to the mylohyoid line.

mylohyoid groove or canal: Groove (indentation) on the medial surface of the ramus of the mandible beginning at the lingula; it houses the mylohyoid artery and nerve.

mylohyoid region: An obsolete term that refers to the area on the lingual surface of the mandible that contains the mylohyoid ridge and the attachment of the mylohyoid muscle. It is part of the alveololingual sulcus.

mylohyoid ridge: Horizontal bony extension on the lingual aspect of the mandibular premolars and molars that is an attachment for the mylohyoid muscle which forms the floor of the mouth.

myofascial pain dysfunction syndrome (MPD): A collection of medical and dental conditions affecting the temporomandibular joint and/or muscles of mastication and other contiguous tissue components. See: Temporomandibular disorders (TMD).

myofibroblast: An isolated cell in connective tissue with projections containing gap junctions to allow for intercellular communication. It shares characteristics of fibroblasts (lacks a surrounding basal lamina) and smooth muscle cells.

myofunctional: Relating to the function of muscles. In dentistry, relates to the role of muscle function in the cause or correction of orthodontic problems or the treatment of muscle-related problems.

myogenous pain: Deep somatic musculoskeletal pain initiating in skeletal muscles, fascial sheaths, or tendons. Myogenous pain associated with temporomandibular disorders has usually been connected to hyperactivity or abnormal contraction of masticatory muscles.

myomonitor: A digital electronic pulse generator expressly designed to provide a bilateral transcutaneous electrical neural stimulus for the stomatognathic system. Developed as a means of applying electrical stimulation for the purpose of providing muscle relaxation as a prerequisite to obtaining an occlusal position and records.

myositis: Swelling or inflammation of muscle tissue induced by the immune system, injury, or infection.

myostatic contracture: Shortening of a muscle resulting from a lack of nerve stimulation and movement.

myotonia: A neuromuscular condition that demonstrates increased muscle irritability and contractility accompanied by an impaired ability of the muscle to relax.

N

N (abbrev.): Newton.

nasal grimace: An oronasal compensatory movement of the tissues of the nares that occurs in response to palatopharyngeal insufficiency.

nasal prosthesis: A prosthesis inserted into the nose to restore those parts of the nose lost due to trauma, amputation, cancer, or burns. See: Nasal reconstruction.

nasal reconstruction: Prosthetic restoration of defects of the nose resulting from surgery, trauma, or congenital etiology.

nasal septal prosthesis: A prosthesis inserted into the nose to occlude or plug a perforation or hole within the nasal septum, also known as a nasal septal button or plug.

nasal spine: The forward prolongation of the left and right maxillae forming a sharp bony extension at the inferior margin of the anterior aperture of the nares.

nasal stent: An intranasal prosthesis used to support the form of the nose; commonly used to increase airflow through the nasal passages and to reduce snoring.

nasal turbulence: Air that is forced through a small opening in the nasal passages causing movement of secretions above the opening resulting in a rustling-like noise.

nasality: The quality of speech sounds when the sounds are produced as a result of the nasal cavity being used as a resonator.

nasion: On the human skull, the point at which the midsagittal plane bisects the intersection between the nasal bones and the frontal bone. It is used as a landmark on cephalometric radiographs.

Nasmyth's membrane: Primary enamel cuticle. A delicate membrane that briefly covers the crowns of newly erupted teeth. Consists of ameloblasts of the reduced enamel epithelium attached to the enamel by a basal lamina.

nasopalatine duct cyst: A developmental, nonodontogenic cyst originating from embryonic remnants within the nasopalatine duct. Also known as an incisive canal cyst.

nasopalatine nerve: A branch from the pterygopalatine ganglion that passes through the sphenopalatine foramen, across the roof of the nasal cavity to the nasal septum, and obliquely downward to and through the incisive canal. It innervates the anterior part of the hard palate and the mucosa of the nasal septum.

nasopharynx: The portion of the pharynx that is superior to the soft palate.

natural color system: Six elementary colors are the basis for the natural color system: white, black, yellow, red, blue, and green. The system uses percentages of individual component colors to determine nuances.

natural tooth intrusion: Apical movement of a tooth produced by an external force. Phenomenon reported in literature as being a complication of connecting a natural tooth to a dental implant with a fixed prosthesis.

navigation: See: Navigation surgery.

navigation surgery: (syn): Computer-aided navigation, implant-guided surgery, navigation, surgical navigation. A surgical modality in which the intraoperative localization of the surgical instrument is fed back visually

Glossary of Dental Implantology, First Edition. Khalid Almas, Fawad Javed and Steph Smith.
© 2018 John Wiley & Sons, Inc. Published 2018 by John Wiley & Sons, Inc.

onscreen in reference to the preoperative diagnostic imaging of the patient by employing patient registration algorithms and motion tracking technology. In implant dentistry, the implant drilling and placement are guided by imaging displaying real-time reconstruction of the intraoperative localization of the dental drill relative to the preacquired CT imaging of the anatomic structures. The dental drill is piloted according to a preplanned drilling path or implant position by means of onscreen direction indicators.

Ncm (abbrev.): Newton centimeters.

Nd:YAG laser (abbrev.): Neodymium-doped yttrium aluminum garnet laser. A solid-state laser containing a Nd:YAG crystal which emits at a wavelength of 1064 nanometers. It is mainly used in soft tissue surgery.

necrosis: The death of cells by unprogrammed methods as opposed to apoptosis, which is a programmed death. Pyknosis (shrunken and hyperkeratosis or darkened basophilic nuclear staining), karyolysis (swollen and pale basophilic nuclear staining), and karyorrhexis (nuclear rupture or fragmentation) are typical events in necrosis of cells. The release of intracellular contents leads to an inflammatory response.

necrotizing ulcerative periodontitis: See: Periodontitis.

negative predictive value: The proportion of negative responses to a diagnostic test for a disease that are accurate indicators of the true absence of the malady in a population. Expressed arithmetically as a proportion which is calculated as the number of true-negative responses divided by the sum of true-negative responses plus false-negative responses, i.e., negative predictive value = TN/(TN + FN).

Neisseria spp.: Gram-negative, nonmotile, microaerophilic cocci found as part of the indigenous oral flora.

neoplasm: A new, abnormal, uncontrolled growth arising from a given tissue. If malignant, can have the capacity to metastasize locally or systemically. When malignant, the disease entity is generically known as cancer.

nerve fiber: See: Fiber.

nerve lateralization: Surgical procedure that repositions the inferior alveolar nerve for the purpose of implant placement without bone augmentation. The buccal cortex surrounding the mandibular canal is removed to allow the repositioning of the nerve. This procedure raises the risk of neuropathies, such as para-, dys-, and/or anesthesia of the inferior alveolar nerve. Because of the high risk of complications, widespread use has not been achieved.

nerve repositioning: (syn): Nerve lateralization, nerve transpositioning. Surgical procedure whereby the course of the inferior alveolar nerve is redirected to allow the placement of longer implants in a mandible with extensive resorption of the posterior ridge.

nerve transpositioning: See: Nerve repositioning.

neuralgia: Neurogenous pain felt along the peripheral distribution of a nerve trunk.

neurapraxia: Mild nerve injury caused by compression or retraction. There is no violation of the nerve trunk and no axonal degeneration. Spontaneous recovery of the motor and/or sensory functions most often occurs within 1–4 weeks from the time of injury.

neuritis: Inflammation of a nerve(s).

neurogenous pain: Pain caused by abnormalities in the structure of nerves that innervate affected areas. Pain can occur with nociception. The pain is frequently described as burning or sharp. A sensation may occur along the pathway of the nerve. While the patient may locate the pain, the apparent area may not be the source, and the severity of the pain is usually more intense than expected given the degree of stimulation.

neuromuscular dysfunction: A collective term for muscle disorders of the masticatory system with two observable major symptoms: pain and dysfunction. Common observations include muscle fatigue, muscle tightness, myalgia, spasm, headaches, decreased range of motion, and acute malocclusion.

neuropathy: An assortment of neuronal pathological conditions that occur as a consequence of trauma, infections, metabolic disorders, or exposure to toxins that induce injury to the nerve axons of the peripheral nervous system. Neuropathy typically induces pain and numbness in the affected area.

neurotmesis: Nerve injury involving a complete severance of the nerve trunk, leading to Wallerian degeneration. Sensory and/or motor functions are impaired. The potential for recovery is remote. In implant dentistry, this may be caused by an incision of the nerve or any of the factors leading to axonotmesis.

neurovascular bundle: Anatomic unit comprising a nerve and its related blood vessels.

neutral zone: The potential intraoral space where denture teeth should be preferably located, so the function of the musculature will not unseat the denture and forces generated by the tongue are counterbalanced by the forces produced by the lips and cheeks.

neutrocclusion: See: Malocclusion.

neutropenia: An abnormal decrease in the number of circulating neutrophils. It may be cyclic in nature.

neutrophil: The predominant polymorphonuclear leukocyte comprising up to 70% of the peripheral white blood cells. It is important in infection and injury repair, and may have impaired function in some forms of early-onset periodontitis.

nevus: 1. A pigmented or nonpigmented lesion on the skin or mucosa, which may undergo malignant transformation. 2. Birthmark; a circumscribed malformation of the skin, especially if colored by hyperpigmentation or increased vascularity. 3. A benign, localized overgrowth.

new attachment: Union of connective tissue or epithelium with a root surface that has been deprived of its original attachment apparatus. New attachment may be epithelial adhesion and/or connective tissue adaptation or attachment and may include new cementum.

Newton (N): Unit of force required to accelerate a mass of 1 kg at a rate of 1 m/s^2; equivalent to 0.2248 lb or 102 g.

Newton centimeter (Ncm): Unit of rotational torque. Work performed by a force of 1 N applied at an arm distance of 1 cm.

Newton meter (Nm): Unit of torque. Work performed by the application of 1 N from a distance of 1 m; equal to 1 J.

nickel-chromium alloy: Dental casting alloys made primarily of nickel 70% and chromium 30% with trace amounts of molybdenum, manganese, silicon, carbon, and aluminum. The greater the nickel content, the more ductile the alloy; however, its strength, hardness, modulus of elasticity, and fusion temperature are adversely affected. Chromium, by its passivation effect, ensures corrosion resistance of the alloy.

nidus: 1. A central point or focus where a morbid process begins. 2. Nucleus or center.

nifedipine: A calcium channel blocker that is antianginal and antihypertensive by depressing the contraction of cardiac and vascular smooth muscle. This increases heart rate and cardiac output, and decreases systemic vascular resistance and blood pressure. A coronary vasodilator drug that may be associated with gingival overgrowth.

night guard: See: Occlusal guard.

Nikolsky's sign: Occurs when the apparently normal, superficial layer of skin or oral mucosa may be rubbed off with slight trauma. Originally associated with pemphigus vulgaris, but can be seen in several bullous conditions.

noble metal: A metal consisting of elements that resist oxidation and corrosion in a moist or humid environment. See: Base metal.

noble metal alloy: A dental casting material that consists of gold, palladium, and silver with lesser amounts of iridium, ruthenium, and platinum. These metal alloys are used for inlays, onlays, complete metal crowns, and backings for ceramic baking.

nociceptive: Caused by or responding to a painful stimulus.

nociceptive pathway: An afferent neural path (conduit) initiating at a peripheral site in the body and ending in the central nervous system's somatosensory cortex where the original peripheral stimulus is perceived as pain.

nociceptor: A sensory receptor preferentially sensitive to noxious or potentially noxious stimuli.

nodule: A small, solid collection of tissue. Similar to a papule, but greater than either 5 mm or 10 mm in both width or depth.

noma: A rapidly progressive, polymicrobial, opportunistic infection occurring in immunocompromised or nutritionally deficient patients. Fusospirochetal organisms have been implicated.

nominal implant length/diameter: The length or diameter of a dental implant as written on the manufacturer's label. See: Actual implant length/diameter.

nonabsorbable: The property exhibited by nonautogenous substances that demonstrate no *in vivo* degradation over time. See: Nonresorbable.

nonadjustable articulator: An articulator that has limited hinge opening and closing arcs about a fixed axis. Casts are arbitrarily mounted without use of a facebow. The maximum intercuspal position is the only reproducible position using this type of articulator. It does not allow for adjustments to duplicate mandibular movements.

nonanatomic teeth: Artificial teeth with occlusal surfaces that are not anatomically correct. These teeth are designed in accordance with mechanical principles and are not intended for anatomic duplication. See: Zero-degree teeth.

nonangled abutment: Prosthetic implant component designed to parallel the long axis of the implant; considered straight to indicate no deviation from the long axis of the implant. Called also nonangulated abutment.

nonarcon articulator: An articulator with the equivalent condylar guidance compartment attached to the lower member and the condyle equivalent hinge axis compartment attached to the upper member.

nonaxial loading: Loading of an implant body that is not along the long axis of an implant body. Compare: Axial loading.

nonbiodegradable: Property of tissue substitute that remains unchanged at the site of implantation, with no dispersion *in vivo*.

noncollagenous matrix protein: Protein presented in the organic matrix of collagen-based calcified tissues together with the supporting collagen meshwork. It contributes to determining the structure and biomechanical properties of the tissues.

nonengaging: Feature of a dental implant or prosthetic component that does not incorporate

an antirotation mechanical design. See: Engaging.

nonfunctional loading: Load placed on an implant that is not generated through normal occlusal function or parafunction; for example, applying load through the tightening of an abutment screw.

nonfunctional side: The side away from which the mandible moves during lateral excursions.

nonhexed: Property of an implant or a prosthetic component that does not incorporate a mechanical design using a six-sided or six-angled hexagonal elevation or shape. A component or a dental implant without a hexagonal connection interface.

nonlamellar bone: See: Bone.

nonocclusal loading: The restoration is not in occlusal contact with the opposing dentition in maximal intercuspal position or in excursions. However, the cheeks, tongue, lips, and food, may touch the restoration. See: Nonfunctional loading, Occlusal loading.

nonresorbable: Materials that do not degrade *in vivo*. See: Nonabsorbable.

nonresorbable membrane: Membrane made of nonabsorbable biomaterial, most often of expanded polytetrafluoroethylene (e-PTFE). Use of a nonresorbable membrane requires a second surgery to remove it from the site. See: Guided tissue regeneration (GTR).

nonrigid connector: A connector that allows a limited movement between the retainer and the pontic components of a fixed partial denture. Its usage is indicated in cases where a single path of insertion cannot be achieved due to nonparallel abutments.

nonrotating abutment: Prosthetic implant component designed to prevent rotation of subsequent component, similar to a natural tooth preparation onto which a restoration or other prosthetic component is placed in a predictable position. A portion of the component incorporates a flat side or similar design to prevent 360° rotation (i.e., spins) of subsequent component.

nonrotating gold cylinder: Attachment element designed so that the interface between the gold cylinder and the transmucosal element does not allow 360° rotation.

nonsteroidal antiinflammatory drug (NSAID): Class of medication with analgesic (nonopioid), antipyretic, and antiinflammatory effects. Its mechanism of action involves the inhibition of the synthesis of prostaglandins from arachidonic acid.

nonsubmerged healing: Implant placement procedure incorporating a transmucosal extension for healing guidance. Special healing cap is required to extend the implant shoulder above the soft tissue level, allowing the suturing of wound margins around the implant neck/healing cap. This approach does not require a second surgical procedure and is often used in posterior implant sites.

nonsubmerged implant: Implant that is placed with a transmucosal element to allow soft tissue healing immediately after initial placement and to prevent the need for a second surgical procedure. Soft tissue healing occurs around the transmucosal element of either a one- or two-piece implant.

nonsubmergible implant: See: One-stage implant.

nonthreaded implant: Implant design that does not incorporate threads circumferentially on the external surface of the implant.

nonuniform rational basis spline (NURBS): A mathematical model commonly used in computer graphics for generating and representing curves and surfaces. It offers great flexibility and precision for handling both analytic (surfaces defined by common mathematical formulae) and modeled shapes.

nonvascularized free graft: Graft harvested solely as an osseous graft and without accompanying vasculature.

nonworking interference: Undesirable tooth contact(s) on the nonworking side of the mandible during excursive movement.

nonworking side: Segment of the dental arch (right or left) that is opposite the side at which the teeth occlude during mandibular function. Also known as balancing side.

nonworking side condyle: The condyle on the nonworking side.

nonworking side interference: Undesirable contacts of the opposing occlusal surfaces on the nonworking side.

normal distribution: Data that has a symmetrical, bell-shaped distribution where the mean, median, and mode are identical.

noxious: A deleterious or harmful substance; not wholesome.

NSAID (abbrev.): Nonsteroidal antiinflammatory drug.

null hypothesis: Hypothesis being tested about a population, typically that no difference exists between the mean values of two groups.

NURBS (abbrev.): Nonuniform rational basis spline.

O

OBJ: Simple data-format file that represents 3D geometry alone: the position of each vertex, position of each texture coordinate vertex, normal, and the faces that make each polygon defined as a list of vertices, and texture vertices.

obligate: Essential; not facultative; limited to a single life condition; able to survive only in a particular environment or to assume only a particular role, as an obligate anaerobe.

oblique fibers: See: Fiber, principal.

oblique slide: See: Cross-sectional slice.

obtundent: An agent or remedy that lessens or relieves sensibility or pain. Soothing, deadening, dulling.

obturator: A structure that closes an opening, such as a prosthetic appliance used to close an opening in the palate.

occlude: 1. To bring together; to shut. 2. To bring or close the mandibular teeth into contact with the maxillary teeth.

occluding jaw record: A registration record of maximum intercuspation.

occluding relation: The jaw relation at which the opposing teeth occlude.

occlusal: Pertaining to the contacting surfaces of opposing maxillary and mandibular posterior teeth, prostheses, or prosthetic baseplates with their associated wax rims.

occlusal analysis: A systematic examination of the masticatory system with special consideration of the effect of occlusion on the teeth and their related structures.

occlusal anatomy, modified: See: Modified occlusal anatomy.

occlusal balance: A condition in which there are simultaneous contacts of opposing teeth or tooth analogues (i.e., occlusion rims) on both sides of the opposing dental arches during eccentric movements within the functional range.

occlusal disharmony: An occlusal scheme that deviates from the ideal interactions of the occlusal contacts and anatomic components of the craniofacial complex.

occlusal embrasure: The interdental space that is coronal to the interproximal contact between adjacent, contacting teeth in the same arch.

occlusal equilibration: The modification of the occlusal form of the teeth with the intent of equalizing occlusal stress, producing simultaneous occlusal contacts or harmonizing cuspal relations.

occlusal force: Force applied to opposing teeth that results from contraction of the muscles of mastication; the force created during mastication via the action of muscles.

occlusal form: The shape on the chewing surfaces of a tooth or a row of teeth.

occlusal guard: (syn): Bite guard, mouth guard, night guard. A plastic removable dental appliance that covers a dental arch separating opposing teeth from each other so that teeth cannot damage each other during parafunctional activity. Called also bite splint.

occlusal harmony: A condition in centric and eccentric jaw relation in which there are no interceptive or deflective contacts of occluding surfaces.

Glossary of Dental Implantology, First Edition. Khalid Almas, Fawad Javed and Steph Smith.
© 2018 John Wiley & Sons, Inc. Published 2018 by John Wiley & Sons, Inc.

occlusal index: Record of the intraoral horizontal maxillomandibular relationship. Facial and/or buccal surfaces may also be recorded for repositioning artificial teeth, pontics, or veneers in the laboratory.

occlusal interference: Any tooth contact that inhibits the remaining occluding surfaces from achieving stable and harmonious contacts.

occlusal load: Force applied to natural or prosthetic teeth, implants, and surrounding structures by the elevator muscles of the mandible. See: Occlusal force.

occlusal load factor: Force factor involved with occlusal or masticatory function and the resultant loading of underlying teeth, implants or bone. See: Occlusal force.

occlusal loading: The restoration is in occlusal contact with the opposing dentition in maximal intercuspal position and/or excursions. See: Nonocclusal loading.

occlusal overload: Application of occlusal loading, through function or parafunction, in excess of what the prosthesis, implant component, or osseointegrated interface is capable of withstanding without structural or biologic damage.

occlusal pattern: The form or design of the masticatory surfaces of a tooth or teeth based on natural, modified anatomic or nonanatomic teeth.

occlusal pivot: A raised area placed on the occlusal surface of a tooth (usually on a molar) that acts as a fulcrum and limits mandibular full closure, thereby inducing rotation of the lower jaw.

occlusal plane: 1. An imaginary plane formed by the incisal edges of the anterior teeth and the occlusal cusps of the posterior teeth. The plane represents the curvature formed by these edges. 2. The surface of wax occlusal rims used for removable partial and complete dentures that simulates the incisal edges of the anterior teeth and the occlusal cusps of the posterior teeth. 3. A flat or curved guide for making dental prostheses that is used to position the incisal edges of the anterior teeth and the occlusal cusps of the posterior teeth.

occlusal prematurity: Any contact of opposing teeth that occurs before the desirable intercuspation.

occlusal pressure: Force applied to the occlusal surfaces of teeth.

occlusal reduction: The amount (in millimeters) of tooth structure removed from the occlusal surface of teeth in order to provide adequate interdental space for a restorative material.

occlusal reshaping: The act of physically recontouring the occlusal surfaces of teeth.

occlusal surface: The anatomic masticatory surface of posterior teeth as outlined by the mesial and distal marginal ridges and the buccal and lingual cusp eminences.

occlusal table: Collective surface anatomy of the posterior teeth inclusive of molar and premolar cusps, inclined planes, marginal ridges, grooves, and fossae.

occlusal trauma: Injury resulting in tissue changes within the attachment apparatus as a result of occlusal force(s). **Primary o.t.:** Injury resulting in tissue changes from excessive occlusal forces applied to a tooth or teeth with normal support. **Secondary o.t.:** Injury resulting in tissue changes from normal or excessive occlusal forces applied to a tooth or teeth with reduced support.

occlusal traumatism: Functional loading of teeth, usually off-axis, that is of sufficient magnitude to induce changes to the teeth (e.g., fractures, wear) or supporting structures. Changes may be temporary or permanent.

occlusal vertical dimension: A vertical measurement of the relationship of the maxilla and mandible when the existing teeth are in maximum intercuspation. See: Vertical dimension.

occlusal wear: The loss of tooth structure caused by attrition or abrasion due to functional and parafunctional contact of opposing teeth.

occlusion: Any contact of opposing teeth. **Centric o.** (acquired centric and habitual occlusion): The maximum intercuspation or contact of the teeth of the opposing arches. **Eccentric o.:** Any relation of the mandibular to the maxillary teeth other than centric occlusion. **Physiologic o.**: Occlusion in harmony with the functions of the masticatory system. **Protrusive o.**: Occlusion of teeth when the mandible is protruded from centric maximum intercuspation. **Retrusive o.**: A biting relationship in which the mandible is more distally placed than in maximum intercuspation. **Traumatic o.**: See: Occlusal trauma.

occlusion analysis: A study of a patient's masticatory system that evaluates how the teeth come together in functional and parafunctional activities. The goal is to discover how all aspects of the system, including teeth, jaws, muscles of mastication, and joints, work together to create either a healthy physiologic occlusion or an unhealthy disease-producing occlusion.

occlusion record: A record of the relationship of the maxilla and the mandible as they occlude in any position.

occlusion rim: A surface that attaches to a denture base that can be used to record the occluding relationship between the maxilla and the mandible and that may facilitate the arrangement of denture teeth as a step toward the creation of a denture.

occlusive membrane: See: Barrier membrane.

ocular implant: Prosthetic conformer placed following enucleation or evisceration of the eye to preserve space for ocular prosthesis.

ocular prosthesis: Artificial human eye or globe.

odontalgia: Toothache; pain in a tooth.

odontoblast: A connective tissue cell of neural crest origin found in the odontoblastic layer of the dental pulp that is responsible for deposition of dentin.

odontogenic: 1. Tooth-forming. 2. Arising in tissues that give origin to the teeth.

odontoma: A developmental anomaly consisting of a calcified mass of enamel, dentin, and cementum that may or may not resemble a tooth.

odontoplasty: The reshaping of a portion of a tooth.

OHIP (abbrev.): Oral health impact profile.

oligodontia: A condition in which fewer than a complete set of teeth are formed; oftentimes the teeth that are present may be smaller than normal

oncogene: A gene controlling cellular proliferation which, when altered through mutation or included in a viral genome, can promote neoplastic transformation or normal cells.

one-part implant: A dental implant in which the endosseous and transmucosal portions consist of one unit which presents a surface without a joint (microgap) to the tissues. See: Two-part implant.

one-piece abutment: An abutment that connects into a dental implant without the use of an additional retaining screw. The abutment can be retained by cement, friction, or screw threads. See: Two-piece abutment.

one-piece implant: A dental implant in which the endosseous and abutment portions consist of one unit. See: Two-piece implant.

one-screw test: A test used to check the fit of a multiple unit screw-retained restoration. One screw is placed in the terminal dental implant abutment. Evaluation is made on the opposite side. If the framework rises or has a ledge, detected clinically or radiologically, the fit is considered inaccurate.

one-stage grafting procedures: Grafting procedures combined with simultaneous implant placement; the remaining bone height must be sufficient for primary stability, and the defect must be self-contained with at least two bone walls. Compare: Two-stage grafting procedures.

one-stage implant: (syn): Nonsubmergible implant, single-stage implant. An endosseous dental implant designed to be placed following a one-stage surgery protocol. The implant is designed with a transmucosal coronal portion. Usually the transmucosal portion and the implant is one piece with no microgap. See: Two-stage implant.

one-stage implant placement: Protocol that involves one surgical procedure for implant placement. In the single stage, the osteotomy site is prepared, the implant is placed, and the transmucosal element exits the soft tissue.

Use of a single-stage implant eliminates the need for a second surgical procedure to expose the coronal portion of the implant.

one-stage surgery: A surgical protocol consisting of placing an endosseous root-form dental implant in bone and leaving it in contact with the oral environment during the healing process, thus eliminating a second surgical procedure. See: Two-stage surgery.

one-stage surgical approach: Category of surgical procedures that can be performed with a single intervention. This group includes standard implant placement with nonsubmerged healing or implant placement with simultaneous bone grafting procedures.

ONJ (abbrev.): Osteonecrosis of the jaw.

onlay graft: A method of attempting to add *de novo* bone to the height or width or other dimension of an existing bony structure, for example, onto the alveolar ridge, by adding autologous or another form of bone or bone-forming substitute subperiosteally onto the native bone.

opacity: The quality or state of a body that makes it impervious to light.

opaque: The property of a material that absorbs and/or reflects all light and prevents any transmission of light.

opaque porcelain: The first porcelain layer applied in the metal-ceramic technique to the underlying metal framework to establish the bond between the porcelain and metal while simultaneously masking the dark color of the metallic oxide layer. Opaque porcelain provides the primary source of color for the completed restoration.

open architecture: A digital process or workflow that can be performed on various digital platforms, as opposed to closed architecture processes. These are workflows that can only be performed on a specific platform. STL is an example of open architecture.

open bite: Lack of contact between opposing teeth in centric occlusion.

open curettage: Curettage facilitated by reflection of a soft tissue flap.

open-ended wrench: Instrument used to apply a torque during removal of an implant mount.

open occlusal relationship: Lack of contact between opposing teeth in centric occlusion.

open-tray impression: syn. Direct impression. Impression technique that uses an impression coping with retentive features around which a rigid elastic impression material is injected. To remove the impression, the impression coping is first unthreaded through an opening on the occlusal surface of the tray. See: Closed-tray impression.

opening movement: The change in position of the mandible as the maxillary and mandibular jaws separate upon opening.

operculum: The flap of mucosa over a partially erupted tooth.

OPG (abbrev.): Osteoprotegerin.

opioid: Morphine-like centrally acting analgesic, the primary medication used to treat moderate to severe pain.

opportunistic infection: An infection that develops in an immune compromised patient that is caused by endogenous, normally non-pathogenic, flora.

opsonin: A substance (e.g., antibody, complement) capable of enhancing phagocytosis.

optical scanners: Devices that use light projection or laser beams to obtain a 3D digital replica of an object.

oral: Pertaining to the oral cavity. See: Lingual.

oral epithelium: The epithelial lining of the oral mucosa which is a stratified squamous epithelium of varying degrees of keratinization.

oral flora: The microbiota of the oral cavity.

oral health impact profile (OHIP): Measurement of people's perceptions of the social impact of oral disorders on their well-being.

oral health-related quality of life: Multidimensional concept assessing how orofacial concerns affect well-being, including functional factors, psychological factors, social factors, and the experience of pain and/or discomfort.

oral hygiene: The maintenance of oral cleanliness. Removal of microbial plaque with brushes, dental floss, and other devices, with the possible adjunctive use of antiplaque agents. Also known as oral physiotherapy and plaque control.

oral implantology: See: Implant dentistry.

oral mucosa: Epithelial lining of the oral cavity continuous with the skin of the lips and mucosa of the soft palate and pharynx. The oral mucosa consists of the following. 1. Masticatory mucosa: mucosa of the gingiva and hard palate. 2, Specialized mucosa: mucosa of the dorsum of the tongue. 3, Lining mucosa: syn. Alveolar mucosa: the remaining mucosa of the oral cavity.

oral orifice: The opening of the oral cavity through the face.

oral prophylaxis: Removal of plaque, calculus, and stains from exposed and unexposed surfaces of the teeth and/or dental implants by scaling and polishing as a preventive measure for the control of local irritational factors.

oral sepsis: Infection of oral origin that causes systemic toxicity.

orbital prosthesis: Artificial replacement of the contents of the human orbit to contain the globe. See: Ocular prosthesis.

organization: The replacement of blood clots by fibrous tissue in a healing wound.

orientation index: Mold or form used as a three-dimensional record to register positions between adjacent structures. See: Index.

orientation jig: See: Abutment transfer device. A laboratory-fabricated device, used to maintain the correct positional relationship of a component when transferring it from the cast to the mouth.

orifice: Any opening, whether by a foramen, a meatus, a perforation, or one which serves as an entrance or outlet to a vessel, canal, or cavity.

O-ring: Retention element resembling a round gasket shape, fitting onto the stud-type patrix of a mechanical attachment. The patrix is soldered or cast to the coping that is cemented into the tooth root.

oroantral fistula: See: Fistula.

orofacial fistula: See: Fistula.

oronasal fistula: See: Fistula.

oropharynx: The portion of the pharynx that lies between the upper edge of the epiglottis and the soft palate.

orthodontic anchorage implant: Endosseous dental implant commonly used as anchorage for orthodontic tooth movement. Osseointegrated interface is exceptionally well suited for use as an orthodontic anchor because of its ankylotic nature. Implant may be miniature or standard sized.

orthodontic implant: Any implant used during orthodontic treatment as anchorage for orthodontic tooth movement. See: Temporary anchorage device (TAD).

orthodontic ligature: See: Ligature.

orthodontics: "The area and specialty of dentistry concerned with the supervision, guidance and correction of the growing or mature dentofacial structures, including those conditions that require movement of teeth or correction of malrelationships and malformations of the related structures and the adjustment of relationships between and among teeth and facial bones by the application of forces and/or the stimulation and redirection of functional forces within the craniofacial complex."

orthognathous: Having a straight profile, neither a protruding nor a receding jaw profile.

orthopantograph: A panoramic radiograph that includes images of the maxilla and mandible on a single extraoral film. Also known as panoramic radiograph.

orthopantomograph: See: Panoramic radiograph.

orthopedic craniofacial prosthesis: An active maxillofacial appliance used to preserve or position the craniofacial osseous sections that are misaligned due to trauma or craniofacial anomalies.

orthopedic implant application: Application of osseointegration to orthopedic procedures such as artificial shoulder or hip replacement.

orthotic device: In dentistry, a bite plate used in treatment of temporomandibular disorders.

osteoradionecrosis: Necrosis of bone following irradiation.

osse(o): (syn): Osteo. Pertaining to bone or containing a bony element.

osseointegrated implant: See: Implant, oral.

osseointegration: The direct contact between living bone and a functionally loaded dental implant surface without interposed soft tissue at the light microscope level. The clinical manifestation of osseointegration is absence of mobility. See: Osseous integration.

osseoperception: Special sensory perception that patients with osseointegrated implants may develop within months following implant placement. A peripheral feedback pathway can be restored, allowing physiologic integration of the implant in the human body and more natural function.

osseous: Bony, pertaining to bone.

osseous coagulum: Mixture of autogenous bone shavings from areas adjacent to the surgical site mixed with blood. Allogeneic, xenogeneic, or alloplastic graft materials may be added to increase volume and delay resorption.

osseous coating: Bone marrow response to osteophilic surfaces.

osseous defect: A reduction or deficiency of the bony architecture around teeth and implants caused by disease or trauma; can be intrabony or interradicular in nature.

osseous dysplasia: A benign fibroosseous lesion in which the periapical bone of vital teeth is replaced first by a fibrous type of connective tissue and then by an osseocementoid tissue.

osseous graft: See: Bone graft.

osseous integration: 1. The apparent direct attachment or connection of osseous tissue to an inert, alloplastic material without intervening connective tissue. 2. The process and resultant apparent direct connection of an exogenous material's surface and the host bone tissues, without intervening fibrous connective tissue. 3. The interface between alloplastic materials and bone.

osseous regeneration: Restoration of original osseous tissue through recapitulation of embryologic events.

osseous rehabilitation: Reestablishment of form and function of deficient osseous tissue, aimed at restitution.

osseous repair: Restoration of form and function of deficient osseous tissue.

osseous restoration: Reestablishment of continuity of osseous tissue, usually restoring form and function.

osseous surgery: rocedures to modify bone support altered by periodontal disease, either by reshaping the alveolar process to achieve physiologic form without the removal of alveolar supporting bone, or by the removal of some alveolar bone, thus changing the position of the crestal bone relative to the tooth root. See: Ostectomy, Osteoplasty, Surgery, osseous.

ossification: 1. The formation of bone or a bony substance. 2. The conversion of fibrous tissue or of cartilage into bone or a bony substance.

ossifying fibroma: See: Fibroma.

osteal: Bony, osseous.

ostectomy: Removal of bone or a portion of bone, usually with rotary instrumentation using a diamond or steel bur to reshape or recontour bone to conform to better bone health by itself or around the neck of a tooth. See: Osteoplasty.

osteitis: Inflammation of bone involving the Haversian spaces, canals, and their branches. **Condensing o.**: 1. Defined as a pathologic growth of maxillomandibular bones characterized by mild clinical symptoms. The bone thickening reflects the impaired bone rearrangement in response to mild infection of dental pulp. 2. A variant of chronic apical periodontitis which represents a diffuse increase in trabecular bone in response to irritation. Radiographically, a concentric radiopaque area is seen around the offending root. 3. A relatively common condition, which manifests as an area of radiopacity in the bone, usually adjacent to a tooth that has a large restoration or pulpal infection. **O. deformans**: a bone disease of unknown cause, characterized by enlargement of the cranial bones and often the maxilla or mandible.Radiographically there may be a cotton-wool appearance. Also known as Paget's disease.

osteo: See: Osseo.

osteoarthritis: (syn): Degenerative joint disease. Chronic degeneration and destruction of the articular cartilage and/or fibrous connective tissue linings of the joint components and disks, leading to bony spurs, pain, stiffness, limitation of movement, and changes in bone morphology. Advanced conditions may involve erosions and disk degeneration with crepitus.

osteoblast: A fully differentiated cell that functions in the formation of bone tissue. Osteoblasts synthesize the collagen and glycoproteins that form the bone matrix, and also produce inorganic salts. With growth, they develop into osteocytes.

osteoblast growth factors: Secreted by mononucleated differentiated cells arising from mesenchymal progenitors and associated with the production of bone by secreting bone matrix and enzymes that facilitate mineral deposition within osteoid matrices.

osteocalcin: A bone-specific protein produced by the osteoblast which may play a role in osteoclast recruitment, found in the extracellular matrix of bone, dentin, and the serum of circulating blood. A marker for bone remodeling or mineralization. This vitamin K-dependent, calcium-binding protein is produced by osteoblasts and is the most abundant noncollagen protein in bone. Because of calcium-binding sites, it plays a role in bone matrix mineralization or in regulation of crystal growth. In addition, its increased serum concentration is a marker of increased bone turnover in disease states (e.g., Paget's disease or postmenopausal osteoporosis). It has a low molecular weight and contains three alpha-carboxyglutamic acid residues per molecule. Called also gamma-linolenic acid (GLA) protein.

osteoclast: A large multinucleated cell that is derived from macrophages. Osteoclasts release cathepsin K, which breaks down the proximal bone mineral matrix, thereby allowing the release of bone morphogenetic proteins that induce osteoblasts to deposit new bone mineral matrix.

osteoclastogenesis: Mechanism of osteoclast generation through differentiation of precursor cells of the hematopoietic lineage induced by regulatory molecules. Calcitropic factors, such as vitamin D3, prostaglandin E2, interleukin-1, interleukin-2, tumor necrosis factor, and glucocorticoid induce receptor activator nuclear factor-kappa ligand (RANKL) expression on osteoblasts. RANKL binding to the RANK expressed on hematopoietic progenitors activates a signal transduction cascade that leads to osteoclast differentiation in the presence of the survival factor colony-stimulating factor 1.

osteoconduction: Bone growth by apposition from the surrounding bone. Process by which a material provides scaffolding along which bone growth can occur. See: Osteoinduction.

osteoconductive: The quality of a graft material which allows it to serve as a scaffold for deposition of osteoid.

osteoconductive graft: Autografts, treated allografts, and bone substitutes that provide a scaffold for osteoid formation.

osteocyte: An osteoblast that has become embedded within bone matrix, occupying a flat oval cavity (bone lacuna). Cells found in bone lacunae send, through canaliculi, slender cytoplasmic processes that make contact with processes of other osteocytes and osteoblasts.

osteodistraction: See: Distraction osteogenesis.

OsteoGen: Proprietary product name for an osteoconductive, nonceramic, synthetic hydroxyapatite that is a bioactive, resorbable graft material used for contouring defects of the alveolar ridge. As new bone is formed, it is resorbed over 6–8 months. It is composed of a mixture of calcium phosphates.

osteogenesis: Formation or creation of bone.

osteogenetic: 1. Forming bone. 2. Concerned in bone formation.

osteogenic: (syn): Osteogenous. Promoting the development and formation of bone, exclusively resulting from the action of osteoblasts.

osteogenic protein: See: Bone morphogenetic protein 7 (BMP-7).

osteoid: The beginning organic matrix of bone. Initial deposit in bone formation starts with the deposition of osteoid, which is secreted by mature osteoblasts at a speed of 1–2 µm per day. When concerned with lamellar bone, a matrix composed of a scaffold of interwoven collagen fibers (mainly type 1) and noncollagenous proteins is sedimented as osteocalcin and bone sialoprotein – unique for the mineralized tissues – as well as osteonectin, osteopontin, and a number of growth factors. The mean thickness of osteoid in lamellar bone formation is 10 µm; when this thickness is reached, mineralization as sedimentation of crystals of carbonated hydroxyapatite ($Ca_{10}(PO_4)_6(OH_2)$) takes place.

osteoinduction: Chemicals, procedures, or materials that have the ability to induce bone formation (osteogenesis) through the recruitment and/or differentiation of osteoblast precursor stem cells and/or recruitment of mature osteoblasts to the area needing bone growth or repair.

osteoinductive: The quality of a biologic adjunct, growth factor, or graft material which leads to differentiation of osteoprogenitor cells into osteoblasts; this potential is often achieved via release of bone-inductive proteins from the material.

osteointegration: Ankylotic anchorage of a titanium implant in living bone to achieve a solid bond.

osteology: The scientific study of bones.

osteolysis: Bone resorption and dissolution, involving the loss or removal of calcium, as part of an ongoing disease process.

osteomyelitis: Infection of bone that is usually caused by bacteria. A long-term infection can lead to bone destruction.

osteon: Cylindrical structure with a diameter of 150–300 µm and a length varying from 2 to 10 µm, composed of concentric lamellae of bone surrounding a Haversian canal with a diameter of 50 µm. In this canal nutritive element, nerves, and connective tissue are present. Between the individual osteons and interstitial lamellae, cementing lines are seen. The longitudinal direction of the osteons is parallel to the axis of the bone. Lamellae are birefringent in polarized light because of changing orientation of the collagen fibers. In the trabecular osteon, the lamellae run parallel to the bone marrow interface.

osteonecrosis: (syn): Bone necrosis. The death or necrosis of bone due to the obstruction of its blood supply. See: Bisphosphonate-related osteonecrosis of the jaw (BRONJ), Osteonecrosis of the jaw (ONJ).

osteonecrosis of the jaw (ONJ): Exposed bone in the mandible, maxilla or both that persists for at least 8 weeks, in the absence of previous radiation or metastases in the jaws. See: Bisphosphonate-related osteonecrosis of the jaw (BRONJ), Osteonecrosis.

osteonectin: A phosphoprotein, found in bone and blood platelets, which binds both collagen and calcium and serves as a regulator of mineralization.

osteopenia: Reduced bone mass due to a decrease in the rate of osteoid synthesis to a level insufficient to compensate for normal bone lysis. It is considered a serious risk factor for the development of osteoporosis.

osteoperiosteal: Relating to bone and the periosteum that covers it.

osteoplasty: Removal or reshaping of the alveolar process with rotary instruments, piezoelectric technology, or hand instruments to accomplish a more physiologic form without removing alveolar bone proper.

osteopontin: Noncollagenous protein with an arginine-glycine-aspartic acid (RGD) tripeptide sequence having specificity for cell surface antigens. It is found in the lamina limitans of the bone surface, possibly playing a role in bone mineralization and attachment of osteoblasts and osteoclasts to bone matrix. It forms a cross-link with fibronectin and is found in cement lines, suggesting a function as a biologic matrix-bonding agent.

osteoporosis: Skeleton pathology distinguished by decreased normal bone mass and mineralized bone density; it is seen most commonly in the elderly.

osteoprogenitor cell: Relatively undifferentiated cell found on nearly all of the free surfaces of bone. Under certain circumstances, these cells undergo division and transform into osteoblasts or coalesce, giving rise to osteoclasts.

osteopromotion: Sealing off of a bone defect from the surrounding soft connective tissue by placement of a mechanical barrier (membrane), thereby creating a secluded space into which only cells from the walls of the bone defect can migrate. Expanded polytetrafluoroethylene (e-PTFE) is the best documented membrane material for promoting bone healing and regeneration by encouraging the biologic or mechanic environment of the healing or regenerating tissues; however, resorbable collagen membranes are equal in value.

osteopromotive: The quality of a biologic adjunct, growth factor, or graft material which, when added to an osteoinductive graft, tends to increase its level of osteoinductivity.

osteoprotegerin (OPG): Produced by osteoblasts, OPG acts as a decoy receptor for RANKL and inhibits osteoclastogenesis and osteoclast activation by binding to RANKL.

osteoradionecrosis (ORN): Necrosis of jaw bone as a late effect of ionizing radiation, which is used in treatment of malignancies of head and neck. It causes vascular changes with reduction in blood flow resulting in hypovascularity, hypocellularity, and hypoxia. Spontaneous necrosis of jaw bone may appear with subsequent ischemic necrosis of the covering mucous membrane and exposure of the necrotic bone to the oral cavity with a secondary invasion of the necrotic bone with microorganisms. Called also radiation-damaged bone and soft tissues.

osteotome: A beveled chisel for use in cutting or preparing bone.

osteotome lift: See: Osteotome technique.

osteotome sinus floor elevation: See: Osteotome technique.

osteotome technique: 1. (syn): Internal sinus graft. A sinus grafting technique whereby the maxillary sinus floor is carefully infractured and the Schneiderian membrane is elevated through an osteotomy prepared and extended in the ridge with an osteotome. 2. The surgical expansion of an osteotomy laterally with or without grafting. See: Ridge expansion.

osteotomy: The intended or desired cutting of a bone; often used to describe the tasks of smoothing, leveling, realigning, or altering external contours of the bone. See: Horizontal osteotomy, Pilot osteotomy.

ostium of the maxillary sinus: Communication between the maxillary sinus and the nasal cavity located at the middle meatus.

outcome, primary: One outcome determined to be the principal result of an experimental study.

outcome, secondary: Outcome other than the primary outcome of a study that is also of interest in the experimental study.

ovate pontic: A pontic that is shaped on its tissue surface like an egg in two dimensions, typically partially submerged in a surgically prepared soft tissue depression to enhance the illusion that a natural tooth is emerging from the gingival tissues.

overbite: Vertical overlapping of the mandibular incisors by the maxillary incisors when the jaws are in centric (habitual) occlusion. See: Vertical overlap.

overclosure: Decreased occlusal vertical dimension.

overdenture: Complete or partial removable denture supported by soft tissue and retained roots or implants to provide support, retention, and stability and reduce ridge resorption.

overgrowth: Excessive enlargement of a part, usually an organ or tissue, due to an increase in size of the constituent cells (hypertrophy), number of constituent cells (hyperplasia), or both.

overhang: Excess of dental restorative material extending beyond cavity margins.

overjet: The horizontal projection of the maxillary incisors beyond the mandibular incisors when the jaws are in centric (habitual) occlusion.

overload: Application of force to an object in excess of the force it was intended or designed to withstand. It has the potential for causing permanent deformation or damage to the structure or its support. See: Occlusal overload.

oxidating surface treatment: Creation of metallic oxides on the surface of metal. In the case of titanium, oxidation occurs immediately upon exposure to air. As a result, dental implants made of titanium are coated with titanium oxides critical for the success of osseointegration.

oxide surfaces: Oxygen-containing compounds and complexes formed at the surface of an absorbent. In the case of titanium dental implants, oxidation of the implant surface creates titanium oxide of various chemical formulas through exposure to air or through treatment of the surface at the time of fabrication.

oxidized surface treatment: Modification of the surface properties of titanium dental implants by alteration of the titanium oxide layer thickness.

oxycodone: Semi-synthetic opioid analgesic, recommended for moderate to severe pain. It may be used as a single agent or combined with products such as acetaminophen, aspirin, or ibuprofen.

oxygen therapy: See: Hyperbaric oxygen therapy (HBOT).

P

P value: Probability that an outcome would occur by chance. P values (probability values) range from 1 (absolutely certain) to 0 (absolutely impossible). A P value equal to or less than 0.05 means that the observed outcome is not likely (≤5%) to be the result of chance.

PACS (abbrev.): Picture archiving and communication system.

Paget's disease: Osteitis deformans. Disease of unknown etiology, characterized by enlargement of the cranial bones and often the maxilla and mandible. Cotton-wool appearance of bone on a radiograph may be a diagnostic feature.

palatal graft: See: Free gingival graft.

palatal groove: A developmental, anomalous groove usually found on the palatal aspect of maxillary central and lateral incisors. Also known as palatogingival groove and palatoradicular groove.

palatal implant: Dental implant placed in the midsagittal area of the maxillary hard palate for use as anchorage in orthodontic treatment. See: Orthodontic implant, Temporary anchorage device.

palatal incompetence: The muscular inability of the soft palate to adequately seal the port between the nasopharynx and the oropharynx during speech and swallowing. Failure to seal this port results in unintelligible speech and nasopharyngeal regurgitation of food and liquids. Conditions that cause palatal incompetence include degenerative nerve diseases, tumors, myasthenia gravis, strokes, cleft palate, polio, cerebral palsy, muscular dystrophy, and araxia. Also known as palatopharyngeal incompetence.

palatal vault: 1. The most superior and deepest portion of the palate. 2. The palatal curvature. 3. Superior surface of the hard palate.

palatogram: A record of the movement of the tongue and soft palate created during function, usually speech.

palatopharyngeal incompetence: Dysfunction of an anatomically intact soft palate resulting in inadequate palatopharyngeal closure. Palatopharyngeal incompetence is usually a result of neurologic or muscular disease or trauma.

palatopharyngeal sphincter: The muscular ring that controls separation of the nasopharynx and oropharynx during swallowing and speech.

palatorrhaphy: Surgical reconstruction of a cleft palate.

palliate: To alleviate symptoms or afford relief from a disease or medical condition.

palliative: Providing relief without effecting a cure.

palpate (palpated; palpating): To examine by manipulation or touch, palpation.

pamidronate: Intravenous nitrogen-containing bisphosphonate used for the treatment of osteoporosis, Paget's disease, and certain cancers affecting bone (e.g., multiple myeloma). Its mechanism of action involves the inhibition of osteoclast migration and maturation.

Glossary of Dental Implantology, First Edition. Khalid Almas, Fawad Javed and Steph Smith.
© 2018 John Wiley & Sons, Inc. Published 2018 by John Wiley & Sons, Inc.

pancytopenia: A significant reduction in blood cells and platelets in circulation.

panoramic radiograph: Tomographic survey radiograph of the maxillofacial complex in two dimensions. Image displays the maxilla and the mandible in its curvature and is produced by conventional tomography. Some X-ray machines allow the image to be obtained in sectors.

panoramic reconstitution: A thin, reformatted section of computed tomography scan data parallel to and following the curvature of the alveolar process as seen in the axial view. See: Axial slice, Cross-sectional slice.

papilla: Soft tissue occupying the interproximal space confined by adjacent crowns in contact. See: Interdental papilla, Interimplant papilla.

- **Circumvallate papilla**: One of 8 or 10 protuberances from the dorsum of the tongue making a V- shaped row anterior to and parallel with the sulcus terminalis. A circular trench having a slightly raised outer wall surrounds each papilla. On the borders of the papilla and on the opposed margins of the vellum are several taste buds.
- **Filiform papilla**: Numerous conical keratinized projections covering most of the dorsum of the tongue. These papillae are mechanical and are not involved in gustation.
- **Foliate papilla**: A series of parallel mucosal projections containing taste buds. They are located on the lateral margins of the tongue just anterior to the palatoglossal fold.
- **Fungiform papilla**: Small, mushroom-shaped elevations on the dorsum of the tongue.
- **Incisive papilla**: An elevation in the soft tissue covering the foramen of the incisive or nasopalatine canal.

papilla preservation: Measure taken to maintain the interdental papillae following tooth extraction to avoid black triangles between an implant and an adjacent tooth or between adjacent implants. This may include an atraumatic extraction, alveolar ridge preservation, and/or respecting certain parameters when placing implants, such as apicocoronal position and interimplant distance.

papilla reformation: The spontaneous reformation of the interproximal papilla following the establishment of a contact point and the management of the interproximal prosthetic papillary space. Also, the reestablishment of the lost interproximal papilla by surgical means.

papilla regeneration: Creating a papilla between an implant and an adjacent tooth or between adjacent implants. This may involve surgical procedures using small rotational pedicle flaps, use of connective tissue grafts, and/or prosthetic techniques to condition periimplant soft tissues. The term is a misnomer, since the papillae flatten in the edentulous space following tooth extraction once the transseptal inserting fibers are lost. A flattened papilla cannot be truly regenerated, but the clinician may optimize its appearance by prosthetic means. The appearance of a papilla is mainly determined by the interdental bone height, which has a documented threshold of approximately 5 mm.

papilla-sparing incision: Incision that does not include the papilla and thus avoids the elevation of these tissues.

papillectomy: Surgical removal of a gingival papilla.

papilloma: A benign epithelial, exophytic, pedunculated, cauliflower-like neoplasm. Viral etiology may be the causative agent.

Papillon–Lefevre syndrome: Palmarplantar hyperorthokeratosis with precocious periodontal destruction in the primary and permanent dentition. Thought to be the result of homozygosity of autosomal recessive genes.

papule: A small, superficial, circumscribed, hard elevation of the skin that does not contain pus.

paracervical saucerization: Progressive bone resorption occurring around the cervical portion of implants. Plausible etiologic factors can include surgical trauma, periimplantitis, occlusal overload, microgap, implant crest module, and compromise of the biologic width. Also, the excavation of tissue to form a shallow shelving depression, usually to facilitate drainage from infected areas of bone. Called also craterization.

paracrestal incision: A crestal incision made away from the middle of the crest of an edentulous ridge, either buccally or lingually. See: Crestal incision, Midcrestal incision, Mucobuccal fold incision.

paracrine: Transfer of chemical compounds such as hormones and growth factors from cell to cell.

parafunction: Abnormal function, as in bruxism or clenching, disordered or perverted function.

parafunctional habit: A detrimental habit characterized by abnormal function often related to occlusion, such as nocturnal bruxism.

parakeratosis: See: Hyperparakeratosis.

parallel (ing) pin: See: Direction indicator.

parallel-fibered bone: Repair bone deposited onto woven bone and old bone surfaces in a healing situation as parallel layers of bone. The collagen fibers run parallel to the surface but are not organized in a lamellar fashion.

parallel-sided implant: (syn): Parallel-walled implant, straight implant. An endosseous, root-form dental implant, with the body of the implant having the same diameter at the coronal and apical ends. The coronal diameter does not necessarily match that of the platform, which may be of a larger diameter.

parallel-walled implant: See: Parallel-sided implant.

parenteral administration: A technique of administration in which the drug bypasses the gastrointestinal (GI) tract (i.e., intramuscular (IM), intravenous (IV), intranasal (IN), submucosal (SM), subcutaneous (SC), intraosseous (IO)).

paresthesia: Morbid or perverted normal sensation, such as tingling or burning. The abnormal sensation is usually caused by injury to a nerve and is sometimes a complication after surgical procedures.

paroxysm: A sharp spasm or convulsion.

paroxysmal trigeminal neuralgia (tic douloureux): A severe paroxysm of pain occurring, usually unilaterally, in the distribution of the trigeminal nerve (especially the second and third divisions). Seen in middle-aged to elderly adults. The pain may be precipitated by a slight stimulus in a "trigger area."

partial anodontia: See: Partially edentulous.

partial coverage restoration: See: Partial veneer crown.

partial denture: Fixed or removable dental prosthesis supported and retained by teeth or implants for the replacement of less than a full complement of natural teeth and related hard and soft tissues. Called also partial prosthesis.

partial dislocation: A condition of the temporomandibular joint characterized by a displaced articular disk and partial displacement of the condylar head from its normal, healthy, resting position. As a result of these pathologic changes, the joint function is disrupted either unilaterally or bilaterally to varying degrees.

partial removable dental prosthesis (PRDP): A dental prosthesis that artificially supplies teeth or other associated structures in a partially edentulous jaw and can be removed and replaced at will.

partial-thickness flap: (syn): Split-thickness flap. A flap resulting from the elevation of epithelium and some connective tissue but not the periosteum, which is left on the bone. See: Full-thickness flap.

partial veneer crown: A nonspecific term that does not distinguish between the partial-coverage crown restoration of the tooth and the partial veneering of an artificial crown.

partially edentulous: State of being without one or more, but not all, of the natural teeth.

particulate autogenous graft: See: Autogenous bone graft.

particulate graft: Graft used in particulate form, which may be an autograft, allograft, alloplast, or xenograft. Particulate grafts differ concerning osteogenic potential, osteoconductivity, hydrophilicity, pore and particle size, and substitution rate.

particulate marrow cancellous bone (PMCB): Graft material obtained from donor sites, such as the iliac crest, with extensive marrow content. PMCB of an autogenous nature is the most osteogenic graft material; the number of multipotential stems cells is especially high.

parulis: A drainage tract seen in attached and/or mucosal gingiva that is associated with an oral abscess of odontogenic origin. Commonly known as a gum boil.

pass principle: A principle that promotes a successful regenerative procedure (originally used for guided bone regeneration, but has recently been expanded to include guided tissue regeneration as well).

passivated surface oxide: Surface treatment of an oxidized implant surface resulting in lower surface energy and increased corrosion resistance. This may be the result of intentional treatment of the surface by the manufacturer or simply exposure to air over time.

passivation: A process by which metals and alloys are made more resistant to corrosion through treatment to produce a thin and stable oxide layer on the external surfaces. See: Depassivation.

passive: 1. Latent, not active, inert. 2. Resistant to corrosion.

passive eruption: See: Eruption, dental.

passive fit: Adaptation of one component to another in a manner that does not impart strain. In dental implant prosthodontics, the creation of passively fitting prostheses is desirable.

passivity: In reference to dental implants, the property of the oxidized layer on the surface of the metal that allows it to not break down under physiological conditions.

patent: Open, not obstructed: the specific unobstructed route in which a removable dental prosthesis (or the precementation stage of a fixed dental prosthesis) may be removed.

pathogen: Any disease-producing microorganism.

pathogenesis: The mechanism by which a disease starts and progresses.

pathogenic occlusion: An abnormal occlusal relationship with the potential to produce pathologic changes in the masticatory system.

pathognomonic: Specifically distinctive, characteristic or symptomatic of a disease. A sign or symptom on which a diagnosis can be made.

pathosis: A disease entity; a morbid condition, the current state of being with disease.

patient assessment: See: Patient evaluation.

patient-based measure: Descriptive term referring to the array of questionnaires, interview schedules and other related methods of assessing health, illness, and benefits of healthcare interventions from the patient's perspective. A patient-based outcome measure that addresses constructs such as health-related quality of life, subjective health status, and functional status; used as a primary or secondary endpoint in clinical trials.

patient evaluation: Process by which a patient's condition is determined. Called also patient assessment.

patient examination: Clinical examination of the patient, including extraoral and intraoral findings.

patient history: Record of the patient's medical and dental histories.

patient motion tracker: An array of active emitters or passive reflectors that are attached to a patient to enable their localization within the operative field by an overhead detector.

patient satisfaction: Individual's perceived fulfillment of a need or want; can be measured by obtaining reports or ratings from patients about services received from an organization, hospital, physician, or healthcare provider.

patient selection: Selection of patients who are appropriate candidates for a particular therapy based on risk assessment, including medical, dental, and anatomic factors, as well as smoking habits and psychologic aspects.

patient-specific abutment: See: Custom abutment.

patrix: The male part of an attachment. See: Attachment, Matrix.

patrix component: The part of an attachment system that is designed specifically to insert and engage the matching receptacle or mate component (matrix) for mechanical retention. Attachment systems that use mechanical retention are available in various designs. See: Attachment system, Ball attachment system, Bar attachment system, Stud-type attachment, Telescopic coping attachment system.

PDGF (abbrev.): Platelet-derived growth factors.

PDL (abbrev.): Periodontal ligament.

pedicle: A narrow base resembling a stalk or stem that connects tissues (e.g., vertebrae) to each other; forms the base of tumors; in dentistry, pedicles are used in grafting procedures. See: Pedicle graft.

pedicle flap: Rotated or laterally moved flap receiving its blood supply from the original base of the flap. It is used to cover an adjacent surgical site or improve the thickness of soft tissue contours. See: Soft tissue augmentation.

pedicle graft: Full- or partial-thickness flap reflected from an area with a base attached to the donor site and in which the free margin is moved. It may be laterally or coronally positioned or rotated to cover an adjacent surgical site or enhance the soft tissue contours. See: Full-thickness flap, Partial-thickness flap.

peer-reviewed journal: Periodical publication for which individuals who are of an academic and/or professional standing equal to that of the author(s) have determined that all articles are of sufficient quality and completeness.

peer-reviewed literature analysis: Analysis of published research reports by individual(s) with expertise similar to that of the author(s).

peg lateral: A permanent maxillary lateral incisor that is tapered and small. Commonly referred to as a baby tooth.

pellucid: Allowing for the passage of light without distortion; transparent.

pemphigoid (cicatricial pemphigoid, benign mucous membrane pemphigoid): A chronic vesiculobullous autoimmune disorder that primarily affects the mucosa in older females; characterized by a subbasalar separation of epithelium from connective tissue; almost all cases have an oral involvement, with the gingiva being the most favored site.

pemphigus: Refers to a group of autoimmune bullous diseases (pemphigus vulgaris, pemphigus vegetans, pemphigus erythematosus) that affects skin and mucous membranes primarily between the fourth and sixth decades of life.

penicillin: Any of a large group of natural or semi-synthetic antibacterial antibiotics derived directly or indirectly from strains of fungi of the genus *Penicillium* and other soil-inhabiting fungi grown on special culture media. They exert a bactericidal and bacteriostatic effect on susceptible bacteria by interfering with the final stages of the synthesis of peptidoglycans, a substance in the bacterial cell wall. They can be classified according to their differing antibacterial spectrum: penicillin G and congeners (penicillin C), antistaphylococcal penicillins (methicillin, dicloxacillin), extended-spectrum penicillins (ampicillin and amoxicillin), and extended-spectrum penicillins with beta-lactamase inhibitors (amoxicillin and clavulanate, ampicillin and sulbactam). See: Amoxicillin, Clavulanic acid.

penicillin-binding proteins (PBPs): Receptor sites (commonly transpeptidase enzymes) for penicillin in its inhibition of bacterial cell wall synthesis; alterations in or formation of new PBPs are major mechanisms of resistance to penicillins. Also known as penicillin-sensitive enzymes (PSEs).

peptidoglycan: Major structural component of bacterial cell walls. Thicker in gram-positive than in gram-negative bacteria. Synthesis is inhibited by the beta-lactam antibiotics.

Peptococcus spp.: Gram-positive, nonmotile, anaerobic cocci occurring in irregular groups or clusters. Frequently found as a part of the subgingival plaque flora and occasionally implicated in oral infections and periodontal diseases.

Peptostreptococcus spp.: Anaerobic, gram-positive cocci that infect the whole body including soft tissues. In dentistry, these organisms can invade the subgingival flora, leading to infection and slow recovery times.

perceived color: Description of color based on various attributes (e.g., names of colors) or based on the senses (e.g., smell, touch, sound).

percentage bone–implant contact: Area of bone in direct contact with the implant surface; usually measured from histologic specimens.

percussion: To strike objects to produce a sound; in dentistry, tapping with fingers or with a medical device on oral structures can allow for diagnoses regarding the state of inflammation, disease onset, or progression or healing.

percutaneous implant: Implant placed and positioned through the skin, e.g., implants placed extraorally for reconstruction of facial structures or those used in the treatment of fractures in buccomaxillofacial and orthopedic areas.

perforation: Inadvertent tear or dehiscence within a flap created during surgery, either by overthinning the mucosa, improper blade direction while making periosteal releasing incisions, or excessive flap retraction.

periabutment: Region surrounding an implant abutment. Usually refers to the soft or hard tissues surrounding the abutment.

periapical: Of or relating to tissues that surround the apex or root (root tip) of a tooth; may include the periodontal ligament or alveolar bone.

periapical radiograph: Radiograph taken intraorally showing the entire tooth from the occlusal plane to the apex. The radiograph should reach 3 mm beyond the structures of the tooth.

pericervical saucerization: (syn): Craterization. Pathologic crestal bone loss due to periimplantitis. Radiographically, the bone loss is cup-shaped or saucer-like around the coronal aspect of the dental implant. See: Periimplantitis.

pericoronal abscess: A pus-producing lesion that forms above the crown of a partially erupted tooth.

pericoronitis: Acute inflammation of the gingiva and/or mucosa surrounding a partially erupted tooth. Also known as operculitis.

pericrestal incision: Incision placed not directly over the crest, but in either a more buccal or lingual location.

periimplant: Around the implant.

periimplant crevicular epithelium: Nonkeratinized epithelium lining the mucosal crevice.

periimplant disease: Collective term for inflammatory reactions in the soft and/or hard tissues surrounding dental implants. See: Periimplantitis, Periimplant mucositis.

peri-implant mucositis: A disease in which the presence of inflammation is confined to the mucosa surrounding a dental implant with no signs of loss of supporting bone.

periimplant soft tissue: Keratinized or nonkeratinized mucosa around an oral implant.

periimplant tissue recession: Location of the receding marginal periimplant tissues apical to the prosthesis–implant interface.

periimplantitis: Inflammation of the soft tissues that surround an osseointegrated implant that results in bone loss.

perimolysis: Erosion of the teeth due to chronic gastric regurgitation of stomach acid.

periodontal: Situated or occurring around a tooth; pertaining to the periodontium. **P. abscess**: See: Abscess, periodontal. **P. bony defects**: Alterations in the morphological features of the bone. Osseous defects may be subcategorized as follows: **Circumferential d.**: A vertical defect that includes more than one surface of a tooth, e.g., a vertical defect that includes the mesial and lingual surfaces of a tooth. **Crater d.**: A cup- or bowl-shaped defect in the interalveolar bone with bone loss nearly equal on the contiguous roots. The facial and lingual palatal walls may be of unequal height. A type of intrabony defect, a crater also may be classified by the number of bony walls (i.e., one-, two-, or three-walled); combination defects also exist. **Funnel-shaped d.**: An intrabony resorptive lesion involving one or more surfaces of supporting bone; may appear moat-like. **Furcation invasion**: Pathologic resorption of bone within a furcation. **Classification of furcation invasions**: **Class I**: Incipient loss of bone limited to the furcation flute that does not extend horizontally. **Class II**: A variable degree of bone loss in a furcation, but not extending completely through the furcation. **Class III**: Bone loss extending completely through the furcation. **Hemiseptal d.**: A vertical defect in the presence of adjacent roots; thus half of a septum remains on one tooth. **Intrabony (infrabony) d.**: A periodontal defect surrounded by two or three bony walls or a combination of these.

periodontal abscess: Pus-producing infection of any periodontal tissue that usually involves the bone and soft tissue surrounding a tooth.

periodontal biotype: Categorization determined by variable biologic or physiologic characteristics of periodontal tissue. To evaluate the periodontal biotype, a periodontal probe can be placed at the facial aspect of the periodontal (or periimplant) sulcus. It is categorized as thin if the outline of the underlying probe can be seen through the gingiva or mucosa, or thick if the probe cannot be seen. **Thick p.b.**: Periodontal biotype characterized by a thick and wide keratinized tissue at the facial aspect of teeth and oral implants. This biotype is prone to pocket formation instead of gingival recession in the presence of periodontal disease. **Thin p.b.**: Periodontal biotype characterized by a thin periodontal tissue at the facial aspect of teeth or oral implants. This biotype is prone to gingival recession following mechanical or surgical manipulation. **Thin-scalloped p.b.**: Classification of periodontium according to its facial aspects, distinguished by a pronounced disparity between the height of the gingival margin on the direct facial and that found interproximally (i.e., noticeable rise and fall of marginal tissue). The underlying bone is usually thin on the facial aspect with dehiscences and fenestrations common.

periodontal bone regeneration: Regeneration of tooth-supporting alveolar bone that includes new cementum and periodontal ligament (PDL) on the root surface of a previously diseased tooth.

periodontal cyst: A developmental odontogenic epithelium-lined cyst that occurs along the lateral root surface of a vital tooth. Also known as a lateral radicular cyst or lateral periodontal cyst.

periodontal disease: General term that includes all pathologic processes that affect the periodontal tissues. They can be restricted to the soft tissues (gingivitis) or involve all the periodontal support tissues (periodontitis) and induce periodontal attachment loss. **Advanced p.d.**: Chronic or aggressive periodontitis characterized by clinical attachment loss of 5 mm or more. Teeth with resorption of more than a third of the supporting alveolar bone constitute advanced or severe disease. See: Periodontitis.

periodontal dressing: A protective material applied over the wound created by periodontal surgical procedures. Also known as surgical dressing

periodontal fiber: See: Fiber.

periodontal intrabony pocket: A periodontal pocket distinguished by its extension into an intrabony periodontal defect.

periodontal ligament (PDL): Specialized fibrous, richly vascular, cellular connective tissue of the periodontium that surrounds the roots of the teeth and is attached to the root cementum, separating it from and attaching it to the alveolar bone. Main functions are to hold a tooth in its socket and to permit tooth mobility and force distribution and absorption by the alveolar process. Called also periodontal membrane.

periodontal maintenance (formerly referred to as supportive periodontal therapy, preventive maintenance, recall maintenance): Procedures performed at selected intervals to assist the periodontal patient in maintaining oral health.

periodontal medicine: The physiological and pathological interplay between the health of the periodontium and the systemic health of the host.

periodontal membrane: See: Periodontal ligament (PDL).

periodontal plastic surgery: Procedures used to reshape the tissues around the teeth or implants to prevent or correct anatomical, developmental, traumatic, or plaque-induced defects of the gingiva, alveolar mucosa, or bone.

periodontal pocket: A pathologic fissure between a tooth and the crevicular epithelium, and limited at its apex by the junctional epithelium. It is an abnormal apical extension of the gingival crevice caused by migration of the junctional epithelium along the root surface.

periodontal probe: Long, thin manual instrument usually blunted at the end and calibrated in millimeters; used to measure the gingival sulcus or pocket depths around a tooth or an oral implant during a periodontal or peri-implant clinical diagnostic examination.

periodontal recession: Marginal soft tissue recession in which the periodontal attachment apparatus (gingiva, periodontal ligament, and alveolar bone) migrates to a point apical to what occurs in a state of health. See: Recession, Gingival recession.

periodontal regeneration: Restoration of lost periodontium, including development of functionally oriented periodontal ligament (PDL), alveolar bone, and gingiva, on the root surface of a previously diseased tooth with *de novo* formation of cementum.

periodontal soft tissue: Nonmineralized periodontal supporting tissue comprising the gingiva and the periodontal ligament (PDL) tissues; usually refers to the gingival tissues.

periodontal space: The space between the tooth root and alveolar bone containing the periodontal ligament.

periodontal suprabony pocket: A periodontal pocket with its deepest point coronal to the alveolar bone.

periodontal surgery: Surgical procedure for treatment of the periodontium. Includes flap elevation for access, guided tissue regeneration (GTR) for narrow and deep intrabony defects, as well as mucogingival procedures for recession and soft tissue corrections around teeth and implants.

periodontal treatment: Surgical or nonsurgical approaches to the treatment of periodontal diseases.

periodontalgia: Pain associated with the periodontal structures.

periodontally accelerated osteogenic orthodontics (PAOO): A surgical intervention performed in conjunction with orthodontic therapy. This procedure is characterized by full-thickness labial and lingual alveolar flaps accompanied by selective labial and lingual corticotomies.

periodontics: That specialty of dentistry which encompasses the prevention, diagnosis, and treatment of diseases of the supporting and surrounding tissues of the teeth or their substitutes; the maintenance of the health, function, and esthetics of these structures and tissues; and the replacement of lost teeth and supporting structures by grafting or implantation of natural and synthetic devices and materials.

periodontist: A dental practitioner who, by virtue of special knowledge and training in the field, is qualified to and limits his/her practice or activities to periodontics.

periodontitis: Inflammation of the periodontal supporting tissues of the teeth from gingiva into the adjacent bone and ligament. Usually a progressively destructive change leading to loss of bone and periodontal ligament.

- **Adult periodontitis**: A rarely used term. In general, patients previously classified as having adult periodontitis are now included under the chronic periodontitis category.

- **Aggressive periodontitis**: A specific type of periodontitis with unmistakably identifiable clinical and laboratory findings that make it sufficiently different from chronic periodontitis to warrant a separate classification. Aggressive periodontitis occurs in patients who are otherwise clinically healthy (except for periodontal disease). Usual features include rapid attachment loss and bone destruction. Patients with aggressive periodontitis generally exhibit amounts of microbial plaque that are inconsistent with the severity of periodontal destruction, phagocyte abnormalities, and increased levels of *Aggregatibacter actinomycetemcomitans* and possibly *Porphyromonas gingivalis.* The generalized form of aggressive periodontitis was formerly referred to as generalized juvenile periodontitis, Aggressive periodontitis usually affects persons younger than 30 years but patients may be older. Normally, there is widespread interproximal attachment loss affecting at least three teeth other than first molars and incisors, and there is a well-defined intermittent nature regarding the destruction of attachment and alveolar bone. The serum antibody response may be lacking or insufficient in response to the infecting agents. Aggressive periodontitis localized form was formerly termed localized juvenile periodontitis. It has many of the common features of aggressive periodontitis generalized form but the onset occurs at puberty. Localized first molar/incisor involvement with interproximal attachment loss has been associated with a first molar and/or incisor and not more than two other teeth. The localized form typically demonstrates a vigorous serum antibody response to infecting agents.

- **Chronic periodontitis**: An infectious disease that presents with inflammation within the supporting tissues of the teeth. Progressive attachment and bone loss are accompanied by pocket formation and/or recession of the gingiva. Chronic periodontitis is the most frequently occurring form of periodontitis. It is found most often in adults but can also occur in young patients. Plaque and calculus accompany chronic periodontitis. The sequence of attachment loss is typically slow; however, periods of fast development may occur. The microbial configuration is not consistent or predictable.
- **Early-onset periodontitis**: A previously used term. See: Aggressive periodontitis.

- **Juvenile periodontitis**: See: Aggressive periodontitis.
- **Necrotizing ulcerative periodontitis**: An infection characterized by necrosis of gingival tissues, periodontal ligament, and alveolar bone. These lesions are often associated with malnutrition, human immunodeficiency virus infection, and immunosuppression.
- **Periodontitis as manifestation of systemic diseases**: Periodontitis, often with onset at a young age, associated with one of several systemic diseases.
- **Prepubertal periodontitis**: A term rarely used to designate the preadolescent existence of periodontitis. These patients are now incorporated under the chronic periodontitis category or the periodontitis associated with systemic diseases category.
- **Rapidly progressive periodontitis**: A previously used term. See: Chronic periodontitis, Agressive periodontitis.
- **Recurrent periodontitis**: A condition in which periodontitis has been successfully treated but then recurs.
- **Refractory periodontitis**: A condition in which one or more forms of periodontitis are unresponsive to treatment despite excellent patient compliance and delivery of periodontal therapy that ordinarily is successful in arresting the progression of periodontitis.

periodontium: The gingiva, alveolar mucosa, cementum, periodontal ligament, and alveolar bone tissues that surround and support the teeth.

periodontology: The scientific study of periodontal tissues in health and disease.

periodontometry: A method for measuring tooth mobility.

periodontopathic: Agents that induce and/or initiate periodontal pathology.

periosteal release: Act of severing periosteal fibers to enhance the mobility of a flap.

periosteal suture: Suturing technique involving the immobilization of a partial-thickness flap, a soft tissue graft, or a membrane by utilizing the subjacent and/or adjacent periosteum.

periosteitis: An inflammatory process involving the periosteum.

periosteum (pl. periostea): The outer membrane of dense irregular connective tissue that covers all bones except the joints of long bones.

periosystemic links: Refers to the impact of periodontal infections on systemic health and the impact of systemic diseases on the periodontium.

periotest: Instrument used to measure the relative mobility of teeth and dental implants. Device utilizes a tapping piston to percuss a tooth or an implant four times per second. Rate of deceleration recorded at the point of contact is measured as the relative stiffness of the tooth or implant. Periotest values range from -08 to +50, with the -08 to +09 range indicating no discernible movement, +10 to +19 just discernible movement, +20 to +29 obvious movement, and +30 to +50 mobile on pressure.

periotome: An instrument used to separate the periodontal ligament fibers in an effort to extract a tooth with minimal trauma and/or loss of alveolar bone.

peripheral ossifying fibroma: Gingival growth which arises from the periosteum or superficial periodontal ligament and may be pedunculated or sessile.

periradicular: Around or surrounding a tooth root.

perleche: An inflammatory process at the corners of the mouth. More commonly known as angular cheilitis. Often caused by fungal or bacterial infection and can be concomitant with decreased occlusal vertical dimension.

permanent dentition: The adult or second set of teeth that remain after childhood.

permucosal: Occurring, passed, performed, or effected through the mucosa.

permucosal extension: See: Healing abutment.

permucosal seal: Junctional epithelium that separates the connective tissues from the outside environment around a dental implant. See: Junctional epithelium.

pernicious: Capable of damaging or destroying body tissues.

petechiae: Red or purple purpuric eruptions measuring <3 mm in diameter each, occurring from minor hemorrhage of skin or mucous membrane.

PG (abbrev.): Proteoglycan.

PGA (abbrev.): Polyglycolic acid.

PGRF (abbrev.): Plasma rich in growth factors. A glycoprotein growth factor, synthesized and released by certain cells, such as platelets; it is involved in wound healing cascade, such as cell division, angiogenesis, cell differentiation, and tissue remodeling.

phagocyte: Inflammatory cells of the mononuclear phagocyte lineage, capable of ingesting foreign or dead cell matter for elimination.

phagocytosis: The process of cellular ingestion and digestion by phagocytes of solid or semi-solid substances, such as other cells, bacteria, bits of necrotic tissue, and foreign particles.

pharmacodynamics: The study of the biochemical and physiological effects of drugs and their action of mechanism in the body. This also includes the effects on actions of other drugs.

pharmacokinetics: Involved with the absorption, distribution, metabolism, and excretion of drugs.

pharmacology: The study of the interaction of chemicals with biological systems.

pharyngeal walls: Boundaries of the nasopharynx and oropharynx.

pharynx (pl. pharynges): A funnel-shaped anatomic landmark composed of musculature that forms a tube which is the pathway for air and food. It is located between the esophagus, nares, and mouth.

phase contrast microscopy: A method of microscopy that takes advantage of varying intensities of light waves passing through transparent objects, thus providing better differentiation of internal structures.

phase 1 bone regeneration: First steps in healing of a bone defect with formation of woven bone and consolidation of particulate grafted bone, if used, by bridges of woven bone.

phenotype: The physical expression of an individual as determined by genetic and environmental influences.

phenytoin (diphenylhydantoin): An anticonvulsant drug used in the control of epilepsy and other disorders. Often associated with gingival overgrowth.

photogrammetry: The practice of determining the geometric properties of objects from photographic images.

PHSC (abbrev.): Pluripotential hematopoietic stem cell. See: Hematopoietic stem cell.

physical elasticity of muscle: An obsolete term referring to the characteristic of muscle tissue to elongate under tensile forces.

physical injury: A wound produced by inappropriate oral hygiene procedures, inadequate dental restorations, poorly designed dental appliances, orthodontic bands and devices, iatrogenic dentistry or parafunctional habits. May be accidental or deliberate.

physical photometer: A device that captures and quantifies physical stimuli in lieu of visual stimuli.

physiologic architecture: See: Architecture.

physiologic occlusion: An obsolete term that refers to occlusion in compliance with the range of motion and function of the masticatory muscles, and temporomandibular joint.

physiologic rest position: Passive state of mandibular musculature in which the muscles are in equilibrium in tonic contraction and the condyles are in a neutral, unstrained position. The dentition is nonoccluding.

physiologically balanced occlusion: An obsolete term that refers to occlusion that is in harmony with the neuromuscular system and the temporomandibular joint. It is typically related to maximum intercuspation that coincides with the centric relation position; there are no interferences from posterior teeth during lateral or protrusive movements of the mandible.

physiology: The scientific study of the functions of living organs and parts and the ways in which they are affected by chemical and physical laws.

pickle: A medium or bath used for cleaning, preserving, maintaining, or processing.

pick-up impression: Impression of seated superstructure on abutments following surgical implant placement and healing. The superstructure is removed in the impression to obtain a cast incorporating contours of the adjacent soft tissues.

picture archiving and communication system (PACS): Medical imaging technology that provides economical storage of, and convenient access to, images from multiple modalities.

pier: An intermediate abutment for a fixed dental prosthesis.

pier abutment: An abutment positioned between adjacent abutments.

piezoelectric bone surgery: Surgical technique using an ultrasonic device operating at a modulated frequency that is designed to cut or grind bone but not damage the adjacent soft tissues.

piezoelectric surgery: Surgery performed using an instrument which generates microvibrating motion via the application of electromagnetic forces on a polycrystal; the microvibration of the metallic tip results in ostectomy and osteoplasty of the bone.

pigmentation: The deposition of coloring matter; coloration or discoloration of a part by a pigment.

pillar: See: Stack.

pilot drill: Drill used to enlarge the coronal aspect of a dental implant osteotomy, thereby directing the path of the subsequent drill.

pilot osteotomy: The initial penetration in the bone by several millimeters with a drill in the sequence of preparing an osteotomy for dental implant placement.

pixel: Abbreviation of picture element: the smallest possible element of a picture. A digital image is defined by a discrete number of pixels arranged in a 2D grid or mosaic. Many very small pixels blend together in the human eye and brain to give the illusion of a continuous, unbroken image.

PLA (abbrev.): Polylactic acid.

place: To set in or position an implant in a desired location. See: Implant placement.

placebo: An inactive substance resembling one having therapeutic value; used in controlled studies to determine the effect of drugs without the influence of bias.

placement torque: See: Insertion torque.

planning software: Computer program specifically designed for use with virtual surgical planning and guided surgery.

plaque: An organized mass, consisting mainly of microorganisms, that adheres to teeth, prostheses, and oral surfaces and is found in the gingival crevice and periodontal pockets. Other components include an organic, polysaccharide-protein matrix consisting of bacterial by-products such as enzymes, food debris, desquamated cells, and inorganic components such as calcium and phosphate.

plaque control: Preventive measures directed to remove/control dental plaque and prevent it from recurring. See: Oral hygiene.

plasma B cell: See: Plasma cell.

plasma cell: Antibody-producing B lymphocyte that has reached the end of its differentiation pathway. Plasma cells are oval or round with extensive rough endoplasmic reticulum, a well-developed Golgi apparatus, and a round nucleus. Principal effector cell involved in humoral immunity. Called also plasmocyte or plasma B cell.

plasma-containing growth factor: Insulin-like growth factor 1 (IGF-1) is the major growth factor derived from human plasma and found in a variety of tissues and organs including bone matrix.

plasma spray: Method of attaching material to the surface of a structure such as an implant body. The coating is produced by heating the sintered coating material in an argon environment at extremely high temperatures (>15 000 °C). The most common plasma spray coatings are titanium and hydroxyapatite plasma sprays. See: Additive surface treatment.

plasma-sprayed implant: Dental implant with a plasma-sprayed surface.

plasmid: A circular DNA molecule that is maintained separately from the cell's chromosomal DNA and is capable of replicating itself. Plasmids are found mainly in bacteria and also in some eukaryotes, and may encode genes for antibiotic resistance.

plaster: A gypsum material that hardens when mixed with water, used for making impressions and casts. See: Dental stone.

plaster of Paris: Calcium sulfate hemihydrate reduced to a fine powder; the addition of water produces a porous mass that hardens rapidly. It has been used extensively for pouring dental impressions and subsequent casts.

platelet: Colorless nonnuclear disk-shaped structure, 2–4 μm in diameter, found in the blood of all mammals. It is derived from fragments of megakaryocyte cytoplasm and released from the bone marrow into the blood. Contains active enzymes and mitochondria and has an important role in blood coagulation by adhering to other platelets and to damaged epithelium. Called also blood platelet, thrombocyte.

platelet gel: A concentrate of platelets derived from a patient's blood and mixed with calcium and thrombin to form a gel which may be used during surgery.

platelet-derived growth factor (PDGF): A glycoprotein carried in the granules of platelets and released during blood clotting; a potent growth factor for cells of mesenchymal origin, including fibroblasts and smooth muscle cells. Growth factors released by platelets initiate connective tissue healing including bone regeneration and repair. They also increase mitogenesis, angiogenesis, and macrophage activation.

platelet-poor plasma (PPP): Preparation obtained from whole blood by differential centrifugation. PPP has a relatively high concentration of fibrinogen and is used for autologous fibrin glue preparation, which is employed in surgeries to obtain hemostasis and glue down flaps.

platelet-rich gel: See: Platelet-rich plasma.

platelet-rich plasma (PRP): (syn): Platelet-rich gel. Autologous preparation derived from whole blood through the process of gradient density centrifugation. Its intended purpose lies in its ability to incorporate high concentrations of growth factors PDGF, TGF-β1, TGF-β2, IGF, VEGF, FGF-1, and fibrin when added to a graft mixture.

platform: (syn): Prosthetic table, restorative platform, seating surface. Refers to the coronal aspect of a dental implant to which abutments, components, and prosthesis may be connected. See: Platform edge.

platform edge: The junction line between the body of a dental implant and its platform. The localization of the platform edge in relationship to the bone crest determines a crestal, subcrestal, or supracrestal positioning of the implant. The edge of the platform and the implant abutment junction may or may not coincide. See: Implant–abutment junction (IAJ), Platform switching.

platform fitting: Implant platform and implant abutment of the same size.

platform shifting: See: Platform switching.

platform swapping: See: Platform switching.

platform switching: (syn): Abutment swapping. The use of an abutment with a diameter narrower than that of the dental implant platform. This switching moves the implant–abutment junction away from the edge of the platform.

pleomorphism: The assumption of various distinct structural forms or shapes by a single organism or species.

plexus: A branching network; chiefly of nerves, lymphatics, or veins.

plunger cusp: A cusp that tends to force food into interproximal areas.

pluripotential hematopoietic stem cell (PHSC): See: Hematopoietic stem cell.

PMCB (abbrev.): Particulate marrow cancellous bone.

PMMA (abbrev.): Polymethylmethacrylate.

pneumatization: Physiologic process that occurs in all paranasal sinuses during the growth period, causing them to increase in volume. See: Sinus pneumatization (maxillary).

pocket: See: Periodontal pocket.

pogonion: The furthermost anterior point on the mandible.

point cloud: A set of vertices in a 3D coordinate system. These vertices are usually defined by X, Y, and Z coordinates, and typically are intended to represent the external surface of an object. Point clouds are most often created by 3D scanners, which automatically measure a large number of points on the surface of an object, and often output

a point cloud as a data file. The point cloud represents the set of points that the device has measured.

polished implant surface: Implant surface intentionally made extremely smooth using abrasives or electrical polishing methods. Compare: Turned implant surface.

polishing cap: Component connected to the apical part of an abutment to protect the base and allow the laboratory technician to polish the prosthesis and abutment without overreducing the base diameter or rounding the edges. Or an abutment analog or implant analog that is connected to the prosthesis and used to protect the intermediate connection surface during dental laboratory finishing and polishing procedures.

polycythemia: An abnormal increase in the proportion of red cells in the blood.

polyglactin: A type of multifilament braided material made of purified lactides and glycosides used to fabricate absorbable sutures or membranes, or surgical mesh.

polyglass: Variety of resin-ceramic composite materials for use as direct restorative materials or as CAD/CAM indirect restorative materials.

polyglycolic acid (PGA): Biodegradable, rigid thermoplastic polymer of glycolic acid and the simplest linear, aliphatic polyester used as a material for the synthesis of absorbable sutures and barrier membranes and as a carrier for bone morphogenetic proteins (BMPs). When exposed to physiologic conditions, PGA is degraded by random hydrolysis and apparently also broken down by certain enzymes, especially those with esterase activity. The degradation product, glycolic acid, is nontoxic and can enter the tricarboxylic acid cycle, after which it is excreted as water and carbon dioxide. A part of the glycolic acid is also excreted by urine. See: Guided tissue regeneration (GTR).

polygon mesh: A collection of vertices, edges, and faces that defines the shape of a polyhedral object in 3D computer graphics and solid modeling. The faces usually consist of triangles, quadrilaterals, or other simple convex polygons.

polylactic acid (PLA): Biodegradable, hydrophobic, thermoplastic, and aliphatic polyester derived from lactic acid. PLA can be processed in fiber and film and has extensive applicability. In the biomedical field, it is used in a number of applications, including sutures, drug delivery devices, membranes, and as a carrier for bone morphogenetic proteins (BMPs). Called also polylactide. See: Guided tissue regeneration (GTR).

polylactide: See: Polylactic acid (PLA).

polymer: Chemical compound or compound mixtures created by molecular reaction to form larger organic molecules containing repeating structural units. A long-chain hydrocarbon. See: Resin.

polymethylmethacrylate (PMMA): Bone cement, a polymer of methylmethacrylate, which polymerizes *in situ* with curing temperatures exceeding 100 °C; completely nonbiodegradable.

polymorphism: Existing in multiple forms or having numerous morphologic types.

polymorphonuclear leukocyte: A type of scavenging white blood cell involved in fighting infections that contains a segmented lobular nucleus and is colorless because of the lack of hemoglobin; eosinophils, basophils, and neutrophils are in this category.

polymorphonuclear neutrophil: See: Polymorphonuclear leukocyte.

polyostotic: Pertaining to or affecting many bones.

polyp: A pedunculated tumor arising from a mucous membrane.

polysulfide: A synthetic rubber used in dental impression materials; it contains chains of sulfur atoms that are anionic or organic in nature.

polytetrafluoroethylene (PTFE): Homopolymer of tetrafluoroethylene (CF_2-CF_2)n that is a nonflammable, tough, inert resin with good resistance to chemicals and heat. Used as a surgical implant material for guided tissue regeneration (GTR), guided bone regeneration (GBR), prostheses such as artificial vessels and orbital floor implants, and for many applications in skeletal augmentation and skeletal fixation. Also used widely in industry, e.g., to insulate, protect, or lubricate apparatuses.

pontic: An artificial tooth on a fixed dental prosthesis that replaces a missing natural tooth, restores its function, and usually fills the space previously occupied by the clinical crown.

porcelain: A ceramic material formed of infusible elements joined by lower fusing materials. Most dental porcelains are glasses and are used in the fabrication of teeth for dentures, pontics and facings, metal ceramic restorations including fixed dental prostheses, as well as all-ceramic restorations such as crowns, laminate veneers, inlays, onlays, and other porcelain-fused-to-metal restorations.

porcelain fracture: The cohesive failure of porcelain. Etiology of the fracture may be imperfections or stresses residual from fabrication, incompatibility with substrate (thermal coefficient of expansion), substructure deformation because of misfit or inadequate structural integrity, or overload caused by occlusion or trauma.

porcelain-fused-to-metal restoration: See: Metal ceramic restoration

porcelain laminate veneer: A thin bonded ceramic restoration that restores the facial surface and part of the proximal surfaces of teeth requiring esthetic restoration.

porous: Property of allowing ingress of fluid or gas within a material or surface; sponge-like quality.

porous bovine-derived hydroxyapatite: See: Bovine-derived anorganic bone matrix.

porous coralline hydroxyapatite: Bone substitute developed from the Porites or Goniopora coral, in which the $CaCO_3$ skeleton of the coral is converted via a hydrothermal process into a hydroxyapatite (HA) substitute with trace levels of beta-tricalcium phosphate. It is nonresorbable but osteoconductive because of the nonending porous structure.

porous surface: See: Plasma-sprayed implant, Sintered (porous) surface.

Porphyromonas gingivalis: A gram-negative, nonmotile, rod-shaped anaerobic bacterium from the phylum Bacteroidetes.

Commonly found in subgingival dental plaque, it is an etiologic agent in the development of chronic periodontal disease. A member of the red complex bacteria.

positional record: Documentation that uses intraoral and extraoral registrations to capture a specified mandibular position.

positioned flap: A flap that is moved apically, coronally, or laterally to a new position.

positive architecture: When the crest of the interdental gingiva or bone is located coronal to its midfacial midlingual margins.

positive predictive value: The proportion of positive responses to a diagnostic test for disease that are accurate indicators of the true presence of the malady in a population. Expressed arithmetically as a proportion calculated as the number of true-positive responses divided by the sum of true-positive responses plus false-positive responses, i.e., positive predictive value = TP/(TP + FP).

post and core crown: A restoration in which the crown and cast post are one unit.

posterior: Located behind; in human anatomy often referred to as caudal; dorsal.

posterior border jaw relation: An obsolete term that refers to the border relationship between the maxilla and the most posterior portion of the mandible.

posterior dentition: Natural teeth or tooth replacements other than the incisors and canines. See: Dentition.

posterior lateral nasal artery: Branch of the sphenopalatine artery which is located close to or within the lateral wall of the nasal cavity (medial wall of the maxillary sinus). Its subdivisions supply the medial and posterior walls of the maxillary sinus. It is one of the three primary arterial suppliers to the maxillary sinus. See: Infraorbital artery, Posterior superior alveolar artery.

posterior superior alveolar artery: Branch of the internal maxillary artery, at the pterygopalatine fossa. This branch descends on the maxillary tuberosity and gives off numerous subdivisions that enter the alveolar process to supply the maxillary sinus membrane and posterior teeth. It is one of the three primary arterial suppliers to the maxillary sinus.

See: Anterior superior alveolar nerve, Infraorbital artery, Posterior lateral nasal artery.

posterior tooth form: The morphologic characteristics of the posterior teeth, including the shape of the tooth and its occlusal surfaces.

postmenopausal atrophy: Deterioration or degradation of tissue, including oral mucosa and bone, that occurs in women after menopause.

postoperative maxillary sinus cyst: See: Secondary maxillary mucocele.

postpalatal seal area: Area of the soft palate located beyond the junction of the hard and soft palate that should be compressed within physiological limits by the post dam part of the maxillary conventional complete denture to achieve an adequate peripheral seal and denture retention.

postsurgical maxillary prosthesis: A maxillofacial prosthesis constructed to correct the intraoral/extraoral defect resulting from maxillary resection due to a tumor or reconstruction of acquired or congenital defects of the maxilla to improve esthetics and function.

postural contraction: The minimal muscular contraction required to maintain mandibular posture.

postural position: Any mandibular position occurring during minimal muscular contraction.

powder bed fusion: Additive manufacturing process that utilizes an inkjet-type printer head that deposits a fluid in a predefined pattern over a layer of powder material. The combination of powder and fluid form a solid structure that can be removed from the powder "bed" after the process is complete. Once removed, the solid object can be further treated to bring about the desired characteristics of strength, hardness, or appearance.

powertome/periotome: An instrument used to separate the periodontal ligament fibers during an atraumatic extraction of teeth minimizing the loss of bone.

PPP (abbrev.): Platelet-poor plasma.

PRDP (abbrev.): Partial removable dental prosthesis.

preangled abutment: See: Angulated abutment.

preangled abutment one piece: The one-piece stock.

preangled abutment two piece: A two-piece stock dental implant abutment that has a preset angle to the long axis of the implant fixture.

preceramic solder: A soldering procedure of the metal framework of a metal-ceramic prosthesis before ceramic build-up at a temperature of 1075–1120 °C.

precious metal: Naturally occurring rare metallic element with a set of physical and chemical properties unrivaled by other materials. It is less chemically reactive than most elements. Examples include gold, platinum, osmium, iridium, palladium, ruthenium, rhodium, and silver.

precision attachment: 1. A retainer consisting of a metal receptacle (matrix) and a closely fitting part (patrix); the matrix is usually contained within the normal or expanded contours of the crown on the abutment tooth/dental implant and the patrix is attached to a pontic or the removable dental prosthesis framework. 2. An interlocking device, one component of which is fixed to an abutment or abutments, and the other is integrated into a removable dental prosthesis in order to stabilize and/or retain it.

prednisolone: An intramuscular and intravenous glucocorticoid with an intermediate half-life. See: Glucocorticoid.

prednisone: An oral glucocorticoid that is the dehydrogenated analog of cortisol. It is used as an antiinflammatory drug, with an intermediate half-life. See: Glucocorticoid.

preemptive analgesia: The use of analgesic medications before the onset of noxious stimuli.

prefabricated: Manufactured in a standardized form or method in anticipation of application.

prefabricated abutment: Prosthetic component manufactured to fit an implant following a design specific to the manufacturer's implant system dimensions.

prefabricated cylinder: A prefabricated component made of a noble alloy, which connects to a dental implant or abutment. A compatible alloy is cast to it to form a custom abutment for a cement-retained or screw-retained prosthesis.

preliminary cast: A cast produced from a preliminary impression for use as a diagnostic tool or special tray construction.

preliminary impression: A negative likeness constructed using a stock tray; the cast produced from this impression is mainly used in diagnosis, treatment planning, or special tray construction.

preload: The tension created in a screw, especially the fluked threading, when tightened. An engineering term used to describe the degree of tightness of a screw, usually in implant dentistry.

premature contact: See: Deflective occlusal contact.

premedication: Medication given prior to an anesthetic or operation.

preoperative cast: A positive likeness of a part or parts of the oral cavity for the purpose of diagnosis and treatment planning. See: Diagnostic cast.

preoperative record: Any record made for the purpose of study or treatment planning.

preoperative wax-up: A dental diagnostic procedure in which planned restorations are developed in wax on a diagnostic cast to determine optimal clinical and laboratory procedures necessary to achieve the desired esthetics and function. Called also diagnostic wax-up, preoperative waxing.

prepable abutment: An abutment that can be prepared and modified from its original manufactured design.

preparation: Planned and executed definitive form of a natural tooth or implant abutment following instrumentation to receive a prosthetic restoration.

preprosthetic surgery: Surgical procedures designed to facilitate fabrication of a prosthesis or to improve the prognosis of prosthodontic care.

preprosthetic vestibuloplasty: Surgical procedure that deepens or lengthens the vestibulum. Several techniques exist, often involving healing by secondary intention or using mucosal or dermal free grafts or split-thickness skin grafts.

prepubertal periodontitis: See: Periodontitis.

press-fit: State of retention of a dental implant at the time of its insertion that results from the slight compression of the oseotomy walls by the implant body. Or joint held together by friction of the parts. Mode of attachment used (either by itself or in conjunction with a screw) by several implant manufacturers for approximating the abutment into the implant body. Also applies to the close adaptation of a root-form (i.e., cylindrical) implant to its osteotomy site at the time of placement.

pressure area: A region of mucosa that is being subjected to excessive pressure from a dental prosthesis.

pressure indicating paste: A material injected or spread on the intaglio surface of the denture to determine the pressure area on the supporting tissue of a dental prosthesis.

pressure necrosis: Cell death due to insufficient local blood supply from pressure. In implant dentistry, it refers to the loss of bone that occurs following the application of excessive pressure by the insertion of a dental implant.

pressure relief: Alteration of the denture-bearing surface of a denture to reduce force on the underlying tissues.

presurgical consideration: See: Patient selection.

pretreatment records: Any records made for the purpose of diagnosis, recording of the patient history, or treatment planning in advance of therapy.

prevalence: Proportion or rate of persons in a population who had a condition at any given time. Compare: Incidence.

preventive: Serving to avert the occurrence of.

preventive maintenance: See: Periodontal maintenance.

Prevotella: Formerly called *Bacteroides* spp. See also *Porphyromonas*. *P. intermedia*: Gram-negative, nonmotile, anaerobic, nonspore-forming bacillus isolated from oral and other body sites. A common inhabitant of the gingival crevice, it has been associated with infections of the head, neck, and pleura. *P. melininogenica*: Gram-negative, nonmotile, anaerobic, rod-shaped bacteria. Formerly called *Bacteroides melaninogenicus*.

primary adhesion: See: Healing by first (primary) intention.

primary bone: See: Bone/Woven bone.

primary closure: Surgical wound closure by close flap adaption and complete coverage of the surgical site. This approach leads to healing by primary intention.

primary implant failure: See: Early implant failure/loss.

primary impression: See: Preliminary impression.

primary maxillary mucocele: Maxillary sinus lesion caused by blockage of the ostium which results in herniation through the sinus walls. See: Secondary maxillary mucocele.

primary pain: Pain proximately associated with a noxious stimulus, versus referred pain, which is nonproximate.

primary soft tissue healing: See: Healing by first (primary) intention.

primary stability: Clinically, implant immobility at the time of surgical placement, resulting from intimate contact of the implant with the bony walls of the osteotomy. Primary stability decreases with time as osseous remodeling occurs. It is distinct from secondary implant stability, which is the result of new bone formation and osseointegration. Compare: Secondary stability.

primary union: See: Healing by first (primary) intention.

primitive bone: See: Bone/Woven bone.

probe: A slender instrument, often calibrated, that is used to explore or measure a wound, body cavity, passage, or periodontal pocket.

probing depth: The distance from the soft tissue (gingiva or alveolar mucosa) margin to the tip of the periodontal probe during usual periodontal diagnostic probing. The health of the attachment apparatus can affect the measurement. **Clinical attachment level**:

The distance from the cementoenamel junction to the tip of the periodontal probe during usual periodontal diagnostic probing.

Relative attachment level: The distance from a fixed reference point on a tooth or stent to the tip of the periodontal probe during usual periodontal diagnostic probing.

process: 1. A bony projection or prominence. 2. Any technical procedure that involves multiple steps. 3. The procedure used to polymerize dental resin in the production of dental prostheses or bases. **Alveolar p.**: The compact and cancellous bony structure that contains tooth sockets that surrounds and supports the teeth.

process jig: See: Analog.

processed denture base: A heat-polymerized, dense, color-stable acrylic foundation that attaches to artificial teeth.

processing analog: syn. Processing jig. A duplicate of either the male or female part of an attachment that is incorporated into a working model.

processing jig: See: Processing analog.

prodrome: An early symptom indicating the onset of a disease or condition.

product liability litigation: Legal proceeding to determine if a specific product resulted in injury, loss, or damage.

profile: An outline image of an object or structure as viewed from the side.

profile of a patient: See: Emergence profile.

profile record: A record or registration of a patient facial profile.

profiler (bone): Bur that removes bone around the platform of a root-form dental implant to allow the connection of components to the implant. Different profiler diameters are used to accommodate a desired component diameter.

profilometer: Instrument used to measure the relative roughness of a particular topography. In dental applications, it is used to measure the relative roughness of implant surfaces.

progenitor cell: Relatively undifferentiated cells that have the capacity for both replication and differentiation and give rise to one or more types of specialized cells. **Mesenchymal p. c.**: See: Mesenchymal stem cell (MSC).

progesterone: A generic term for naturally occurring steroid hormones containing a prename nucleus; secreted from the corpus luteum and placenta; a lute hormone; implicated in hormonal and pubertal gingivitis.

prognathic: A forward relationship of the mandible and/or maxilla to the skeletal base in which either of the jaws (usually the mandible) protrudes beyond a imaginary line in the sagittal plane of the skull.

prognathism: The condition of a protruded position of the maxilla and/or mandible in relation to the face.

prognosis: A prediction as to the progress, course, and outcome of a disease.

progressive loading: Concept of gradually increasing the amount of functional load applied to a newly integrated dental implant or implants by modifying the design and the material of the prosthesis. Based upon the assumption that the Wolff Law applies to the bone adjacent to newly osseointegrated dental implants. See: Wolff Law.

progressive mandibular lateral translation: The lateral positional change of the mandible as the nonworking condyle translates along the articular eminence.

progressive maxillary sinus hypoplasia: An uncommon clinical entity that represents a persistent decrease in sinus volume resulting from centripetal retraction of the maxillary sinus walls.

progressive systemic sclerosis (scleroderma): A chronic disorder of unknown cause characterized by progressive fibrosis of skin and multiple organs, and by vascular insufficiency. Oral structures become indurated and stiff; radiographically, the periodontal ligament spaces may be thickened.

projected pain: The sensation of pain at an area remote from the site of origin.

prophylaxis: The use of measures to prevent the onset of disease. **Antibiotic p.**: The administration of antibiotics to patients without evidence of infection to prevent microbial colonization and thus avoid or

reduce subsequent postoperative complications.
Oral p.: Preventing gingivitis through the removal of bacterial plaque, materia alba, calculus, and extrinsic stain from the teeth and roots performed by a dentist or hygienist. See: Periodontal maintenance.

Propionibacterium spp.: Gram-positive, nonmotile, anaerobic, rod-shaped, slow-growing bacteria primarily isolated from subgingival plaque. *P. propionicus:* Gram-positive, nonmotile, facultative, rod-shaped bacteria found primarily in subgingival plaque. Formerly called *Arachnia propionica.*

proportional limit: The measurement of stresses that is the point beyond which deformation is not directly proportional to the load being applied.

proprioception: Perception of movement and spatial orientation of the body or parts of the body. In the oral cavity, the periodontal ligament possesses refined mechanoreceptors that provide highly sensitive neural feedback. This perception is lost or damaged following tooth extraction. It has been proposed that osseoperception of dental implants exists, although on a much lower level than proprioception of natural teeth.

proprioceptor: Sensory nerve terminal that mediates signals related to movement and position of the body and its parts.

prospective study: Study planned in advance of data collection. Considered to be more reliable than retrospective studies, because potentially confounding variables can be better controlled when the study question is known before data is collected. Compare: Retrospective study.

prostaglandins: A family of fatty acids, unsaturated carboxylic acids, generated by arachidonic acid metabolism via the cyclooxygenase pathway. They are produced by most cells and are potent regulators of a number of biological processes. Their production is inhibited by aspirin, ibuprofen, and other inhibitors of cyclooxygenase.

prosthesis (pl. prostheses): 1. A fabricated, artificial replacement of a missing part of the human body. 2. A device to improve or alter function of a damaged or missing body part.

3. A device used to help achieve a desired surgical outcome.

prosthesis bar, dolder: See: Dolder bar.

prosthesis construction: Fixed or removable orodental, maxillofacial, or cranial prosthesis. See: Restoration.

prosthesis, temporary: A fixed or removable restoration which will eventually be replaced with a more permanent device.

prosthetic: Concerning prosthetics or a prosthesis.

prosthetic joint: Artificial replacement for a natural joint. Usually indicated as the result of arthritic degeneration or trauma in a natural human joint.

prosthetic platform: See: Platform.

prosthetic retaining screw: Prosthetic component serving as a retention screw; used to connect the prosthetic component to the mesostructure or to a transmucosal element.

prosthetic screw: A threaded fastener used to connect a prosthesis to a dental implant, an abutment, or a mesostructure.

prosthetic space: See: Crown height space.

prosthetic table: See: Platform, Occlusal table.

prosthetics: The art and science of supplying missing parts of the human body.

protein: Any of a group of complex organic compounds which contain carbon, hydrogen, oxygen, nitrogen, and usually sulfur, the characteristic element being nitrogen. Proteins, the principal constituents of the protoplasm of all cells, are of high molecular weight and consist essentially of combinations of alpha-amino acids in peptide linkages. Twenty different amino acids are commonly found in proteins, and each protein has a unique, genetically defined amino acid sequence which determines its specific shape and function. Their roles include enzymatic catalysis, transport and storage, coordinated motion, nerve impulse generation and transmission, control of growth and differentiation, immunity, and mechanical support.

proteoglycan (PG): Extracellular and cell surface macromolecules derived from a class of glycoproteins of high molecular weight occurring primarily in the matrix of connective tissue and cartilage. Proteoglycans are composed of a protein core with sites for the attachment of one or more polysaccharide chains, particularly glycosaminoglycan; they assemble polysaccharides rather than proteins in their side chains. PGs function in cell adhesion, growth, and organization of the extracellular matrix.

protocol: Precise and detailed set of instructions or directions for performing a study. The instructions state what the study will do and how and why it will be performed. It explains how many subjects will be included, who is eligible to participate (i.e., inclusion and exclusion criteria), what and how often study agents or other interventions will be performed, what controls and tests will be included, what information will be gathered, and how the information will be analyzed.

protooncogene: A gene in the normal human genome that appears to have a role in normal cellular physiology and is often involved in regulation of normal cell growth and proliferation.

protrusion: Indicating teeth or other maxillary and mandibular structures that are positioned anterior to the normal or to the generally accepted standard.

protrusive: Thrusting forward; adjective denoting protrusion.

protrusive deflection: The displacement of the mandible from the midline during the protrusive movement of the mandible; the symptomatic restriction of mandibular movement.

protrusive deviation: The amount of protrusive deflection during protrusive movement of the mandible. Protrusive deviation indicates interference during movement.

protrusive interocclusal record: A registration of the mandibular movement relative to the maxilla during forward movement of the condyles in the temporal fossa.

protrusive jaw relation: A jaw relation resulting from an anterior positioning of the mandible.

protrusive movement: Mandibular movement anterior to centric relation.

protrusive occlusion: An obsolete term referring to an occlusion that results when the mandible is advanced anterior to centric maximum intercuspation.

provisional abutment: See: Temporary abutment.

provisional cementation: The cementation of an interim or final restoration with a weak luting agent such that the restoration can be easily removed at a future date.

provisional implant: Endosseous implant made to smaller dimensional specifications with narrow widths. Can be used for a defined period of time (i.e., immediate, temporary, and/or transitional) or to support a transitional prosthesis. See: Mini-implant, Transitional implant.

provisional prosthesis: Fixed, removable, or maxillofacial tooth- or implant-supported prosthesis designed for limited-term use.

provisional prosthesis/restoration: See: Interim prosthesis/restoration.

provisional restoration: See: Provisional prosthesis.

provisional splint: An interim device that stabilizes mobile teeth during diagnostic or therapeutic procedures. Also known as an interim splint.

provisionalization: Act of planning and fabricating a prosthesis amenable to alteration and use for a limited time period. See: Provisional prosthesis.

proximal: 1. Nearest or adjacent to the reference point. 2. Situated near a point of origin, the midline or attachment. 3. In dentistry; the tooth surface adjacent to another tooth.

proximal wedge: A periodontal surgical procedure for removal of excessive soft tissue mesial or distal to a tooth or teeth in an arch. See: Wedge procedure, Distal wedge.

PRP (abbrev.): Platelet-rich plasma.

pseudomembrane: A thin, adherent, gray-white exudative layer that forms over mucosa. It appears as a false membrane and is composed of necrotic cells, debris, and bacteria. Pseudomembranes are seen in necrotizing ulcerative periodontitis.

pseudopocket: A deepening of the gingival crevice resulting primarily from an increase in bulk of the gingiva without apical migration of the junctional epithelium or destruction of the periodontal ligament and alveolar bone.

pseudopocket space: The gingival crevice containing the periodontal ligament.

pseudopocket syndrome: A collection of symptoms and clinical signs characteristic of periodontal diseases such as inflammation, loss of the gingiva, tooth mobility, etc.

pseudopocket traumatism: See: Occlusal traumatism.

psychophysical: A term referring to the relationship between physical stimuli and sensory perception of the physical stimuli.

psychophysical color: A measurement of color stimuli by scientifically defined values, such as tri-stimulus coordinates.

pterygoid implant: A root-form dental implant that has its origin in the region of the former second maxillary molar and its end-point encroaches in the scaphoid fossa of the sphenoid bone. The implant follows an intrasinusal trajectory in a dorsal and mesi-ocranial direction, perforating the posterior sinusal wall and the pterygoid plates.

pullout force: Force needed to displace an implant along its long axis and opposite from its direction of placement.

pullout strength: Mechanical testing method used to determine the relative resistance to removal of a dental implant. The test may be used immediately following implant placement to determine primary implant stability or at various times following placement and during the healing period. Determines the relative advantages (or disadvantages) of various shapes, materials, and surface textures for dental implants.

pulp: Richly vascularized and innervated connective tissue found at the inner core of a tooth called the pulp cavity. The pulp is divided into the coronal aspect (coronal pulp) and root aspect (radicular pulp).

pulp capping: The placement of a material or medicament to serve as a barrier to protect the pulp and promote healing of the pulpal tissues. Pulp capping is accomplished either directly or indirectly.

pulp vitality tests: Tests used to determine whether the pulp of a tooth is without vitality, inflamed, or within normal limits of health. The different tests include electrical stimulation, thermal stimulation, or the more invasive cutting into dentin with a bur to determine sensitivity.

pulpectomy: Complete extirpation of the coronal and radicular pulp.

pulpitis: A state of inflammation of the dental pulp that can be reversible or nonreversible.

pulpotomy (pulp amputation): The surgical removal of the coronal portion of a vital pulp to preserve the vitality of the remaining radicular portion.

pulsed mode: Type of operation in which the laser emits radiation energy in the form of pulses.

pumice: Sand-like volcanic glass that is used as a polishing agent in dentistry. Different sized particles proceeding from coarser to finer are used to progressively smooth a hard surface. Materials polished may include natural tooth structure, acrylic, and other restorative materials.

punch technique: See: Tissue punch technique.

pure titanium: See: Titanium (Ti).

purpura: Hemorrhage into the tissues with resultant large discoloration (greater than 2 mm in diameter) that does not blanch on pressure. Initial discoloration is red/purple, but later it becomes brown-yellow as it fades away.

purulent: Accompanied by or containing pus.

pus: A generally viscous, yellowish-white fluid formed in infected and inflamed tissue consisting of white blood cells, cellular debris, necrotic tissue, and bacteria.

pustule: A reaction of tissue to infection that results in a small superficial elevation caused by the collection of pus under the skin.

pyogenic: Pus-producing substance or agent.

pyogenic granuloma: See: Granuloma.

pyorrhea: A description of periodontal disease, not in common use.

pyramidal fracture: A complex of fractures of the midfacial bones involving the upper jawbone. The main fracture lines meet above the nasal bones and form a triangular section detached from the skull.

Q

quadrant: One of the four sections into which the dental arches can be divided, as determined by an imaginary midline between the central incisors, dividing each dental arch into two halves.

quality of life: See: Oral health-related quality of life.

quartz: The second most abundant mineral in the earth's continental crust. It is an extremely hard material made up of a continuous framework of SiO_4.

quinolones: A class of synthetic, broad-spectrum antibacterial agents that exhibit bactericidal action.

Glossary of Dental Implantology, First Edition. Khalid Almas, Fawad Javed and Steph Smith.
© 2018 John Wiley & Sons, Inc. Published 2018 by John Wiley & Sons, Inc.

R

R value: A two-dimensional roughness parameter calculated from the experimental profiles after filtering. R_a: The arithmetic average of the absolute value of all points of the profile, also called central line average height. R_t: The maximum peak-to-valley height of the entire measurement trace.

RAD (abbrev.): Radiation absorbed dose, a unit of absorbed dose of ionizing radiation equivalent to an energy of 100 ergs per gram of irradiated material.

radiation: In dentistry, usually refers to ionizing radiation. The energy that comes from a source of unstable atoms, which have excess energy, is then passed through tissue, producing charged particles called ions. These unstable ions are radioactive and become stable by release of energy, which can be in the form of electromagnetic radiation, such as X-rays, or particulate rays, such as gamma rays.

radiation-damaged bone and soft tissues: See: Osteoradionecrosis (ORN).

radiation shield: A prosthesis used during radiation treatment that protects adjacent areas of tissue not meant to be radiated from ortho-voltage during treatment of malignant lesions of the head and neck area. Also known as a radiation positioner.

radiation source prosthesis: A prosthesis made for a specific patient to aid in the trajectory and targeting of radiation to an anatomic site in order to treat a tumor at that site.

radicular: Pertaining to the root of a tooth and its adjacent structures.

radiodensity: The relatively opaque white appearance of dense materials or substances on radiographic imaging studies.

radiograph: An image generated on a sensitive surface (sensor) by a form of radiation other than visible light, specifically, an X-ray or gamma ray picture.

radiographic guide: See: Radiographic template.

radiographic marker: A radiopaque structure of known dimension or a material incorporated in, or applied to, a radiographic template to yield positional or dimensional information.

radiographic prosthesis: Prosthesis that represents the position of missing teeth and dentoalveolar tissues for radiographic imaging. Structure or marking that directs the motion or positioning of something. It is used to transfer the intended position of the implant from the diagnostic cast to the patient and to record its relationship to the underlying bone.

radiographic template: Acrylic resin guide used by the surgeon to direct placement of an implant into its proper position. It is based on the information from two-dimensional panoramic radiographs or three-dimensional computed tomography (CT) or digital volume tomography (DVT) images to achieve optimal implant body placement within the available bone and to preserve vital structures.

radiology: Medical specialty directing medical imaging technologies for the diagnosis and possible treatment of diseases.

Glossary of Dental Implantology, First Edition. Khalid Almas, Fawad Javed and Steph Smith.
© 2018 John Wiley & Sons, Inc. Published 2018 by John Wiley & Sons, Inc.

radiolucent: Relatively more penetrable by electromagnetic radiation, with relatively little attenuation by absorption. In radiography, radiolucent materials appear to have shades of gray to black on radiographs.

radionecrosis: Osteonecrosis induced by radiation. It can occur in patients who have undergone radiotherapy because of a malignant process in the ear, nose, and throat (ENT) or other maxillofacial region.

radiopaque: Relatively less penetrable by electromagnetic radiation; In radiography, radiopaque materials appear light or white on the exposed radiograph.

radiopaque marker: Marker made of metal or any radiopaque material (e.g., radiopaque filling material) that is placed into the mouth before taking radiographs. Detected in the radiograph, the markers help to interpret the image mostly for length, angulation, or localization assessment.

ramus: Bilateral posterior vertical extensions of the mandibular body. At the superior border, each ramus ends in two processes: the coronoid, which is anterior, and the condyle, which is separated posteriorly by a deep concavity. See: Mandibular ramus.

ramus endosteal implant: A dental implant that is inserted at least partially into the ramus of the mandible.

ramus frame endosteal implant: A dental implant design comprising a horizontal intraoral supragingival bar-shaped abutment and bilateral posterior endosseous segments that pass through the soft tissues and enter the ramus on each side of the mandible. An anterior segment also passes through the soft tissue covering the symphysis and enters the symphyseal bone. These implants are typically constructed from one piece of metal, although two or five endosteal sectional implant segments can be placed and connected with fitted parts after placement of the individual segments. See: Implant, oral.

ramus graft: An autogenous bone graft harvested from the lateral aspect of the ascending ramus of the mandible. The graft is mostly cortical bone. See: Alveolar ridge augmentation, Bone graft, Mandibular block graft.

ramus implant: Type of blade implant placed into the anterior border of the ramus of the mandible.

random assignment: Process of assigning study participants to experimental or control groups at random, such that each participant has an equal probability of being assigned to any given group. This method of assignment helps to prevent bias in a study.

randomized controlled trial: A prospective study of the effects of a particular procedure or material, in which subjects are randomly assigned to either of two groups: test or control. The test group receives the procedure or material, while the control group receives a standard procedure, or material, a different test procedure or a placebo.

randomization: See: Random assignment.

range: Statistical measure of dispersion. Distance between the highest and the lowest values of distribution.

range of motion: A measurement of the degree to which a joint may be extended or flexed. A measurement describing the degree to which the temporomandibular joint may move as in opening or demonstrating lateral or protrusive excursions.

rank sum test: Comparison of two groups on the median values of the response variable. Called also Wilcoxon rank sum test.

RAP (abbrev.): Regional acceleratory phenomenon.

raphe: 1. An area marking the line of union. 2. A fibrous area where paired muscles meet.

rapid manufacturing: See: Solid freeform fabrication (SFF), Stereolithography, Three-dimensional printing.

rapid prototyping: The automatic construction of physical objects using solid freeform fabrication. It takes virtual designs from computer-aided design (CAD) or animated modeling software, transforms them into thin, virtual, horizontal cross-sections and then creates each cross-section in physical space, one after the next, until the model is finished. See: Stereolithography, Three-dimensional printing.

rapidly progressive periodontitis: See: Periodontitis.

raster graphics image (bitmap): A dot matrix data structure representing a generally rectangular grid of pixels, or points of color, viewable via a monitor, paper, or other display medium.

ratchet: Instrument with a mechanism consisting of a metal wheel operating with a catch that permits motion in only one direction. Used with threaded implants to facilitate final implant seating.

RBM (abbrev.): Resorbable blast media.

reactive bone: See: Bone, Wolff's Law.

reamer: Tool designed to finish the mating surface of a metal cylinder/coping, specifically the screw seat interface.

reattachment: A periodontics term that describes the reconnection of epithelial and/or connective tissues to the surfaces of roots or bone after the connection is disrupted by surgical or other means. Not to be confused with new attachment.

rebase: A dental laboratory process by which the entire base material of an existing removable prosthesis, but not the teeth, is replaced.

recall appointment after implantation: Scheduled dental visits after endosseous implants have been placed in a patient.

recall maintenance: See: Periodontal maintenance.

receptor activator of nuclear factor-kappa B ligand (RANKL): A 317-amino acid peptide, member of the tumor necrosis factor (TNF) superfamily, that stimulates osteoclast differentiation and activity as well as inhibiting osteoclast apoptosis. It is expressed by osteoblast-stromal cells, fibroblasts, and activated T cells. In the bone tissue, RANKL binds directly to its receptor (i.e., receptor activator of nuclear factor-kappa B [RANK]) on the surface of osteoclasts or preosteoclasts, stimulating both the differentiation of osteoclast progenitor cells and the activity of mature osteoclasts. It exists as either a 40–45 kD cellular, membrane-bound form or a 31 kD soluble form derived by cleavage of the full-length form at position 140 or 145. It also has a number of effects on immune cells, including activation of c-Jun N-terminal kinase (JNK) in T cells, inhibition of apoptosis of dendritic cells, induction of cluster formation by dendritic cells, and proliferation of cytokine-activated T cells.

receptor site: A biologic site where molecular binding occurs.

recession: The migration of the marginal soft tissue to a point apical to the cementoenamel junction of a tooth or the platform of a dental implant. **Gingival r.**: Migration of the gingiva to a point apical to the cementoenamel junction.

recipient site: (syn): Host site. The receiving area into which a graft or transplant material is placed.

reciprocal: A designed reality in which a force from one part of a prosthetic device is opposed by a different part of the device.

reciprocal click: Related clicking sounds from the temporomandibular joint, which occur during opening and closing movements.

reciprocation: A condition where lateral forces from a retentive clasp moving over the height of the contour of a tooth or crown are opposed by an another (reciprocal) clasp that engages a guiding plane.

recombinant DNA: Deoxyribonucleic acid (DNA) sequences produced in a laboratory by joining genetic material from multiple sources.

recombinant DNA: Genetically engineered deoxyribonucleic acid that has been altered by joining genetic material from two different sources (usually different species). Deoxyribonucleic acid that has been modified by deletion or addition of genetic information.

recombinant human bone morphogenetic protein (rhBMP): Osteoinductive protein produced by recombinant DNA technology.

reconstruction: Restoration of an anatomic organ or structure to its original appearance and function. In dentistry, it is the restoration or replacement of a tooth, teeth, or portion of a jaw or craniofacial structure using an artificial prosthesis. See: Alveolar reconstruction, Prosthesis.

reconstructive surgery: 1. The use of surgical procedures to restore or correct a body part to a more normal appearance or function.

2. To improve a body part from an existing deficiency or abnormality caused by congenital defects, trauma, infection, tumors, or disease.

record: Information or data recorded in any medium (e.g., handwriting, print, tapes, film, microfilm, microfiche, any electronic form). It provides evidence of what was planned, the treatment provided, and the results. See: Clinical record.

record base: A denture base that supports material that is used to document the positional correlation of the maxilla to the mandible.

record rim: Material placed on an interim denture base that may be used to establish and record the positional relationship between the maxilla and mandible; it may also be used to establish the position of teeth. Also known as an occlusal rim.

records, legal requirements for maintaining: Laws that specify the length of time for which records must be kept.

recurrence: Reappearance or return, as of inflammation or disease that has been successfully treated.

recurrent periodontitis: See: Periodontitis.

reduced interarch distance: A vertical dimension that allows for overclosure. Compared with the proper relationship, there is a reduced interridge distance when the maxillary and mandibular teeth are in contact and an extreme interocclusal distance when the mandible is at a position of rest. Also known as overclosure.

reduction: Using surgical or manual methods to correct a dislocation or fracture, thereby restoring it to its normal anatomic relationship.

reentry: Second surgical procedure to place an implant in a staged approach, such as alveolar ridge augmentation or sinus grafting procedures. It can be combined with the removal of an inert biomaterial (e.g., nonresorbable membranes or bone graft fixation screws). Can also be performed to improve, enhance, or evaluate results obtained from the initial operation. See: Stage two surgery.

reference plane locator: A component of a facebow system used to transfer a reference plane from the patient to an articulator.

reference scan: Technique of scanning an object, such as a diagnostic wax-up or prepreparation dentition. This is used as a template for the fabrication of an identical object.

referred pain: Pain felt in a site in the body different from the diseased or injured location where the pain would be expected.

referred symptoms: Symptoms perceived in tissues distant to and unrelated to the true diseased site.

reflectance: The measure of the fraction of radiant energy that is reflected from a surface.

reflection: The elevation and folding back of all, or part, of the soft tissue to expose the underlying structures. See: Surgery, periodontal.

refractory: Persistent; patients or sites that continue to demonstrate disease after appropriate therapy.

refractory cast: A cast made of a material that will not deteriorate at the high temperature used in casting.

refractory die: A die made of a material that will not deteriorate at the high temperatures used during firing or casting procedures.

refractory mold: A mold made from refractory material into which metal is cast.

refractory periodontitis: See: Periodontitis.

refractory prosthodontic patient: A patient in whom it is difficult to achieve prosthetic success even when the appropriate prosthesis is provided. The patient may not be able to follow directions or lacks adaptability to prosthodontic treatment.

regenerate: (syn): Distraction zone. The tissue that forms between gradually separated bone segments in distraction osteogenesis.

regenerate maturation: The completion of mineralization and remodeling of the regenerate tissue.

regeneration: Reproduction or reconstitution of a lost or injured part to its original state. See: Repair. **Guided tissue r.**: A surgical procedure with the goal of achieving new bone, cementum, and PDL attachment to a periodontally diseased tooth, using barrier devices or membranes to provide space maintenance, epithelial exclusion, and wound stabilization. **Periodontal r.**: Restoration of lost or diminished periodontal tissues including cementum, periodontal ligament, and alveolar bone.

regenerative medicine: Field of medicine concerned with developing and using strategies to repair or replace damaged, diseased, or metabolically deficient organs, tissues, and cells via tissue engineering, cell transplantation, artificial organs, and bioartificial organs and tissues.

regenerative therapy for alveolar ridge defect: Use of barrier membranes for guided bone regeneration (GBR) to provide a more predictable restoration of form. This method often permits placement of implants simultaneous to defect restoration.

regional acceleration phenomenon (RAP): Increase in all metabolic activities in a soft or hard tissue (including modeling and remodeling activity in the skeleton) that is initiated by a provocative stimulus (e.g., fracture, crush injury). Typical RAP is induced by periosteal stimulation. A local response to a stimulus in which tissues form 2–10 times more rapidly than the normal regeneration process. The duration and intensity of RAP are directly proportional to the kind and amount of stimulus and the site where it was produced.

registration: (syn): Co-registration. A preliminary procedure in navigation surgery in which the patient is synchronized against the preacquired imaging scan by the use of fiducial markers.

registration (bite): A record of the occlusal relationship between the maxillary and mandibular jaws.

regression: Class of procedures for predicting the values of a response variable when the value of one or more explanatory variables is known.

rehabilitation: Restoration to a former state of appearance, well-being, and function using artificial replacements. See: Osseous rehabilitation, Restoration.

reimplantation: The act of replacing a tooth in the same alveolar socket from which it had been removed, either surgically or as a result of trauma.

Reiter's syndrome: A condition of unknown cause, usually seen in young men, characterized by urethritis, arthritis, conjunctivitis, and mucocutaneous lesions.

rejection: An immunological response to incompatibility in transplanted tissues and organs mediated by both cellular and humoral immunity; may lead to destruction of the transplanted tissue or organ.

releasing incision: An incision made at a right or oblique angle to the main incision to relieve tension on a mucoperiosteal flap and allow more flap reflection than the original incision allows.

relief: Placement of a measured amount of space in an area under a denture base or removable partial framework to eliminate tissue contact or pressure or to make room for impression material.

relief area: A delineated space created on the tissue surface of a removable dental prosthesis to eliminate contact with the tissue.

reline: To replace the base material on the tissue side of a removable dental prosthesis with new base material to correct the adaptation of the base to the tissue. Compare: Rebase.

remission: A diminution or abatement of the signs and/or symptoms of a disease; also the period during which such diminution occurs.

remodel: The ongoing process by which bone is resorbed and replaced in a dynamic steady-state process that maintains the health of bone.

remodeling (bone): The turnover of bone in small packets by BMUs (basic multicellular unit of bone remodeling).

remount cast: A cast made to facilitate remounting the prosthesis on an articulator. Frequently done to refine occlusion.

remount index: Record of the definitive position of maxillary occlusal surfaces on the articulator for remounting restorations (usually complete dentures) on the articulator for occlusal refinement.

remount procedure: A process in which prostheses are replaced on an articulator after fabrication to refine occlusion.

remount record: Record of positional registration of maxillary occlusal surfaces to be affixed to the lower member of an articulator for occlusal refinement following complete denture prosthesis processing. See: Remount index.

remount record index: A record made on an articulator component to allow remounting of the maxillary cast after processing.

removable dental prosthesis: 1. Any dental prosthesis that replaces some or all teeth in a partially dentate arch (partial removable dental prostheses) or edentate arch (complete removable dental prostheses). It can be removed from the mouth and replaced at will. 2. Any dental prosthesis that can be readily inserted and removed by the patient. The means of retention for such prostheses include tissue-retained RDP, tooth-retained RDP, implant retained RDP, or tooth and implant-retained RDP.

removable denture: See: Removable prosthesis.

removable prosthesis: A restoration that is removable by the patient. The restoration may be partial arch (removable partial denture, RPD) or complete arch (removable complete denture, RCD). See: Denture, Fixed prosthesis.

removal torque: Rotational force required to remove an implant from its osteotomy. See: Reverse torque value (RTV).

removal torque value (RTV): syn. Reverse torque value. Measure of the rotational force needed to rupture the bone–implant interface of a root-form implant.

repair: Healing of a wound by tissue that does not fully restore the architecture or function of the part that was lost. See: Regeneration.

replantation, tooth: The replacement of a totally luxated (accidentally or intentionally) tooth into its socket.

replica: Prosthetic component or element made as a duplicate in every dimension of a specific surgical and/or prosthetic component. A replica can be incorporated in dental laboratory procedures to facilitate making an accurate master cast and/or accurate

prosthesis. It can also be incorporated into a model for the purpose of patient education. See: Analog.

repositioning: The changing of any relative position of the mandible to the maxillae, usually altering the occlusion of the natural or artificial teeth.

repositioning splint: An intraoral maxillofacial prosthesis constructed to temporarily or permanently alter the relative position of the mandible to the maxillae.

resection: Excision (removal) of some portion of the jaw, tooth root, or other maxillofacial structure. Typically done for the treatment of pathology.

residual abscess: A persistent lesion that remains from a prior infection. It often presents with a radiolucent area.

residual bone: Fraction of mandibular or maxillary bone that remains after the teeth are removed or lost.

residual ridge: Portion of the alveolar ridge that remains after the alveoli have disappeared from the alveolar process, following extraction of teeth.

residual ridge crest: The most superior portion of the residual ridge.

residual ridge resorption: The phenomenon of diminishing volume and density of the residual ridge after the teeth are removed. See: Ridge atrophy.

resilient attachment: A special attachment intended to give a combination tooth and soft tissue-borne removable dental prosthesis sufficient flexure to allow for its placement without introducing unnecessary stress on the abutments.

resin: Organic substance that forms a plastic material following polymerization initiated by heat or chemical activation. It is usually transparent or translucent, not water soluble, and named according to chemical composition, physical structure, or means of activation or curing. See: Acrylic resin, Autopolymerizing resin, Composite resin, Epoxy resin, Heat-curing resin.

resin-bonded splint: A fixed splint made of heavy wire, fibrous resin materials and/or cast metal that is bonded to the labial or lingual surface of natural teeth with an acid etch technique. It is used to stabilize traumatically displaced or periodontal compromised teeth.

resin crown: A resin restoration that restores a clinical crown without a metal substructure.

resistance: Ability of a human, organism, or inert material to resist the damaging effects of chemical, microbiological, or mechanical agents.

resistance form: The features of a tooth preparation that enhance the stability of a restoration and resist dislodgment along an axis other than the path of placement.

resolution: 1. In dentistry or medicine, the return to health or improvement of a pathologic state. 2. In digital imaging, a pixel that is the smallest recognizable point found in the master image.

resonance frequency analysis (RFA): Determination of the relative stiffness of an implant within the bone via attachment of a resonance frequency transducer containing two piezoceramic elements to an implant. One piezo element is excited by an electrical signal, and the resulting vibration is measured by the second element. The higher the resulting frequency (in kHz), the stiffer the implant-to-bone connection. The device records the resonance frequency arising from the implant–bone interface (change in amplitude over induced frequency band).

resorbable: The ability of an autogenous graft to dissolve physiologically. Natural or synthetic material that can be removed by a cellular process, osteoclasts, or foreign body giant cells and macrophages. See: Bioabsorbable.

resorbable barrier membrane: See: Resorbable membrane.

resorbable blast media (RBM): Particles of a resorbable abrasive used to produce a specific surface topography of a dental implant.

resorbable membrane: Membrane made of absorbable natural or synthetic materials used to avoid a second surgery for its removal. After implantation in the body, membranes are degraded by enzymatic activity (collagen membranes) or by hydrolysis (polylactic acid and co-polymers of polylactic and polyglycolic acids membranes).

resorbed maxilla: Extensive resorption of the alveolar process of the maxilla leads to a nearly complete loss of trabecular bone. Remaining as an alveolar process, it is then almost only a cortical plate, often forming the bottom of the sinus and the nasal cavity.

resorption: The progressive loss of soft or hard tissue due to physiologic or pathologic processes. **Bone r.**: Bone loss due to osteoclastic activity. **Cavernous r.**: Bone loss of the alveolar processes of the maxilla and/or mandible due to osteoclastic activity, either physiologically or pathologically, resulting in hollow spaces within the maxilla and/or mandible. **External r.**: Resorption that initially affects the external surface of a tooth. It may be classified as inflammatory or replacement, or by location as cervical, lateral or apical. It may or may not invade the pulp. **Idiopathic r.**: Loss of calcified tissues for no obvious reason. **Inflammatory r.**: A pathologic loss of cementum, dentin and bone resulting in a defect in the root and adjacent bone. **Internal r.**: A pathologic process initiated in the pulp characterized by loss of dentin and possibly cementum. It may or may not perforate to the external root surface and is best managed by removal of the vital pulp followed by conventional root canal therapy. **Replacement r.** (ankylosis): A pathologic loss of cementum, dentin and periodontal ligament with the ingrowth of bone into the resulting defect. There is a union of bone to cementum and/or dentin and loss of mobility.

rest jaw relation: An obsolete term for the relationship of the mandible to the maxilla when the patient is in an upright relaxed position and proper physiologic interocclusal distance exists between the teeth as the condyles are resting in the glenoid fossae.

rest position, physiologic: The postural position of the mandible when an individual is resting comfortably in an upright position and the associated muscles are in a state of minimal contractual activity. Also known as postural position.

rest seat: Area prepared on a tooth surface or restoration to support vertical or lateral occlusal forces.

rest vertical dimension: Distance measured between a predetermined point on the maxilla and mandible when the mandible is in physical rest position. One point is on the middle of the face or nose and the other point is on the lower face or chin. See: Vertical dimension.

restoration: Material or prosthesis used to restore or replace teeth, parts of jaws, or craniofacial structures. See: Acrylic restoration, Osseous restoration, Prosthesis.

restorative dentistry: Branch of dentistry concerned with the replacement or reconstruction of a tooth or teeth and their supporting structures altered or lost through trauma, surgery, disease, or congenital etiology.

restorative phase: Portion of patient treatment concerned with the diagnosis, treatment planning, and provision of prosthetic therapy.

restorative platform: See: Platform.

retained impression coping: Impression coping fixed intraorally either through frictional fit or by being screwed into position. Immediately after removal of the impression, it remains intraorally.

retainer: Device used to stabilize teeth in the desired position; it is usually an orthodontic appliance.

retaining screw: A threaded fastener that secures a prosthetic reconstruction to an abutment or a mesostructure. See: Abutment screw, Prosthetic retaining screw.

retention: Capacity of a prosthesis or dental restoration to maintain its intended position in function. For a removable prosthesis, the resistance to displacement in the designed path of insertion.

retention arm: Extension of metal or plastic arm to add stability to a dental prosthesis.

retention form: The feature of a tooth preparation that resists dislodgment of a crown in a vertical direction or along the path of placement.

retention of the denture: An obsolete term that refers to denture retention obtained by utilizing bony undercuts covered with tissue.

retentive element: Portion of a prosthetic component that is the cylinder-to-implant position, directly in contact with the implant.

rethreading: Repair of the damaged internal threads of a root-form dental implant using a tap instrument.

reticular fiber: See: Fiber.

retraction cord: Slender woven or twisted string-like fabric (usually cotton or similar material) used to retract gingival or mucosal tissues for the exposure of prepared tooth or abutment margins prior to impression making. It is usually impregnated with an appropriate substance to stiffen the cord and provide vasoconstriction.

retractor: Instrument used to hold soft tissue away from bony structures in order to visualize an area during surgery or to photograph an area.

retrievability: Capacity of a prosthesis, dental restoration, attachment, or screw to be removed without compromising its structure.

retrofilling: Apical reflection of soft tissue and bone to expose the root tip where a preparation is made and filled with material to seal a root canal.

retrognathic: Position of the mandible in relationship to the maxilla where the mandible is retruded from its normal position.

retrognathism: Position of mandible and/or maxilla that is posterior to its normal craniofacial relationship. Typically refers to the mandible.

retrograde periimplantitis: See: Implant periapical lesion.

retromolar implant: Endosseous dental implant placed in the mandibular retromolar area for the purpose of protraction or retraction of the dentition. See: Orthodontic implant, Temporary anchorage device.

retromolar pad: Mass of freely movable, nonkeratinized mucosal tissue located posterior to the retromolar papilla of the most distal tooth in the mandible.

retromylohyoid area: An obsolete term referring to the area located lingual to the retromolar tissue pad extending inferiorly toward the floor of mouth and distally to the retromylohyoid curtain.

retrospective study: A study designed to observe events that have already occurred. See: Prospective study.

retruded contact: The contact that occurs during the closure of the mandible in its most retruded path of closure.

retruded contact position: The occlusal relationship that occurs when the mandible and the condyles are in their most retruded position. This position may be more retruded than the position referred to as centric relation.

retrusion: Movement of the mandible directed posteriorly.

retrusive: A mandibular position that may be more distal than that described as maximum intercuspation.

Retrusive jaw relation: A jaw position resulting from a posterior positioning of the mandible.

reverse architecture: When the crest of the interdental gingiva or bone is located apical to its midfacial and midlingual margins. See: Architecture.

reverse articulation: Positioning of the mandibular teeth that is more buccal than normal relative to the maxillary teeth, such that the fossae of the mandibular teeth articulate with the buccal cusp of the maxillary teeth. See: Cross-bite occlusion.

reverse articulation teeth: Artificial teeth that are shaped to allow for the buccal cusp of the maxillary teeth to be arranged in the central fossae of the mandibular teeth.

reverse curve: When viewed in the sagittal plane, the occlusal plane position as outlined by the cusp tips and incisal edges of the teeth is curved upward.

reverse torque test (RTT): Experimental procedure in which an implant is subjected to unscrewing to determine the relative strength of attachment between the implant and bone. It is usually done on a comparative basis between differing implant surface topographies or roughness. It is assumed that the reverse torque value (RTV) will increase as the process of osseointegration progresses. RTT of implants to a torque of 20 Ncm has also been described as a method for determining the success of machined surfaced, threaded implants in clinical situations.

reverse torque value (RTV): Resulting value of the torsional force required to unscrew an implant body from its osteotomy. It is assumed that RTV would increase as osseointegration progresses during the healing phase. See: Reverse torque test (RTT).

reversible hydrocolloids: Gels that solidify by cooling and return to a flowable state when the temperature is increased.

reversible splint: A device used for, or method of, splinting or fixing teeth that does not change or alter the structure of the involved teeth.

revolutions per minute (RPM): Speed at which a shaft turns. It is recorded as the number of complete (360°) revolutions the shaft makes in a minute.

RFA (abbrev.): Resonance frequency analysis.

rhBMP (abbrev.): Recombinant human bone morphogenetic protein.

rhinosporidiosis: In immunocompromised individuals, this disease is caused by *Rhinosporidium seeberi*, which is a *Candida* species responsible for oral mycoses and may cause oral infections (thrush) in AIDS patients or other debilitated humans. *Candida* species are designated as "opportunistic" pathogens since they are often found as members of the normal oral flora.

ribbon: See: Articulating tape.

ribonucleic acid (RNA): Polymer composed of ribonucleotides; three types of RNA function in translation of information from genes (DNA) to proteins. In some viruses, RNA is also the genetic material. **Messenger RNA** (mRNA): RNA that mediates the transfer of genetic information from the coding region of a gene to ribosomes. It serves as a template for protein synthesis. **Ribosomal RNA** (rRNA): RNA component of the ribosome that provides a mechanism for translation of messenger RNA (decoding) during protein synthesis. **Transfer RNA** (tRNA): RNA that transports an amino acid to the ribosome, according to the code specified in the messenger RNA (mRNA), for incorporation into a polypeptide during protein synthesis.

ridge: The remainder of the alveolar process after tooth extraction. See: Alveolar process, Alveolar ridge, Residual ridge.

ridge atrophy: Decrease in volume of a ridge due to resorption of bone.

ridge augmentation: A procedure used to increase the size, shape, or quality of an edentulous dental ridge or space that has typically lost ideal contour after loss of the dentition (or failure to develop dentition). See: Alveolar ridge augmentation, Edentulous ridge.

ridge crest: The most highly contoured part of an edentulous dental ridge.

ridge defect: A deficiency in the contour of an edentulous ridge. The deficiency can be in the vertical (apicocoronal) and/or horizontal (buccolingual, mesiodistal) direction.

ridge expansion: Surgical widening of a residual ridge in the lateral direction (buccolingually) with osteotomes and/or chisels, to accommodate the insertion of a dental implant, and/or bone graft.

ridge lap: The surface of an artificial tooth that has been shaped to accommodate the residual ridge. The tissue surface of a ridge lap design is concave and envelops both the buccal and lingual surfaces of the residual ridge.

ridge lap design: Tissue-contacting surface of an artificial tooth prepared to accommodate the residual ridge contour on the facial, buccal, and lingual or palatal aspects. A fixed or removable prosthesis incorporating such features may be designated a ridge lap-designed restoration.

ridge mapping: Penetration of anesthetized soft tissue with a graduated probe or caliper at several sites and transposing the information to a diagnostic cast. The shape of the residual ridge is reproduced by trimming back the stone of the cast to the corresponding depth of soft tissue. See: Bone sounding, Ridge sounding.

ridge preservation: A surgical procedure aimed at preventing ridge collapse and preserving ridge dimension after tooth extraction, typically done for purposes of implant site development. Involves the use of hard and/or soft tissue biomaterials and/or membranes.

ridge relationship: The positional relationship of the mandibular residual ridge to the maxillary residual ridge.

ridge resorption: Refers to the loss of bone in an edentulous area. See: Residual ridge.

ridge slope: An obsolete term referring to the angulation established by the crest of the mandibular ridge extending from the posterior region toward the anterior area relative to the inferior border of the mandible.

ridge sounding: (syn): Bone sounding, sounding. Penetration of anesthetized soft tissue in order to determine the topography of the underlying bone. See: Ridge mapping.

ridge splitting: A surgical procedure involving the use of one or more corticotomies in order to mobilize one or more bony segments for purposes of expanding an atrophic edentulous ridge in a faciolingual dimension. See: Ridge expansion.

rigid connector: Part of a removable prosthesis that connects its parts or, in regards to a fixed prosthesis, a portion of the device that connects the retainer to a pontic in such a manner that no movement can occur.

rigid fixation: Clinical term that implies absence of observed mobility, process of becoming fixated or rendered immobile, inflexible; applicable to a prosthesis or prosthesis component.

rigidity: Stiffness or inflexibility of an object.

ring artifact: Phenomenon that occurs due to inaccurate calibration or failure of one or more detector elements in a CT scanner. It occurs close to the isocenter of the scan, and is usually visible on multiple slices at the same location. It is a common problem in cranial CT and CBCT.

ringless investment technique: A method of investing such that no containment is used that may restrict expansion. A paper or plastic cylinder may be used that is less restricting than a metal cylindrical casting ring.

risedronate: Oral nitrogen-containing bisphosphonate used for the prevention and treatment of osteoporosis and treatment of Paget's disease. Its mechanism of action involves the inhibition of osteoclast formation and activity.

risk assessment: The process by which qualitative or quantitative assessments are made, regarding the likelihood of adverse events occurring as a result of exposure to specified health hazards or absence of beneficial influences.

risk determinant: A risk factor that cannot be modified, i.e., genetic factors, gender, age.

risk factor: Environmental, behavioral, or biologic factor that increases the likelihood of developing disease; identified through longitudinal studies and confirmed to be present before the onset of disease, i.e., smoking, diabetes, pathogenic bacteria.

risk indicator: A probable risk factor that has not been confirmed by longitudinal studies.

RNA (abbrev.): Ribonucleic acid.

Rochette bridge: (Alain L. Rochette, French physician and dentist): a resin-bonded fixed dental prosthesis incorporating holes within the metal framework and lutes to the lingual aspect of teeth adjacent to an edentulous space that replaces one or more teeth. See: Resin-bonded prosthesis.

roentgen ray: 1. Radiation emitted from a tube that results from striking an anode with electrons emitted from a heated cathode. 2. Radiation resulting from the excitation of the innermost orbital electron within an atom.

root: The part of a tooth that is typically covered by cementum and is found in the more apical portion. Attached to it is usually a periodontal ligament that allows for connection to the adjacent bone.

root canal: The space within the root of a tooth containing connective tissue, nerves, and blood vessels, and connecting the pulp chamber with the apex of the root.

root concrescence: The fusion of roots of adjacent teeth. See: Root.

root-form endosteal dental implant: An implant used in dental applications that is placed into the bone and has some degree of similarity to a natural root. See: Implant, oral.

root fracture: A fracture, split, or breaks in the otherwise solid part of a tooth that is typically covered by cementum and is found in the more apical portion (root of the tooth).

root fragment: A portion of the root, usually the root tip, retained in the jaws following the incomplete extraction or incomplete resorption of the primary tooth. See: Root.

root fusion: The connection of roots of a multirooted tooth.

root planing: A treatment procedure designed to remove cementum or surface dentin that is rough, impregnated with calculus, or contaminated with toxins or microorganisms. See: Scaling.

root preparation: The use of chemical or mechanical means to remove contaminants from a root to improve wound healing.

root proximity: Closeness of roots of adjacent teeth typically associated with inadequate interdental tissue.

root resection: Removal of a portion or all of a tooth's root.

root resorption: Loss or blunting of some portion of a root, sometimes idiopathic, but also associated with orthodontic tooth movement, inflammation, trauma, endocrine disorders, and neoplasia.

root retention: Preservation of a root, frequently endodontically treated, after the coronal portion has been removed in order to support a prosthesis or preserve the alveolar ridge.

root submergence: Process of covering a tooth's root with soft tissue.

rotated (rotational) flap: A gingival flap which is moved laterally from a donor site while rotating around a pivot point, maintaining a blood supply through the base of the flap. Used for root coverage and ridge augmentation procedures.

rouge: A material made of ferric oxide and binding agents used for polishing and thereby imparting luster to a surface.

rough implant surface: Implant surface with a varying degree of macro- and microirregularity in contrast with a machined or polished, smooth surface. A rough implant surface is generally considered to be superior to a smooth or polished surface in its ability to osseointegrate from both the rate of integration and the relative surface area of bone-implant contact (BIC). Surface roughness of implants can be categorized into three basic levels: minimally rough, 0.5–1 μm; moderately rough, 1–2 μm; and rough, greater than 2 μm.

rough surface: See: Textured surface.

round bur: Circular bur used to mark a site for an osteotomy or to decorticate bone. It may also be used in the outline of a lateral window access for the purpose of sinus grafting.

RPD (abbrev.): Removable partial denture (now termed a partial removable dental prosthesis).

RPI (abbrev.): Rest, proximal plate, and i-bar; the clasp components of one type of partial removable dental prosthesis clasp assembly.

RPM (abbrev.): Revolutions per minute.

RTT (abbrev.): Reverse torque test.

RTV (abbrev.): Removal torque value (reverse torque value).

Ruffini receptor: Highly sensitive nerve ending of the periodontium in close approximation with collagen fibers that allow refined proprioception around teeth.

ruga (pl. rugae): Anatomic ridges of soft tissue that are frequently present on the surface in the anterior portion of the hard palate.

runt-related transcription factor 2 (runx2): See: Bone morphogenetic protein (BMP), Core-binding factor alpha 1 (CBFα1).

S

S value: A three-dimensional roughness parameter calculated from topographical images. **S$_a$**: The arithmetic average of the absolute value of all points of the profile. It is a height descriptive parameter. **S$_{cx}$**: A space descriptive parameter. **S$_{dr}$**: The developed surface area ratio.

saccharolytic: The ability of some microorganisms to catabolize carbohydrates.

saddle pontic: A pontic with a broad concave faciolingual area of contact with the residual ridge. It is also known as a ridge lap pontic. This type of pontic is known to be uncleanable and results in tissue irritation at the area of contact with the ridge mucosa.

sagittal: Situated in the plane of the cranial sagittal suture or parallel to that plane. See: Sagittal plane.

sagittal axis: An imaginary anteroposterior line around which the mandible may rotate when viewed in the frontal plane.

sagittal plane: The anteroposterior plane or section parallel to the long axis of the body.

saliva: The secretions of the major and minor salivary glands.

salivary pellicle: The rapid formation of an acquired, organic, acellular deposition of salivary and gingival crevicular fluid proteins, on a clean surface, exposed to the oral environment.

sandblasted implant surface: Implant surface that has been treated by exposure to silica sand particles propelled under high pressure, thus creating a rough surface texture. See: Rough implant surface.

sandblasted, large-grit, acid-etched (SLA) **implant surface**: A surface treatment that improves surface roughness to enhance osseointegration through greater bone–implant contact (BIC) as well as an increased rate of osseointegration.

sandblasting: Act of modifying or roughening the surface of an implant body by propelling silica sand onto the surface at high velocity under high pressure.

sanitary pontic: A trade name originally designed as a manufactured convex blank with a slotted back. The name was used occasionally as a synonym for a hygienic pontic, wherein the pontic does not contact the residual ridge.

saucerization: Part of surgical treatment for osteomyelitis in which an essentially closed cavity is opened to the surface by excavation, converting the cavity into a saucer-like defect.

scaffold: A three-dimensional biocompatible construct (may be seeded with cells) that serves as a framework on which tissue can grow. It may or may not be biodegradable.

scaffold tissue engineering: Appropriate three-dimensional material with pores and an interconnected pore network with proper surface for attachment, proliferation, and differentiation. It has matching mechanical properties and is bioresorbable with controllable degradation.

scaler: Instrument for removing calculus or other deposits from the surface of teeth or oral implants. **Sonic s.**: An instrument vibrating in the sonic range (approximately 6000 cps) that, accompanied by a stream of water, can be used to remove adherent deposits from teeth. **Ultrasonic scaler**: An instrument vibrating in the ultrasonic range (approximately 25 000–30 000 cps) which, accompanied by a stream of water, can be used to remove adherent deposits from teeth.

scaling: Instrumentation of the crown and root surfaces of the teeth to remove plaque, calculus, and stains from these surfaces. See: Root planing.

scallop: To shape, cut, or finish in scallops; segments or angular projections forming a border.

scalloped implant: A root-form implant design that has the level of the implant-abutment junction elevated interproximally to accommodate the papilla–crestal bone relationship.

scan body: Scannable object used to accurately translate the position of an implant into a digital file for use in the digital design of an implant abutment. The scan body serves the same purpose in digital design that the impression coping serves in the traditional impression and model technique.

scanographic template: A radiographic template utilized for CT scanning. See: Radiographic template.

scar: Area of fibrous tissue resulting from the biologic process of wound repair that replaces normal tissues destroyed by injury or disease. Called also a cicatrix.

scatter radiation: Any radiation that is not absorbed by the target tissues. This radiation may pass through or be deflected by the tissue. The unabsorbed radiation may then collide with nearby objects or personnel.

scene file: A file format that contains objects in a strictly defined language or data structure; it would contain geometry, viewpoint, texture, lighting, and shading information as a description of the virtual scene. The data contained in the scene file is then passed to a rendering program to be processed and output to a digital image or raster graphics image file.

Schneiderian membrane: (syn): Sinus membrane (maxillary). Layer of pseudostratified ciliated columnar epithelium cells lining the maxillary sinus. See: Perforation.

Schneiderian membrane perforation: See: Maxillary sinus membrane.

scleroderma: See: Progressive systemic sclerosis.

sclerosis: An induration, thickening, or hardening of a body part, usually induced by a chronic inflammatory reaction or by hyperplasia of interstitial fibrous connective tissue. When found in the jaws, it is depicted by an increased calcification as found in condensing osteitis.

screw: A threaded fastener used to adjoin two mating parts. See: Abutment screw, Prosthetic screw, Retaining screw.

screw design: Common design for cylindrical endosseous dental implants; the screw shape allows for increased primary stability. The time of placement and the screw threads may provide additional load-carrying capacity, although this has not been shown to be significant clinically.

screw endosteal dental implant: A sterile device that is placed into the jaw bones for the attachment or retention of a tooth or teeth and whose configuration is similar to a screw; it may be hollow or solid, and normally consists of the fixture and the abutment.

screw fracture: The breakage of a prosthetic screw.

screw implant: Threaded root-form dental implant, which can be parallel-sided or tapered. See: Root-form implant, Threaded implant, Screw-type implant.

screw joint: Interface or junction of two prosthesis components connected by a screw.

screw loosening: A prosthetic complication whereby a screw loses its preload, causing the loosening of a restoration or abutment.

screw preload: Clamping or stretching force that occurs across the interface of implant components being attached together via screw tightening. See: Preload.

screw tap: See: Tap, Tapping.

screw tightening: Act of turning a screw into its receptacle until resistance is met, resulting in increased tightness of the screw. See: Preload.

screw, teflon-coated: Implant/prosthesis retention screw that has been modified with a polytetrafluoroethylene (PTFE) surface coating. See: Screw.

screw-retained: The use of a screw for retention of an abutment or a prosthesis. See: Cement-retained.

screw-type implant: An implant with threading on the surface, resembling a screw shape, sometimes referred to as screw-shape. See: Threaded implant.

SCTG (abbrev.): Subepithelial connective tissue graft.

scurvy: Malnutrition caused by a dietary deficiency of vitamin C. Oral manifestations may include ulcerations, mucosal hemorrhage, and gingival enlargement.

SD (abbrev.): Standard deviation.

SE (abbrev.): Standard error.

sealing screw: Healing component used to cover the coronal portion of the implant or as part of a transmucosal healing component that seals the occlusal portion of that component. See: Healing abutment.

seating surface: See: Platform.

sebaceous: Relating to or resembling fat or sebum; oily; fatty; discharging fat or a grease-like oil substance.

second moment principle: See: Moment of inertia.

second stage dental implant surgery: 1. For eposteal dental implant surgery, the term refers to the procedure involving placement of the eposteal framework fabricated after the first stage implant surgery. 2. For endosteal dental implant surgery, after surgical reflection, the occlusal aspect of the dental implant is exposed, the cover screw is removed, and either the interim or definitive dental implant abutment is placed. After this, the investing tissues are (when needed) sutured.

secondary adhesion: See: Healing by second (secondary) intention.

secondary closure: Misnomer, since the general goal of surgery is to have close flap adaptation and complete closure of the surgical site, and hence healing by primary intention. However, in certain situations, incomplete closure is indicated, which leads to healing by secondary intention. See: Healing by second (secondary) intention.

secondary crown: See: Telescopic crown.

secondary implant failure: See: Late implant failure.

secondary maxillary mucocele: syn. Postoperative maxillary sinus cyst. Maxillary sinus lesion caused by previous trauma or surgery which divides the sinus into two compartments. The cyst is derived from the antral epithelium and mucosal remnants that were previously entrapped within the surgical site. See: Primary maxillary mucocele.

secondary occlusal trauma: The effects induced by occlusal force (normal or abnormal) acting on teeth with decreased periodontal support.

secondary stability: Implant stability within its prepared bony site, created by osseointegration and the formation of new bone subsequent to loss of the bone initially in contact with the implant at the time of placement. This delayed clinical implant immobility may follow osteotomy site augmentation with bone substitutes and/or healing adjuncts. Compare: Primary stability, secondary union. See: Healing by second (secondary) intention.

second stage dental implant surgery: 1. Regarding eposteal dental implant surgery, it is the surgical procedure involving placement of an eposteal framework constructed from the first-stage implant surgery impression. 2. Regarding endosteal dental implant surgery, it involves the surgical reflection of soft tissue to uncover the superior (tabletop) aspect of the dental implant, the cover screw is removed, and either the healing collar or the interim or definitive dental implant abutment is placed. After this, the relevant tissues are sutured in place as needed.

second stage permucosal abutment: See: Healing abutment, Transmucosal abutment.

second stage surgery: See: Stage two surgery.

secretion: The formation and release of a product by glandular activity.

sectional impression: A process of capturing, in segments or parts, any anatomic area using a material that will produce a negative likeness of the area of interest.

sedation, conscious: A minimally depressed level of consciousness induced for anxiolysis and fear management that allows the patient to independently maintain an airway and respond appropriately to physical stimulation and verbal commands.

sedative: An agent, usually a drug, that produces physiologic changes to soothe, lessen irritability, and allay excitement and activity in the apprehensive patient.

seesaw model (of prosthesis loading): Model describing the mechanical loading aspects of implants or teeth arranged linearly.

segmental defect: Resulting defect following removal of jaw segments in tumor patients.

Seibert classification: A system of three categories used to describe the form of a residual alveolar ridge.

- **Class I defect**: Loss of tissue width in the facial-lingual or buccal-lingual direction but there is adequate ridge height.
- **Class II defect**: Loss of ridge height but adequate ridge width.
- **Class III defect**: Loss of both ridge height and width.

selective grinding: Alteration of the occlusal forms of teeth to improve occlusal function and to decrease or redirect occlusal forces to the teeth.

selective laser sintering (SLS): Additive manufacturing technique that uses a high-power laser (e.g., a carbon dioxide laser) to fuse small particles of plastic, metal (direct metal laser sintering), ceramic, or glass powders into a mass that has a desired 3D shape.

Selenomonas sputigena: Gram-positive, anaerobic, rod-shaped bacteria, mainly from subgingival plaque, that displays a tumbling motility.

self-curing resin: Autopolymerizing resin.

self-separating plaster: An obsolete term for an impression plaster that disintegrates in hot water.

self-tapping: Ability of certain implant profile designs to cut their own threads into the osteotomy walls at the time of implant placement. A self-tapping implant may be screwed into the osteotomy without first having to pretap the thread grooves.

semi-adjustable articulator: An articulator that allows adjustments to replicate typical mandibular movements. See: Articulator, Class III.

semi-precious metal alloy: An alloy made of both base and precious metals. No specified ratio of components distinguishes one group of semi-precious alloys from another.

sensitivity: A state of abnormal responsiveness to stimulation. **Clinical s.**: Clinical sensitivity, also called tooth sensitivity or dentin hypersensitivity, is the experience of a sensation ranging from mild discomfort to shooting pain caused by the exposure of susceptible teeth to thermal (cold or hot) stimuli. **Statistical s.**: The ability of a diagnostic test to detect a disease, when present, in a diseased population. Sensitivity = true positives divided by the sum of true positives plus false negatives, or TP/(FN + TP).

sensory function evaluation: Clinical evaluation that tests sensory function.

sensory mapping: The process of evaluation and delineation of a cutaneous, mucous, or gingival area presumably affected by an altered sensation or dysesthesia.

separating medium: 1. A coating used to keep one surface from adhering to a second surface. 2. A material applied on an impression that aids removal of the cast once it has set (hardened).

sepsis: Unsafe quantities of pathogenic microorganisms or their products in blood or tissues.

septicemia: Systemic disease initiated by the presence of pathological microorganisms or their toxins in the blood.

septum: Lining or wall separating two cavities or chambers within the body. **Maxillary sinus s.**: Cortical bone wall within the maxillary sinus that divides the maxillary sinus floor partially or completely into two or more chambers. Extent of a septum can vary. It is most common in edentulous maxillae, usually located between the second premolar and first molar region, and may cause complications during sinus floor elevation procedures. Called also Underwood septum.

sequestration: The process whereby necrotic bone separates from native healthy bone and forms a sequestrum.

sequestrectomy: Removal of a sequestrum by surgical means.

sequestrum: An island of nonvital bone that is separated from native healthy bone.

sessile: Having a wide base of attachment; lacking a stem; not pedunculated.

set screw: Type of retention or attachment screw that is made in smaller dimensions and used to connect a suprastructure and a mesostructure with lingual or palatal horizontal access. Sometimes it is configured as a metal tube with an internally threaded bore and screw system in which prefabricated components are incorporated into the mesostructure and suprastructures.

setting expansion: The dimensional increase that occurs concurrent with the hardening of various materials, such as plaster of Paris, dental stone, die stone, and dental casting investment.

sextant: Generally, the sixth part of anything. In dentistry, it is a one-sixth subdivision of the dental arches. The anterior sextants are composed of the incisor teeth and canines; the posterior sextants are composed of the premolar and molar teeth.

SFF (abbrev.): Solid freeform fabrication.

shade: The color selected for a coronal or gingival portion of a dental prosthesis (crown, bridge, or implant restoration).

Sharpey connective tissue fibers: Terminal portions of principal fibers that insert into the cementum of a tooth. These collagenous fibers pass from the periosteum and are embedded in the outer circumferential and interstitial lamellae of bone. Called also bone fibers.

shear stress: Stress caused by a load (two forces applied toward one another but not in the same straight line) that tends to slide one portion of object over another. See: Stress.

shelf, buccal: Cortical bony surface of the mandible extending from the alveolar ridge to the external oblique line in the vestibular region.

shell crown: 1. An artificial full-veneer crown swaged from metal plate. 2. An artificial crown that is adapted like a shell or cap over the remaining clinical crown of a tooth; the space between the crown and the shell is filled with cement. Called also cap crown.

shellac base: A record base constructed using a shellac-based wafer that has been adapted to the cast with heat.

shim stock: A thin strip (8–12 μm) of polyester film used to mark or confirm the point(s) of contact on natural teeth, artificial teeth, or a restoration. It is used to facilitate occlusal and proximal contact adjustment.

shoulder finish line: A finish line design for tooth preparation in which the gingival floor meets the external axial surfaces at approximately a right angle.

sialadenitis: Salivary gland inflammation.

sialagogue: Any substance or agent that promotes the secretion and flow of saliva.

sialolith: A salivary stone (calculus).

sialoprotein: Noncollagenous protein with a molecular weight of approximately 33 000 kDa that contains the arginine-glycine-aspartic acid (RGD) tripeptide sequence, characteristic for attachment proteins, which interact with cell surface integrins. It has a high calcium-binding potential and binds tightly to hydroxyapatite (HA) as well as to cells.

sialorrhea: Salivary flow greater than the normal rate.

sign: An objective indication of disease discoverable by the clinician upon evaluation of the patient. See: Symptom.

signaling molecule: Molecules that participate in intracellular and intercellular mechanisms involved in chemical transmitting of information between cells. Such molecules are released from the cell sending the signal, cross over the gap between cells, and interact with receptors in another cell, triggering an intracellular signaling cascade that results in a cellular response to the impulse.

signed rank test: Nonparametric form of the paired t test for comparing two samples.

silent sinus syndrome (SSS): Rare clinical entity characterized by unilateral enophthalmos and hypoglobus secondary to thinning and inward bowing of the maxillary sinus roof in the absence of signs or symptoms of intrinsic sinonasal inflammatory disease. The obstruction of the ostium of the ostiomeatal complex results in hypoventilation of the maxillary sinus.

silica: Silicon dioxide occurring in crystalline, amorphous, and usually impure forms (as quartz, opal, and sand, respectively).

silicone: Polymeric organic silicon compound in which some or all of the radical positions that could be occupied by carbon atoms are occupied by silicon. Used for heat- or water-resistant lubricants, binders, and insulators.

simple fracture: A linear bony fracture that is not in communication with the exterior.

simple joint: A joint in which only two bones articulate.

simple regression: Predicts the value of a single response variable from a given value of a single explanatory variable.

simulation: Imitative representation of the functioning of one system or process by means of the functioning of another. For example, in radiology, it could be an image obtained with the same source-to-skin distance, field size, and orientation as the diagnostic beam for visualization of a treated area on a radiograph.

simultaneous implant placement: Implant placement with a simultaneous bone-grafting procedure.

single-stage implant: Misnomer used for an implant that is placed with a one-stage procedure. See: One-stage implant.

sintered (porous) surface: A dental implant surface produced when spherical powders of metallic or ceramic materials become a coherent surface layer with the metallic core of an implant body. Porous surfaces are characterized by pore size, pore shape, pore volume, and pore depth, which are affected by the size of the spherical particles used and the temperature and pressure conditions of the sintering chamber.

sintering: Heating a powder below the melting point of any component such as to permit agglomeration and welding of particles by diffusion alone, with or without applied pressure.

sinus: A cavity or hollow space in a bone or other tissue such as the air-filled paranasal sinuses or dilated channels for venous blood in the cranium or liver.

sinus augmentation: See: Maxillary sinus floor elevation, Maxillary sinus floor graft.

sinus disease: Pathology of the maxillary sinus.

sinus elevation: See: Sinus graft.

sinus elevator: Spoon-like instrument used to elevate the Schneiderian membrane.

sinus graft: (syn): Maxillary antroplasty, sinus augmentation, sinus elevation, sinus lift, subantral augmentation. Augmentation of the antral floor with autogenous bone and/or bone substitutes to accommodate dental implant insertion. See: Maxillary sinus floor elevation, Maxillary sinus floor graft.

sinus grafting technique: See: Lateral window technique, Maxillary sinus floor elevation, Maxillary sinus floor graft, Osteotome technique.

sinus lift: See: Sinus graft.

sinus lift surgery: Misnomer used to describe surgical techniques for maxillary sinus floor elevation. See: Maxillary sinus floor elevation.

sinus lining: See: Schneiderian membrane.

sinus membrane (maxillary): See: Schneiderian membrane.

sinus perforation: Oroantral fistula following tooth extraction or perforation of the maxillary sinus membrane during a sinus grafting procedure.

sinus pneumatization (maxillary): Maxillary sinus enlargement. With aging, and especially after loss of maxillary teeth and reduction of masticatory forces acting on the maxilla, the sinus walls get gradually thinner as a result of the increase in size of the maxillary sinus.

sinus tract: A communication between a pathologic space and an anatomic body cavity.

sinusitis (maxillary): Inflammation of the sinus. Signs include sensitivity of teeth to percussion, fever, and facial swelling. Symptoms include nasal congestion, postnasal discharge, facial pain/headache, rhinorrhea, halitosis, popping of ears, and muffled hearing. Inflammation of the maxillary sinus arises from bacterial, viral, fungal, allergic, or autoimmune origin. While acute sinusitis is usually caused by infection with a single type of bacterium or virus, chronic sinusitis is usually caused either by allergies or by infection with several types of bacteria. Infections may be of either dental or otolaryngeal origin.

site development (implant): process by which the quantity and quality of soft and/or hard tissues are augmented at a site prior to dental implant placement.

Skalak models of prosthesis loading: Biomechanical models created by Richard Skalak explaining implant loading by forces applied to an attached rigid prosthesis.

skin: Two-layered outer integument or covering of the body, consisting of the dermis and the epidermis and resting upon the subcutaneous tissues. The outer ectodermal epidermis is more or less cornified and penetrated by the openings of sweat and sebaceous glands, and the inner mesodermal dermis is composed largely of connective tissue and is richly supplied with blood vessels and nerves. Called also cutis.

skin-penetrating implant: Endosseous implant placed in an extraoral site requiring skin penetration for prosthesis attachment as opposed to wet-surfaced gingiva or mucosa. Maintenance of adequate hygiene in the skin penetration area can be problematic. See: Percutaneous implant.

skull simulator: Dummy of a skull to elucidate anatomy and execute phantom surgery.

SLA (abbrev.): Sandblasted, large-grit, acid-etched; stereolithography.

sleeper implant: Nonfunctioning endosseous implant retained in bone and covered by mucosa for subsequent exposure and/or use or bone conservation.

slough: Necrotic tissue in the process of separating from viable portions of the body.

SLS (abbrev.): Selective laser sintering.

SM (abbrev.): Subtractive manufacturing.

smear: A thin daub of blood, pus, or extraneous matter on a glass slide stained and mounted for study under the microscope.

smile: Expression of the face in which the lip commissures are elevated to connote pleasure, approval, or joy.

smile line: Imaginary line following the contour of the upper lip in the act of smiling. The contour of the lower lip generally parallels the curvature of the incisal edges of the maxillary anterior teeth. In arranging maxillary artificial teeth, the incisal-occlusal plane parallels the smile line to project a pleasing appearance. See: Lip line.

SNA angle: Acronym for sella-nasion-a point; in analysis of a cephalometric radiograph, an angle that indicates the relationship of the maxillary basal arch to the anterior cranial base. It denotes whether the maxilla is in a normal, prognathic, or retrognathic position.

snap impression: See: Preliminary impression.

socioeconomic factors: Issues included when describing the relationship between financial activity and social life.

socket: Any opening or hollow that forms a holder for something, e.g., a tooth. See: Alveolus, Extraction socket.

socket graft: See: Ridge preservation.

socket preservation: See: Extraction socket.

socket seal: A minimally invasive form of ridge augmentation in which a soft tissue autograft is used to cover an augmented socket. Commonly used for esthetic and functional pontic site development.

soft splint: 1. A dental device (appliance), fabricated from a resilient material such as flexible acrylic or vinyl, which covers the upper, lower, or both arches to protect them from trauma or disclusion. An athletic mouth guard is an example. Unlike its hard counterpart, this appliance is used only for short-term indications because of its lack of durability. 2. A characteristic of a portion of an occlusal splint; generally, resilient acrylic placed on the intaglio surface for comfort or increased retention.

soft tissue: Any noncalcified tissue. In periodontics, usually refers to the oral mucous membranes including the gingiva.

soft tissue augmentation: Grafting procedure aimed at increasing soft tissue volume.

soft tissue cast: A cast with the implant laboratory analog platform surrounded by an elastic mucosa-simulating material.

soft tissue defect: Defect of soft tissue that may include scarring from previous surgeries, inadequate soft tissue margins, or inadequate soft tissue volume related to an underlying bone defect following trauma or infection.

soft tissue graft: See: Acellular dermal allograft, Connective tissue graft, Subepithelial connective tissue graft.

software-based planning: The use of preoperative computed tomography or cone beam computed tomography imaging with computer software for the diagnosis and planning of dental implant placement and restoration. Information derived from the planning can be used in navigation surgery or the generation of a surgical or stereolithographic guide. See: Stereolithographic guide, Surgical guide.

solder: A fusible metal alloy used to unite the edges or surfaces of two pieces of metal; something that unites or cements.

solder joint: Interface of adjacent metallic surfaces united with appropriate metal alloys to produce a continuous unit.

soldering index: 1. Using a heat-stable investment material to form a refractory cast in order to capture the exact orientation of the units to be soldered that were retrieved via a pick-up impression. 2. Fixing the relative positions of units to be soldered through a rigid connecting material. Fixation of this type is often used in conjunction with an implant analog master cast to accurately capture implant prosthetic unit positions on their respective fixtures.

solid freeform fabrication (SFF): (syn): Additive fabrication, layered manufacturing. A collection of techniques for manufacturing solid objects by the sequential delivery of energy and/or material to specified points in space to produce that solid.

solid screw: A root-form threaded dental implant of a circular cross-section without any vents or holes penetrating the implant body.

somatoprosthesis: Artificial body part.

somatoprosthetics: The science of artificial replacement of missing or deformed parts of the body with medical-grade silicone, glass, and/or acrylic. Often these prostheses are anchored to the body through the use of osseointegrated implants with clips, snaps, or magnets.

sonicate (sonicated, sonicating, sonication): Application of sound energy to agitate particles in a solution. Often used to create air bubbles through cavitation in order to disrupt microorganisms.

sonics: An instrument vibrating in the sonic range (approximately 6000 cps) that, accompanied by a stream of water, can be used to remove adherent deposits from teeth.

sounding: Serial measurement of the thickness of intraoral soft tissue in order to map the topography of the underlying bone. See: Ridge sounding, Bone sounding.

spacemaking: Property of surgical site capable of maintaining a space under a membrane for the purpose of guided bone regeneration (GBR). This may be provided by (1) defect morphology in either three-wall or two-wall defects; (2) use of bone grafts or substitutes to support the membrane; (3) membrane itself, which is rigid and stable enough to maintain a secluded space below; (4) using a reinforced membrane to avoid membrane collapse.

spark erosion: See: Electric discharge method (EDM).

spasm: A sudden, involuntary, generally painful contraction of a muscle, or groups of muscle fibers.

spatula: A flat-bladed instrument used for mixing or spreading materials.

spatulation: The manipulation of material with a spatula to produce a homogenous mass.

speaking space: The dynamic air space between intraoral structures (e.g., the incisal or occlusal surfaces of the opposing teeth) during speech.

specialized oral mucosa: See: Oral mucosa.

specificity: The ability of a diagnostic test to detect the absence of a disease in a healthy population. Specificity = true negatives divided by the sum of true negatives plus false positives, or TN/(FN + TN). True positives are correct positive diagnoses; false negatives are incorrect negative diagnoses. Diagnostic tests with high specificity are often used to confirm the presence of a malady first suggested by a highly sensitive but less specific screening test. See: Sensitivity.

specimen: A representative sample removed from the whole for analysis in order to make a diagnostic or histologic characterization.

spicule: A slight, pointed, needle-like body, such as a small piece of bone. In dentistry, a bony fragment may be loose or attached to the maxilla or mandible after a tooth extraction.

spiral cone beam computed tomography: See: Cone beam computed tomography (CBCT).

spiral drill: Cutting instrument with a three-dimensional continuous curving surface around a shaft used to create cylindrical openings in bone.

spirochete: General term for any microorganism of the order Spirochaetales. This spiral, gram-negative, highly motile bacterium is characterized by a flexible cell wall. It is markedly increased in number in diseased periodontal pockets. The major genus in diseased periodontal tissues is *Treponema*. See: *Treponema denticola.*

splint: 1. In dentistry, the connection of two or more teeth into a nonmobile unit by means of fixed or removable restorations or appliances. 2. In physiology, protracted muscle spasms that impede or prevent movement. 3. A rigid or flexible device that maintains in position a displaced or movable part; also used to keep in place and protect an injured part.

splinting: Joining of two or more teeth or implants into a rigid or nonrigid unit by means of fixed or removable restorations or devices. See: Cross-arch stabilization.

splinting, of abutments: The joining of two or more teeth into a rigid unit.

splinting, of muscles: Prolonged muscle spasms that inhibit or prevent movement of a joint or appendage.

split-cast method: 1. Technique for mounting indexed casts on an articulator to facilitate their removal and replacement on the instrument in the same relationship. 2. Method of checking an articulator's ability to accept or be adjusted to a maxillomandibular occlusal record.

split-cast mounting: A technique of mounting casts where the base of the dental cast is grooved and indexed to the mounting ring's base. The procedure allows for verification of the mounting accuracy, ease of removal, and precise replacement of the casts.

split-crest technique: See: Ridge expansion, Alveolar ridge augmentation, Split-ridge technique for alveolar ridge augmentation.

split-ridge technique: See: Partial-thickness flap, Split-thickness flap.

split-thickness graft: A transfer of a partial-thickness (depth-wise) skin or mucous membrane tissue composed of epithelium and a portion of the dermis to a site distant from the site of origin.

spongy bone: See: Trabecular bone.

spontaneous fracture: Breakage of bone occurring without any apparent external damage or trauma. Also called pathologic fracture. The fracture may be caused by osteoporosis, osteosarcoma, or other necrotic condition.

spoon denture: An obsolete term for a claspless maxillary interim removable dental prosthesis that has a spoon-shaped palatal resin base. The resin base is limited to the central portion of the palate and therefore does not contact the lingual surfaces of the maxillary teeth. Frequently, it is used during periodontal treatment because the design of the resin base does not contact the teeth, so it permits surgical procedures and does not promote plaque collection around the teeth.

sporadic: Single, scattered; not epidemic; occurring at isolated geographical and/or temporal loci, especially when referring to a disease.

sprue: 1. The channel or hole through which plastic or metal is poured or cast into a gate or reservoir and then into a mold. 2. The cast metal or plastic that connects a casting to the residual sprue button.

sprue button: The material remaining in the reservoir of the mold after a dental casting.

sprue former: A wax, plastic, or metal pattern used to form the channel or channels allowing molten metal to flow into a mold to make a casting.

SPT (abbrev.): Supportive periodontal therapy. See: Periodontal maintenance.

square impression coping: Impression coping designed as a square when viewed in cross-section. The height varies as does the manufacturer's design; it may include indentations (i.e., concavities or convexities) along the length of the square. See: Impression coping.

SSS (abbrev.): Silent sinus syndrome.

stability: Property of a material, implant, prosthesis, or dental restoration to maintain an intended physical position or state when subjected to forces disturbing its equilibrium, e.g., resistance to displacement of a prosthesis or restoration in the horizontal plane. See: Primary stability, Secondary stability.

stabilization: The seating of a fixed or removable denture so that it will not tilt or be displaced under pressure. See: Bicortical stabilization, Cross-arch stabilization, Bilateral stabilization, Stability.

stabilize: 1. To make firm, steadfast, stable. 2. To hold steady, as to maintain the stability of any object by means of a stabilizer.

stack: Vertically aligned and assembled combination of a prosthetic restoration, abutment, and implant.

staged protocol: A treatment sequence where one procedure is performed, followed by another at a later time.

stage one surgery: (syn): First-stage surgery. A surgical procedure that consists of placing an endosseous dental implant in bone and suturing the soft tissues over the implant, thereby submerging the implant for healing.

stage two surgery: Following stage one surgery, the uncovering or reopening of an implant site at a later date by a small gingival excision or tissue punch to remove the healing screw and replace it with an abutment.

staggered implant placement: See: Tripodization.

staggered offset: Positioning of multiple implants (minimum of three) such that the implant bodies are not in a linear relationship; the purpose is to increase the mechanical stability of the resulting assembly. See: Tripodization.

standard abutment: Machined titanium, cylindrical abutment used to support a screw-retained prosthesis. See: Hybrid prosthesis.

standard deviation (SD): Measure of the dispersion or variability of a set of values. Defined mathematically, it is the square root of the variance of these observations. By definition, approximately 68% of the values in the normal distribution (or bell-shaped curve) fall within 1 SD on either side of the mean. If the SD exceeds one half the mean, the data is not normally distributed.

standard error (SE): Measure of the dispersion of the possible differences between samples of two populations, usually the difference between the means of the samples.

standard tessellation language (STL): File format native to the stereolithography CAD software created by 3D Systems. This format is supported by many other software packages and is widely used for rapid prototyping and computer-aided manufacturing. An STL file describes only the surface geometry of a 3D object without any representation of color, texture, or other common CAD model attributes.

standard of care: The level of care that reasonably prudent healthcare providers in the same or a similar locality would provide under similar circumstances.

Staphylococcus aureus: Aerobic bacteria characterized as being gram-positive and nonmotile that present as cocci, chains, clusters, or pairs; frequently found in the nares, gingiva, and sputum; appear as a white, pink, or red area on the skin.

Staphylococcus epidermidis: Aerobic bacteria characterized as being gram-positive, nonmotile, and spherical in nature; frequently found in the supragingival plaque; they can cause infection in compromised hosts.

staple implant: See: Transosseous implant.

static: In a state of rest or equilibrium; not dynamic; pertaining to that which is stationary.

static loading: Situation where a dental implant is subject to a force which is constant in magnitude and direction (e.g., during its use for orthodontic anchorage). See: Dynamic loading.

statistical significance: See: Null hypothesis, P value.

statistics: A collection of numerical facts pertaining to a subject; the science that deals with collection, organization, and analysis of such facts.

stay plate: A temporary partial denture that is used while a patient's gums and supporting bone are healing after tooth removal. It replaces the missing tooth or teeth and can help the patient with chewing and speaking until a more permanent solution is achieved. A stay plate also helps maintain the patient's appearance and keeps the remaining teeth in the same arch from shifting.

steam cleaning: Using pressurized steam, debris is removed from objects; in dentistry, this process is used to remove debris from a restoration, framework, or dental prosthesis.

stem cell: Primary undifferentiated cell that retains the ability to produce an identical copy of itself when divided (self-renew) and differentiated into another cell type.

stenosis (pl. stenoses): A narrowing in the diameter of a passage; may occur by constriction, occlusion, or inflammation. *Adj*: stenotic.

stent: Prosthesis used to hold grafts together or to maintain patency of orifices, vessels, or ducts; in dentistry; a prosthetic device used to prevent movement of hard and soft tissues to promote healing and protect from infection.

stepped implant: Specific implant shaft design that incorporates concentric steps that narrow in width toward the apex of the implant.

stereognosis: Ability to perceive the weight and form of an object by touch.

stereolithographic guide: A drilling guide generated via computer-aided manufacturing (CAM), according to information derived from software-based planning, used for dental implant placement *in vivo*.

stereolithographic model: A three-dimensional reconstruction of the maxilla or mandible generated via computer-aided manufacturing (CAM) according to information derived from software-based planning.

stereolithography (SLA): syn. Three-dimensional modeling. A rapid manufacturing and rapid prototyping technology for creating a three-dimensional model by using lasers driven by CAD software from information derived from a CT scan. It is used for surgical planning and the generation of a stereolithographic guide. Also known as 3D printing, optical fabrication, photo-solidification, solid freeform fabrication, and solid imaging.

stereophotogrammetry: A method to estimate the 3D coordinates of points on an object. These are determined by measurements made in two or more photographic images taken from different positions. Common points are identified on each image. A line of sight (or ray) can be constructed from the camera location to the point on the object. It is the intersection of these rays (triangulation) that determines the 3D location of the point.

sterile: Complete absence of all microbial life, including transmissible agents (e.g., fungi, bacteria, viruses, spore forms) on a surface, contained in a fluid, in medication, or in a compound, such as biological culture medium.

sterile technique: Surgical procedure performed under sterile conditions. It takes place under hospital operating room conditions and follows operating room protocol for set-up, instrument transfer and handling, and personnel movement. Surgical scrubs, head covers, shoe covers, and sterile gowns are worn. See: Clean technique.

sterility: All forms of viable microbial life are nonexistent.

sterilization: A term referring to any process that eliminates or kills all forms of microbial life.

steroid hormones: A large family of biologically important hormones containing a tetracyclic (cyclopentanophenanthrene) nucleus. Steroid hormones are generally synthesized from cholesterol and are able to pass through the cell membrane.

Stillman's cleft: A localized V-shaped or slit-like indentation or recession at the midline of the gingival margin of a tooth. It may extend several millimeters toward the mucogingival junction or even to or through the junction.

stimulator, interdental: A device designed for massage of interproximal soft tissues.

stimulus: An agent or action that elicits a physiologic activity or response within the oral tissues.

stipple: The process of producing a stippled appearance of the attached gingiva or its artificial replacement.

stippling: The pitted orange-peel appearance of the attached gingiva, which is considered a structural characteristic of a healthy gingiva.

STL (abbrev.): Standard tessellation language.

stock tray: A metal or plastic prefabricated impression tray used principally for preliminary impressions; available in several standardized sizes and shapes. Compare: Custom tray.

stoma (pl. stomata or stomas): Any surgically constructed opening made for drainage or other purposes.

stomatitis: Inflammation of the mucosal tissues of the oral cavity. **S. medicamentosa**: Eruptive lesions of the oral mucosa resulting from the ingestion of a systemic allergen, usually a medication. **S. venenata**: Lesions caused by exposure to contact allergens.

stomatology: The study of the structures, functions, and diseases of the mouth.

straight abutment: See: Nonangulated abutment, Parallel-sided implant.

strain: Change in dimension of an object when subjected to an external force (stress).

Streptococcus spp.: Gram-positive, nonmotile, facultative bacteria that represent a major group of oral bacteria. Normal constituent of plaque, but also associated with streptococcal diseases elsewhere in the body. **S. intermedius**: Gram-positive, facultative cocci that have been associated with refractory periodontitis. **S. mitior**: Formerly called *Streptococcus viridans*. Gram-positive, nonmotile, aerobic, spherical bacteria that form chains and are isolated from the human respiratory tract and from certain clinical conditions. including infective endocarditis. **S. mitis**: Gram-positive, nonmotile, aerobic cocci that tend to form chains and are found in dental plaque. It is difficult to define *S. mitis* as it does little physiologically and is antigenically heterogeneous. It is often defined by exclusion. **S. oralis**: Gram-positive, nonmotile, facultative cocci found primarily in plaque of healthy individuals or in healthy sites in individuals with periodontal disease. **S. sanguis**: Gram-positive, nonmotile, aerobic cocci that form chains and are found in dental plaque. Also isolated from blood cultures of patients with subacute bacterial endocarditis. *S. sanguis* is grouped into types I and II.

stress: Force or load applied to an object. See: Bending stress, Compressive stress, Shear stress, Tensile stress, Torsion stress.

stress-bearing region: Areas of the maxillary or mandibular jaws that are capable of supporting a denture prosthesis. This represents the residual ridge, buccal shelf area, and retromolar pad for the mandibular arch and the residual ridge and the palate for the maxillary arch.

stress bending: Load applied to a structure that tends to deform. For an implant, bending stress deforms the long axis of the implant body. See: Nonaxial loading.

stress concentration: A location in a subject or a system where there is a remarkably higher stress compared with other areas or points in response to a particular load.

stress director: Any device, appliance, or system that redirects the occlusal forces of the stomatognathic system.

stress distribution: The pattern of distribution of stress seen when a load is applied to an object or series of objects. For example, the stress distribution in bone associated with an implant-supported restoration depends on the number and location of implants, the design of the prosthetic super-structure, and the anatomy of the surrounding bone.

stress shielding: Situation, particularly in orthopedic joint replacement, in which an implant is stiffer than the bone in which it is placed. Under loading, the implant bears the load and the surrounding bone undergoes disuse atrophy. The shaft of the implant shields the bone from functional loading.

stripped thread: Screw (or internal screw channel) that has lost its thread architecture because the screw was inserted and tight-ened incorrectly or because the screw was pulled from its channel without unscrewing.

stripping: Removal of the surface of an object; the act of creating a stripped thread. See: Stripped thread.

stroma: The connective tissue that forms the framework of an organ, gland, or structure.

structured-light 3D scanner: Scanning device for measuring the three-dimensional shape of an object using projected light pat-terns and a camera system.

stud-type attachment: See: Ball attach-ment, Ball attachment system, O-ring.

study cast: See: Diagnostic cast.

stylus tracing: A planar tracing showing the marginal movement of the mandible as it is scribed on a plate attached to an arch by means of a stylus device attached to the opposing arch. The shape produced depends on the location of the marking point relative to the tracing table during marginal mandib-ular movement.

subantral augmentation: Augmentation of the antral floor with autologous bone or bone substitutes to provide a host site for dental implants. Called also sinus lift, anthroplasty. See: Sinus graft.

subacute: Denotes a phase of disease between the acute and chronic stages.

subcondylar fracture: A fracture located below the condylar head and within the lim-its of the condylar neck.

subcrestal implant placement: See: Crestal implant placement.

subdermal implant: See: Mucosal insert.

subepithelial connective tissue graft (SCTG): Surgical transplantation of har-vested autogenous connective tissue to a recipient area for the purpose of epithelial keratinization, to gain root coverage, to improve esthetics, and/or correct ridge deficiencies.

subgingival calculus: Calculus formed apical to the gingival margin; often brown or black, hard, and tenacious. Also known as seruminal calculus.

subgingival margin: The restoration mar-gin or tooth preparation finish line that is located apical to the free gingival margin.

sublingual: Below or beneath the tongue.

sublingual artery: A branch of the lingual artery, with distribution to the extrinsic mus-cles of the tongue, the sublingual gland, and the mucosa of the region, and with anasto-moses to the artery of the opposite side and the submental artery. The sublingual artery arises at the anterior margin of the hyoglos-sus and runs forward between the genioglos-sus and mylohyoideus to the sublingual gland. It supplies the gland and gives branches to the mylohyoideus and neighbor-ing muscles, as well as to the mucous mem-brane of the floor of the mouth and lingual gingiva.

sublingual fossa: A shallow concavity on the lingual surface of the mandible above the mylohyoid line that accommodates the sub-lingual gland.

subluxation: In reference to the temporo-mandibular joint, an incomplete dislocation or misalignment of the condyle in its fossa.

submerged healing: Implant placement with complete primary soft tissue closure, requiring a second surgical procedure to expose the implant and initiate prosthetic restoration following healing.

submerged implant: A dental implant cov-ered by soft tissue, and isolated from the oral cavity.

submergible implant: Implant that is sub-merged beneath the oral mucosa at time of surgical placement. See: Two-stage implant placement.

submucosal insert: See: Mucosal insert.

subnasal elevation: Rarely performed surgical technique to enhance anterior bone height in the anterior maxilla. Surgically, it can be compared with a sinus floor elevation; instead of elevating the maxillary sinus membrane, the nasal mucosa is elevated.

subocclusal connector: A nonrigid interproximal connector placed apical to and not in alignment with the occlusal plane.

subocclusal surface: An obsolete term for a segment of a tooth's occlusal surface that is beneath the level of the occluding portion of the tooth.

subperiosteal dental implant: A type of dental implant placed beneath the periosteum that rests on the surface of the bone with abutments that protrude through the oral mucosa and are used to support a dental prosthesis. See: Implant, oral.

subperiosteal dental implant abutment: That portion of the implant that protrudes through the mucosa into the oral cavity for the retention or support of a crown or a fixed removable denture. See: Abutment.

subperiosteal dental implant substructure: The component of a subperiosteal implant located beneath the periosteum that provides support for a dental prosthesis via abutments that protrude through the oral mucosa. Also known as the implant body.

subperiosteal dental implant superstructure: Dental prosthesis metal framework that is supra-gingival in location and provides support for artificial teeth and/or denture base material that fits onto the subperiosteal implant abutments.

subperiosteal fracture: A bony fracture occurring beneath the periosteum, without displacement.

subperiosteal implant: Implant designed to rest on the surface of bone, under the periosteum. It consists of a customized casting, made of a surgical-grade metal or alloy. Permucosal abutments, posts and intraoral bars are designed for prosthetic retention. Three types may be distinguished.

(1) Complete subperiosteal implant, used in a completely edentulous arch. (2) Unilateral subperiosteal implant, located on one side of the posterior mandible or maxilla. (3) Circumferential subperiosteal implant, that bypasses remaining teeth or implants.

substantivity: Duration of time a chemical is in contact with a particular substrate; protracted release of a chemical. Related to clearance of a chemical.

subtracted implant surface: Implant surface created through removal of material by exposure to acid, abrasives, or electrolysis. Subtractive process generally creates roughness intended to enhance cell proliferation and osseointegration.

subtracted surface: See: Subtractive surface treatment.

subtraction radiography: Manipulation of a radiograph photographically or digitally where background images are eliminated to highlight areas for comparison.

subtractive manufacturing (SM): Conventional machining is a form of subtractive manufacturing, in which a collection of material-working processes use power-driven machine tools, such as saws, lathes, milling machines, and drill presses. These are used with a sharp cutting tool to physically remove material to achieve a desired geometry.

subtractive surface treatment: (syn): Subtracted surface. Alteration of a dental implant surface by removal of material. See: Additive surface treatment, Textured surface.

succedaneous dentition: See: Dentition, Permanent dentition.

success criterion: Condition established to determine whether data have satisfied their objectives and met the requirements for success.

success rate: The percentage of successes of a procedure or device (e.g., dental implant) in a study or clinical trial according to success criteria defined by the study protocol. See: Survival rate.

sulcular epithelium: (syn): Crevicular epithelium. The nonkeratinized epithelium of the mucosal sulcus surrounding dental implants and teeth.

sulcular fluid: See: Gingival fluid.

sulcular incision: (syn): Intracrevicular incision, Intrasulcular incision. Cut made directly into the gingival or periimplant sulcus, reaching the alveolar bone crest and following the contours of the teeth or dental implants.

Summer osteotome technique: See: Maxillary sinus floor elevation, Osteotome technique.

supereruption: The eruption of teeth beyond the normal occlusal plane.

supernumerary: More than the routine or normal number.

superstructure: The upper (most superior) part of a fixed or removable dental prosthesis of which the replacement teeth and associated gingival/alveolar structures are part.

supporting cusps: Those cusps of teeth that contact the fossae of the opposing teeth to support centric occlusion. In the normal adult tooth arrangement, these are the palatal cusps of the maxillary posterior teeth, the facial cusp.

supportive periodontal therapy (SPT): See: Periodontal maintenance.

suppuration: Formation or discharge of pus; associated with an acute or chronic infection.

supracrestal implant placement: See: Crestal implant placement.

supraeruption: Eruption of a tooth or teeth above the standard occlusal plane.

supragingival: 1. Located above the gingival tissue. 2. Portion of a natural or artificial tooth structure that is coronal to the gingival crest.

supragingival calculus: Calculus formed coronal to the gingival margin; usually formed more recently than subgingival calculus. Also known as salivary calculus.

surface alteration: Modification of an implant surface by additive or subtractive surface treatment. See: Additive surface treatment, Subtractive surface treatment.

surface bonding: Additive surface applied to the implant body.

surface characteristics (implant): The topography of a surface is defined in terms of form, waviness, and roughness. Roughness describes the smallest irregularities in the surface, while form relates to the largest structure or profile. Waviness and roughness are often presented together under the term texture. Two types of dental implant surfaces are usually distinguished: machined and textured.

surface roughness: Qualitative and quantitative features of a dental implant surface determined two-dimensionally by contact stylus profilometry (See: R value) or three-dimensionally by a confocal laser scanner (See: S value). See: Surface characteristics (implant).

surface tension: A property of liquids in which the exposed surface tends to contract to the smallest possible area, as in the spherical formation of drops. This is a phenomenon attributed to the cohesion between the molecules of the liquid.

surface translocating bacteria (STB): Gram-negative, motile, rod-shaped bacteria that have a gliding movement and are found in dental plaque. They include *Campylobacter rectus*, *Eikenella corrodens*, and *Capnocytophaga spp.*

surface treatment: Modification to the implant surface, either structural or chemical, which alters its properties. It may be additive or subtractive in nature.

surfactant: An agent that acts on the surface to reduce interfacial surface tension between two liquids or between a liquid and a solid.

surgery: 1. That branch of medical science concerned with the treatment of diseases or injuries by means of manual or operative methods. 2. The procedures performed by a surgeon. **Implant s.**: Procedures concerned with the placement, uncovering, and removal of implants and the repair or modification of associated hard or soft tissues. **Mucogingival s.**: A surgical procedure indicated to correct or enhance the thickness or amount of, or change the position of, mucogingival tissue. **Osseous s,**: A surgical procedure intended to achieve long-term periodontal health by osteoplasty or ostectomy to reshape and recontour the alveolar bone resulting in physiologic form and contour of the alveolar bone and overlying soft tissues.

surgical bed: Surgically prepared site, ready to receive an implant, bone graft, or soft tissue graft.

surgical curettage: See: Curettage

surgical dressing: See: Periodontal dressing.

surgical guide: A guide, derived from the diagnostic wax-up, used to assist in the preparation for and placement of dental implants. It dictates drilling position and angulation. See: Surgical prosthesis, Surgical template.

surgical implant: Device made from a non-living material and surgically placed into the human body where it is intended to remain for a significant period of time to perform a specific function.

surgical indexing: Record used to register the position of an implant at stage one or stage two surgery.

surgical navigation: Computer-aided intra-operative navigation of surgical instruments and operation site, using real-time matching to the patient's anatomy. During surgical navigation, deviations from a preoperative plan can be immediately observed on the monitor.

surgical occlusion rim: An occlusion rim used for recording the maxillomandibular relationship and for guidance in positioning replacement or denture teeth.

surgical prosthesis: Any ancillary prosthesis intended for a short-term application that can be inserted at the time of surgery.

surgical splint: An ancillary appliance used to maintain tissues in a new position after surgery. It is commonly used to reset normal occlusal relations during a period of immobilization. The appliance is frequently designed to make use of existing teeth and/or alveolar processes as points of anchorage to help stabilize broken bones during the healing phase. Often patient's existing prosthesis can be used with modification to serve this purpose.

surgical stent: Named for the dentist who first described their use, Charles R. Stent. Such ancillary prostheses are used to apply pressure to soft tissues to facilitate healing and prevent cicatrization or collapse. Syn. Columellar stent, periodontal stent, skin graft stent.

surgical template: 1. A guide conforming to the tissue surface and used for surgically shaping the alveolar process. 2. A guide for the surgical placement of implants in the correct position and angulation in the alveolar bone. 3. A guide for establishing proper occlusion during orthognathic surgery.

survival rate: Percentage or estimated percentage of subjects in which a given censored event (e.g., implant failure, prosthesis failure) has not occurred during a time period measured from a given starting point. It is usually used to describe the percentage of implants that remain in the mouth over a specified period of time. See: Kaplan–Meier analysis.

suture: 1. The material (synthetic or natural, resorbable or nonresorbable) used in closing a surgical or traumatic wound. 2. The act or process of uniting the tissues at a surgical or traumatic wound site using suture material.

suturing: The process of uniting the tissues separated by either a traumatic or a surgical wound in a specific manner using an appropriate material.

swage: Any tool used for shaping metal by striking with a hammer or sledgehammer. Or to shape a material by hammering or adapting it onto a die with a swage instrument.

symphysis (pl. symphyses): 1. A type of cartilaginous joint that connects opposing bony surfaces with a plate of fibrocartilage. 2. The immovable dense bony connection between the right and left halves of the adult mandible at the midline.

symptom: Any characteristic of a disease or medical condition that is subjectively perceived.

syndrome: A group of signs and symptoms of disordered function related to one another by means of some anatomical, physiological or biochemical peculiarity. Does not include a precise cause of illness but provides a framework for investigation and management.

syngeneic graft: See: Isograft.

synovial fluid: A viscid fluid secreted by the synovial membrane found inside joint cavities.

synovial membrane: The articular membrane consisting of specialized endothelial cells that have the ability to produce a fluid that fills the joint cavity.

synthetic bone: See: Alloplast, Bone substitute.

synthetic bone material: See: Bone substitute.

synthetic graft: See: Alloplast, Bone substitute.

synthetic graft material: See: Bone substitute.

system (implant): 1. A product line of implants with specific design, surgical protocol, instrumentation, and matching prosthetic components. An implant system may represent a specific concept, inventor, or patent. See: Configuration. 2: ISO 10451 definition: "Dental implant components that are designed to mate together. It consists of the necessary parts and instruments to complete the implant body placement and abutment components."

systematic review: Process of systematically locating, critically appraising, and synthesizing evidence from scientific studies, using appropriate statistical techniques, to draw conclusions based on data summaries and report what is known and not known.

T

T cell: Thymus-dependent lymphocytes that are spherical cells of the lymphoid series and among the principal cells involved in the cell-mediated immune response.

t test: Statistical test often used to compare two groups on the mean value of a continuous response variable. The test is used when the variables have normal distribution.

table, occlusal: The occlusal surface of posterior teeth (premolars and molars).

tack: (syn): Fixation tack. Metal or bioabsorbable pin with a flat head used to secure the position of a barrier membrane in guided bone regeneration.

TAD (abbrev.): Temporary anchorage device.

Tannerella forsythia: A gram-negative, nonmotile, rod-shaped anaerobic bacteria from the phylum Bacteroidetes. Commonly found in subgingival dental plaque, it is an etiologic agent in the development of chronic periodontal disease.

tantalum (Ta): Malleable metal used in the past to fabricate plates, wires, and disks for implantation; atomic number 73 and atomic weight 180.948.

tap: (syn): Threader, Thread former. 1. Bone tap: device used to create a threaded channel in bone for a fixation screw or prior to the insertion of a dental implant into an osteotomy. 2. Metal tap: an instrument made out of a hard metal, used for rethreading damaged internal threads of a dental implant.

tape: See: Articulating tape.

taper: In dentistry, the amount of convergence of opposing external surfaces of a tooth or tooth preparation. The extension of lines representing the external walls form the angle of convergence of a tooth or teeth for a prosthesis.

tapered implant: An endosseous, root-form dental implant, with a wider diameter coronally than apically. The sides of the implant converge apically. It may be threaded or nonthreaded.

tapered impression coping: Impression coping designed to narrow toward the occlusal surface; varies in length.

tapping: The process of creating a threaded channel in bone with a bone tap, for the placement of a fixation screw or prior to the insertion of a dental implant in an osteotomy. Also known as pretapping.

taurodontism: A variation in tooth form affecting some or all of the primary and secondary molars, marked by elongation of the body of the tooth so that the pulp chambers are large apicoocclusally and the roots are reduced in size.

TCP (abbrev.): Tricalcium phosphate.

team approach: Multidisciplinary combination and collaboration of care and/or therapy providers in the restorative management of a patient whose treatment involves dental implants.

teflon compression ring: Prosthetic component made of polyoxymethylene intended to provide resilience between the implant and the prosthesis. This ring is placed between the transmucosal element and the prosthesis. See: Intramobile connector.

teflon scaler: See: Implant scaler.

Glossary of Dental Implantology, First Edition. Khalid Almas, Fawad Javed and Steph Smith.
© 2018 John Wiley & Sons, Inc. Published 2018 by John Wiley & Sons, Inc.

telangiectasia: Permanent dilation of blood vessels near the surface of the skin or mucous membranes that results in small focal red lesions that are commonly seen on the nose, cheeks, and chin. Also called angioectasias or spider veins.

telescopic coping: A thin cast cover fabricated for a prepared tooth or implant abutment, which acts as an undersubstructure for a prosthesis.

telescopic coping attachment system: Retentive mechanism that employs a frictional fit between the matrix and patrix components. External surface of the patrix mirrors the internal surface of the matrix and fits within the confines of the matrix for a frictional, passive fit. See: Telescopic coping.

telescopic crown: A secondary or artificial crown that fits over a fixed or nonremovable prosthesis, such as a primary crown, coping, bar, or any other suitable rigid support for the dental prosthesis.

telescopic denture: See: Overdenture.

temporomandibular articulation: Ginglymoarthrodial-type articulating joint involved in the bilateral connection of mandibular condyles to the temporal bone. Anatomic structures comprising the joint are the anterior part of the glenoid cavity of the temporal bone, its articular eminence, and the mandibular condyle; the ligaments supporting the joint are the temporomandibular, capsular, sphenomandibular, stylomandibular, and articular disk or meniscus. The joint facilitates mandibular movements involving depression and elevation, as well as forward, backward, and lateral combinations.

temporomandibular disorders (TMD): A collection of medical and dental conditions affecting the temporomandibular joint (TMJ) and/or muscles of mastication and other contiguous tissue components. Includes myofascial pain-dysfunction syndrome (MPD), meniscal displacement with or without reduction (internal derangement), degenerative joint disease (osteoarthritis), rheumatoid arthritis, and other disorders of systemic origin, facial growth disharmonies, traumatic injuries, and neoplasms.

temporomandibular joint (TMJ): The joint that connects the head of the condyloid process of the mandible and the mandibular fossa of the temporal bone via an articular disk; allows rotational and sliding movement of the mandible by a sliding hinge mechanism.

temporomandibular joint hypermobility: Pathologically excessive mobility of the temporomandibular joint commonly associated with internal disk derangement.

template: 1. A pattern, mold, or gauge used as a guide to form a piece being made. 2. A curved or flat surface pattern that is used as an aid in arranging teeth.

temporary abutment: (syn): Temporary cylinder. Abutment used for the fabrication of an interim restoration. The interim restoration may be cemented on the temporary abutment or the temporary abutment may be incorporated in the interim restoration, enabling it to be screw-retained.

temporary anchorage device (TAD): Mini-screw, osseointegrated palatal or retromolar dental implant, placed to control tooth movement during orthodontic treatment.

temporary cement: See: Cement.

temporary cylinder: See: Temporary abutment.

temporary healing cuff: See: Healing abutment.

temporary prosthesis: See: Prosthesis.

temporary prosthesis/restoration: See: Interim prosthesis/restoration.

tensile strain: Elongation/original length × 100%.

tensile stress: Stress caused by a load (two forces applied away from one another in the same straight line) that tends to stretch or elongate an object. See: Stress.

tension: The state of being stretched, strained, or extended.

tension-free flap closure: The capacity of a surgical flap to be passively repositioned into its original position, and to maintain that position without the intervention of an operator or the placement of sutures.

tension-free wound closure: Wound closure that can be obtained without flap tension. Underlying periosteum may need to be released to provide coverage of an augmented site. See: Releasing incision.

tent pole: A mechanical device fixed to the surface of the bone used to elevate a barrier membrane. See: Tenting.

tent pole procedure: Operation in which the anterior part of an atrophic mandible is exposed by an extraoral approach; periosteum and soft tissues are elevated to expose the superior aspect of the mandible. Dental implants are placed by tenting the soft tissue matrix to prevent graft resorption. Particulate autogenous bone chips are onlayed under the periosteum and around the implants.

tenting: The adjustment of a barrier membrane to create a space between the membrane and the bone. Tenting screws, poles, or titanium reinforcement assist in the creation of that space.

tenting screw: A metal screw used in guided bone regeneration to support a barrier membrane, thus maintaining a space under the membrane for bone regeneration.

teratogenesis: The production of birth defects in a fetus or embryo, often by a drug.

terminal jaw relation record: A record of the mandible in relation to the maxilla in the terminal hinge position.

tessellation: The division of a surface into smaller polygons, yielding a higher level of detail.

test group: See: Experimental group.

test, chi-square: See: Chi-square test.

tetracycline: Group of wide-spectrum antibiotics seldom used in treatment of oral infections but may be used for rhinogenic infections. Some are natural (i.e., isolated from certain species of *Streptomyces*) and others are produced semi-synthetically. Tetracyclines and their analogs inhibit protein synthesis by their action on microbial ribosomes and have antimatrix metalloproteinase (MMP) activity. All have similar toxic and pharmacologic properties, differing mainly in their absorption and suitability for various modes of administration. They are effective against a broad range of aerobic and anaerobic gram-positive and gram-negative bacteria, as well as Rickettseae, Chlamydiae,

and Mycoplasmas. Because of the binding to calcium, it is not advisable to use tetracyclines in the treatment of infections in children.

tetracycline bone labeling: Permanent labeling of osteoid (bone matrix) as it mineralizes in a two-phase process. With up to 80% of complete mineral uptake regulated by osteoblasts, the remaining 20% is regulated by osteocytes. The osteoid zone is separated from the mineralized part of the bone by a layer called the mineralization front. This layer is able to bind tetracycline, resulting in a permanent fluorescent line.

texture mapping: Method for adding detail, surface texture (a bitmap or raster image), or color to a computer-generated graphic or 3D model.

textured surface: A surface that has been altered or modified from its original machined state. A dental implant surface can be altered by addition or by reduction.

texturing: Process of increasing the surface area. See: Textured surface.

TGF (abbrev.): Transforming growth factor.

TGF-β (abbrev.): Transforming growth factor beta.

therapeutic prosthesis: An appliance that assists in the treatment of periodontal disease.

therapy: Treatment of disease.

thermal expansion: Heat-induced expansion of a material or substance.

thermoplastic: A property of a material that allows it to be softened by the application of heat and returned to the hardened state on cooling; thermoplasticity.

thick flat periodontium: See: Periodontal biotype.

thin scalloped periodontium: See: Periodontal biotype.

thread: Grooves cut into the walls of a cylinder making it a screw (positive) or a screw channel (negative). These structures guide the insertion and removal of a screw or bolt. Also, the act of inserting a screw or bolt into its receiving channel.

thread angle: The angle between the flanks, measured in an axial plane section.

thread crest: The prominent part of a thread, whether internal or external.

thread depth: The distance between the major and minor diameter of the thread.

thread flank: The portion of a screw thread that joins the thread root to the screw crest.

thread-former: See: Tap.

thread lead: The distance a screw thread advances axially in one turn.

thread path: The conduit in the internal aspect of a screw access hole which guides the threads of a component. Also, the pathway created by a bone tap in an osteotomy, which directs a dental implant during insertion.

thread pitch: The distance from a point on the screw thread to a corresponding point on the next thread measured parallel to the axis.

thread root: The bottom of the groove between the two flanking surfaces of the thread, whether internal or external.

thread run out: The end section of a threaded shank that is not cut or rolled to full depth providing the transition between the fastener shank and full-depth threads.

threaded implant: An endosseous, root-form dental implant, with threads similar to a screw. It is also known as a screw-shaped implant. It may be parallel-sided or tapered.

threader: See: Tap.

three-dimensional guidance system for implant placement: A computed tomography (CT) scan is performed to provide image data for a three-dimensional guidance construct for implant placement. A guide is a structure or marking that directs the motion or positioning of something, thus in implant dentistry this term should not be used as a synonym for surgical implant guide. A radiographic guide is rather used as a positioning device in intraoral radiography. See: Radiographic prosthesis.

three-dimensional imaging: See: Computed tomography (CT).

three-dimensional implant: An endosseous dental implant that is inserted laterally, from the facial aspect of an edentulous ridge.

three-dimensional layering: See: Stereolithography.

three-dimensional modeling: See: Stereolithography.

three-dimensional printing: A category of rapid prototyping technology. A three-dimensional object is created by layering and connecting successive cross-sections of material from information derived from a CT scan. It is used for surgical planning and the generation of a surgical guide. See: Stereolithography.

thrombocyte: See: Platelet.

thrombocythemia: An abnormal increase in the number of circulating platelets.

thrombocytopenia: A decrease in the number of circulating platelets.

Ti: Symbol for titanium.

Ti-6Al-4V: See: Titanium alloy.

tibia: The inner and larger bone of the leg below the knee. It articulates superiorly with the femur and head of the fibula and inferiorly with the talus. It may serve as a source for bone grafting.

tibial bone graft: A bone graft harvested from the proximal tibia. The graft is mostly cancellous.

tibial bone harvest: Extraoral source of autogenous cancellous bone harvested from the lateral proximal tibia, which can be performed in an ambulatory setting under intravenous sedation. This procedure is rarely used in daily practice.

tic: A spasm; involuntary contraction or twitching, usually of the facial and shoulder muscles.

tinfoil: 1. Paper-thin metal sheeting usually of a tin-lead alloy or aluminum (a misnomer). 2. A base-metal foil used as a separating material between the cast and denture base material during flasking and polymerizing.

tinnitus: A noise in the ears, often described as ringing or roaring.

tinted denture base: Coloration of a denture base to resemble the natural appearance of oral mucosal tissues.

tissue: Composed of cells of a given degree of specialization, differentiation, maturation, and a characteristic intercellular substance. Although the intercellular substance may comprise the major volume, tissues are primarily classified according to the predominating types of cells they contain. **Bone t.**: consists of 70% mineral and 30% organic material. Hydroxyapatite (HA) comprises

95% of the mineral and the other 5% comprises complex salts with magnesium, fluorine, sodium, potassium, and chlorine. The organic part consists of 98% matrix, where collagen type I comprises 95% and noncollagenous proteins 5%. The remaining 2% of organic material are the cells, osteoblasts, osteocytes, osteoclasts, and lining cells.

tissue bank: Centers for acquiring, characterizing, and storing human organs or tissue for future use by other individuals. It may also designate storage of information about tissues (e.g., bone bank, skin bank).

tissue-borne: See: Tissue-supported.

tissue conditioner: Elastomeric material with limited flow properties used to massage abused or healing soft tissues. Usually a modified acrylic resin consisting of a polymer (e.g., ethyl methacrylate or co-polymer) and an aromatic ester-ethyl alcohol mixture.

tissue conditioning: Process of restoring health to oral stress-bearing soft tissues following surgical or mechanical trauma using the occluding prostheses to transmit continuous stress of force and motion to the basal-seat tissues. A tissue conditioner is often used.

tissue displaceability: The quality of tissue that allows it to be displaced to a position not achieved by the natural and relaxed state; different tissues allow for varying degrees of displacement.

tissue displacement: Alteration in form or position of tissues that can occur when pressure is applied; this may alter the accuracy of oral tissue impressions during impression taking.

tissue engineering: A technique to utilize a combination of cells, signaling molecules, and scaffolds in an effort to regenerate tissues, thereby restoring biological function and structures. Combination of principles of life and engineering sciences used to develop materials and methods to repair damaged, lost, or diseased tissue. It is also used to create entire tissue and organ replacements.

tissue-integrated prosthesis: Screw-connected, fixed or removable, orodental, maxillofacial restoration retained by osseointegrated endosseous implants. Term was originally proposed by Brånemark and colleagues (Sweden) and intended for a full-arch prosthesis fabricated for an edentulous arch.

tissue integration: Interdigitation of soft or hard tissues with an implant biomaterial.

tissue punch: A sharp circular instrument of different diameters used to create an incision in the soft tissue. See: Tissue punch technique.

tissue punch technique: Circular incision made in the soft tissue over a submerged dental implant, manually or mechanically, of a diameter similar to the implant platform. This results in the exposure of the implant by the removal of a circular piece of soft tissue. See: Stage two surgery. Also, the excision of a circular piece of soft tissue to access the underlying bone surface for implant placement. See: Flapless implant surgery, Tissue punch.

tissue recession: Drawing away of a tissue from its normal position (e.g., gingival recession). See: Gingival recession, Periimplant tissue recession.

tissue registration: An obsolete term for the process of recording the shape of tissues with a material such that distortion does not occur.

tissue-supported: (syn): Tissue-borne. Supported by the soft tissue of the edentulous alveolar ridge.

titanium-reinforced expanded polytetrafluoroethylene membrane: Expanded polytetrafluoroethylene (e-PTFE) membrane reinforced by an attached titanium structure that allows increased rigidity when performing guided bone regeneration (GBR) procedures.

titanium (Ti): An element that has qualities making it biocompatible, bioinert, and nontoxic.

titanium alloy: A biocompatible medical alloy used for the fabrication of dental implants and their components. Its physical properties are superior to most commercially pure titanium. The most common titanium alloy used for the fabrication of dental implants is Ti-6Al-4V, which contains approximately 90% titanium, 6% aluminum, and 4% vanadium. See: Commercially pure titanium, Titanium.

titanium mesh: A flexible titanium grid used in bone augmentation procedures to assist in maintaining a predetermined volume for bone regeneration during healing.

titanium oxide: Naturally occurring compounds of titanium and oxygen in various configurations. Chemical formula for titanium oxides are: TiO, TiO_2, $Ti2O_3$, and $Ti3O_5$. Titanium oxide occurs naturally on the surface of titanium when it is exposed to air, and it is critical to osseointegration between living bone and a titanium implant.

titanium plasma sprayed (TPS): A process involving high-temperature deposition of titanium powders that are totally or partially melted and then rapidly resolidified, forming a dense or porous coating. See: Plasma sprayed.

titanium reinforced: A material that is reinforced by a titanium structure for increased rigidity.

titanium root-form implant: See: Endosseous implant.

titanium skin-penetrating implant: See: Percutaneous implant.

TMD (abbrev.): Temporomandibular disorders.

TMJ (abbrev.): Temporomandibular joint.

tolerance: 1. The ability to endure or be less responsive to a stimulus over a period of continued exposure. 2. The power of resisting the action of a poison or of taking a drug continuously or in large doses without injurious effect. 3. Decreasing response to continued use of the same dose of a drug.

tomogram: A radiograph that demonstrates images at various depths based on a method of moving the film during exposure.

tomograph: An apparatus that is used to create a tomogram. The machine allows for the movement of the film in one direction, while the source of radiation moves in an opposite direction to produce images at a targeted depth within the tissues.

tomography: Imaging by sections or sectioning. See: Computed tomography (CT), Cone beam computerized tomography (CBCT).

tongue thrusting: The infantile pattern of suckle swallow in which the tongue is placed between the incisor teeth or alveolar ridges during the initial stages of deglutition, resulting sometimes in an anterior open occlusion, deformation of the jaws, and/or abnormal function.

tonus, muscle: The slight continuous contraction of muscle that aids in the maintenance of posture and in the return of blood to the heart.

tooth arrangement: The art of placing teeth into determined ideal positions on a denture base so as to achieve the desired results related to esthetic and functional objectives. Trial placements are frequently done allowing for further movement to enhance the initial results.

tooth borne: See: Tooth supported.

tooth color selection: To choose an appropriate shade of a tooth or teeth so as to harmoniously match the needs of a patient.

tooth extraction: Removal of a tooth or teeth.

tooth extrusion: The tendency of a tooth to continue the state of eruption. It can be excessive when the forces that naturally limit eruption are not present. Also known as overeruption.

tooth form: The characteristics of the curves, lines, angles, and contours of various teeth that permit their identification and differentiation. See: Anterior t. f., Posterior t. f.

tooth fracture: Breakage of natural tooth or polymer-based or ceramic prosthetic tooth.

tooth preparation: Shaping a tooth to accept a restoration; this may involve the removal of decayed and/or healthy enamel, dentin, and/or cementum.

tooth selection: Choosing the size, color, and shape.

tooth-size discrepancy: Teeth that are not within normal size parameters compared with the rest of the arch or opposing arch.

tooth supported: A term used to describe a dental prosthesis or part of a prosthesis that depends entirely on the natural teeth for support.

tooth-supported base: The base of a prosthetic device that is completely supported by adjacent teeth.

tooth-supported denture: See: Overdenture.

toothbrush trauma: Damage to the teeth and/or adjacent soft tissues as a result of aggressive tooth brushing.

topical: Surface application, restricted to a surface area.

topography: The description of an anatomical surface region, surface characteristic.

topology: Study of those properties of geometric forms that remain invariant under certain transformations, such as bending or stretching. Whatever type of geometry is used, NURBS, or points, edges, and faces create it. The way these components are connected together and the flow around the 3D object is the topology.

torque: 1. A force that produces rotation or torsion. 2. A measurement of an instrument's capacity to do work or to continue to rotate under resistance to rotation. It is expressed in Newton centimeters (Ncm). Compare: Moment.

torque controller: Device that limits the potential torque that can be applied to an object; generally considered to be a safety mechanism. See: Torque driver.

torque driver: Instrument used to apply torsional force to an object; generally includes a wrench and a method of gauging the torque being applied.

torque gauge: See: Torque indicator.

torque indicator: Device that registers the torsional force being applied; usually registered as Newton meters, centimeters, or foot pounds. See: Torque driver.

torque wrench: Device designed to apply a tightening force (i.e., torque) with a self-limiting feature to prevent over- or under-tightening. It may be manual or electric. See: Torque driver.

torsion stress: Stress caused by a load that tends to twist an object. See: Stress, Torque.

torus (pl. tori): Rounded protruding bony projection found at the maxillary midline of the hard palate or on the mandible's lingual surface in the premolar/molar region. Often bilateral. **T. mandibularis**: A bony exostosis on the lingual aspect of the mandible, generally in the premolar/molar region; commonly bilateral. **T. palatinus**: A bony protuberance occurring at the midline of the hard palate.

toughness: The ability of a material to resist fracture when stressed.

toxicity: The degree to which a substance can damage an organism. The reaction can be localized or systemic and the response level depends on the toxin's dose, rate of release, route of administration, duration of exposure, and specific characteristics.

toxin: A poisonous substance produced by an organism or within living cells. A poison of animal, vegetable, or microbial origin.

TPS (abbrev.): Titanium plasma sprayed. See: Plasma spray.

trabecula: Interconnected bony spicules in cancellous bone.

trabeculae of bone: Anastomosing bony spicules in cancellous bone forming a meshwork of intercommunicating spaces filled with connective tissue.

trabecular bone: Trabecular cancellous bone consists of bone trabeculae, thin plates or spicules with thickness ranging from 50 µm to 400 µm. Trabeculae are interconnected in a honeycomb, nonending, porous system. The pattern of the trabeculae is oriented according to mechanical stress to ensure maximal adaptation to a given stress pattern. See: Cancellous bone.

tranquilizer: A drug that may be used to reduce anxiety and tension. Major tranquilizers are generally used for treatment of psychoses (aka antipsychotic drugs). Minor tranquilizers are prescribed for reduction of anxiety, irritability.

transcranial oblique radiograph: A radiographic view of the temporomandibular joint taken by projection from a superior position on the opposing side of the skull.

transcutaneous electrical neural stimulation: Application of intermittent electrical stimulation through the skin to nearby nerves for the purpose of relieving pain.

transdermal: A technique of administration in which the drug is administered by patch or iontophoresis through skin.

transduction: Process by which genetic material (DNA) is transmitted from one bacterial cell to another via a bacterial virus (phage), thereby changing the genetic constitution of the second organism.

transepithelial: Going through or across the epithelium.

transepithelial abutment: The dental implant abutment that passes through the epithelium and attaches to the dental prosthesis. Called also the dental implant abutment.

transfer coping: A thin, metallic, acrylic resin or other covering or cap used to position a die in an impression.

transfer (implant) impression: See: Closed-tray impression.

transfer index: Core or mold used to record and/or register the relative positions of teeth, anatomic structures, or implants to one another. The fabrication material is rigid and stable, so that the index can be used to transfer the three-dimensional information accurately. See: Index.

transfer jig: See: Transfer index.

transforming growth factor (TGF): Any of several proteins secreted by transformed cells that stimulate growth of normal cells, although not causing transformation. TGF-alpha or TGF-A is a 50-amino acid polypeptide which binds to the epidermal growth factor receptor (EGFR) and also stimulates growth of microvascular endothelial cells. TGF-beta or TGF-B exists as several subtypes, all of which are found in hematopoietic tissue and promote wound healing.

transforms: The process of changing the geometric shape and form of a 3D digital object by manipulating polygonal vertices, points, and lines of the surface mesh structure.

transillumination: The passage of light through body tissues for the purpose of examination.

transit dose: Measurement of the amount of primary radiation that has transmitted through (beyond) the patient and is in line with the transmission axis of the central ray.

transitional contour: The shape that exists at the point where a dental implant abutment and the corresponding dental implant body meet or join.

transitional denture: A removable dental prosthesis serving as an interim prosthesis to which artificial teeth will be added as natural teeth are lost and that will be replaced after postextraction tissue changes have occurred. A transitional denture may become an interim complete dental prosthesis when all the natural teeth have been removed from the dental arch. Called also complete denture.

transitional implant: (syn): Provisional implant. Dental implant used during implant therapy to support a transitional fixed or removable denture. It is usually an immediately loaded narrow diameter implant, which may be removed at a later stage of treatment.

transitional prosthesis: Prosthetic restoration designed to facilitate the progression of patient treatment from one phase to another. Called also conversion prosthesis.

transitional prosthesis/restoration: A temporary prosthesis to replace a missing tooth or teeth during the course of treatment.

transitional restoration: See: Transitional prosthesis.

translation: 1. Movement of the condyle–meniscus complex of the temporomandibular joint over the articular eminence. 2. The movement of a tooth (bodily movement) through alveolar bone without change in inclination.

translucency: Having the appearance between complete opacity and complete transparency; partially opaque.

transmandibular implant: See: Mandibular staple implant, Transosseous implant.

transmucosal: Passing through or across the oral mucosa.

transmucosal abutment: Any piece that connects an implant to the oral cavity through the soft tissue.

transmucosal healing: See: Nonsubmerged healing.

transmucosal loading: The pressure exerted through the soft tissue on a submerged dental implant, usually by a removable denture.

transosseous implant: (syn): Transosteal implant. 1. A dental implant that completely penetrates through the edentulous ridge buccolingually. 2. A dental implant that completely penetrates through the parasymphyseal region of the mandible, from the inferior border through the alveolar crest. See: Mandibular staple implant.

transosteal: Transition of an object through the internal and external cortical plates of bone into and beyond the oral cavity mucosa.

transosteal dental implant: 1. A dental implant that penetrates both cortical plates and passes through the full thickness of the alveolar bone. 2. A dental implant composed of a metal plate with retentive pins to hold it against the inferior border of the mandible that supports transosteal pins that penetrate through the full thickness of the mandible and pass into the mouth in the parasymphyseal region. Called also staple bone implant, mandibular staple implant, transmandibular implant.

transosteal implant: See: Transosseous implant.

transplant: Removal of tissue from one person's body and placing it in another person's body or the removal of tissue from a donor site in one's own body and placing it in another location.

transport segment: In distraction osteogenesis, the sectioned and moving segment of alveolar bone that has been surgically prepared for alveolar distraction osteogenesis. See: Alveolar distraction osteogenesis.

transseptal fiberotomy: See: Gingival fiberotomy.

transudate: Exudate fluid that passes through a tissue surface or membrane; usually associated with inflammation.

transverse horizontal axis: An imagined line about which the mandible rotates within the sagittal plane.

transversion: Displacement of a tooth from its proper numerical position in the jaw.

trap: See: Bone trap.

trauma: A wound or injury, whether physical or psychological.

trauma reconstruction: Surgical and/or prosthetic reconstruction of the craniofacial complex, alveolar ridge, and/or teeth by means of bone grafting, implant placement, and soft tissue reconstruction.

traumatic occlusion: See: Occlusal traumatism.

traumatism: The damaged physical state resulting from an injury or wound. See: Occlusal traumatism.

traumatogenic: Having the ability to produce injury.

traumatogenic occlusion: An obsolete term for a malocclusion that can injure the occlusal tooth surface or supporting bone and/or soft tissue structures.

treatment: See: Adjunctive treatment.

treatment denture: A temporary dental prosthesis used to support and retain tissue during the healing phase in preparation for construction of the definitive prosthesis. See: Interim prosthesis.

treatment plan: The sequence of procedures planned for the treatment of a patient after diagnosis.

treatment planning: Organization and sequencing of treatment procedures and providers (e.g., surgeons, prosthodontists) following patient diagnosis.

trephine: 1. Surgical act of creating a circular opening. 2. Hollow rotary circular instrument that removes a disk or cylinder of bone or tissue; it can be used to create a trough around an endodontic post to assist in its removal from a natural tooth or to remove a dental implant from bone.

trephine drill: Hollow drill used to remove a disk or cylinder of bone or other tissue.

Treponema denticola: Long, thin, corkscrew-like, gram-negative, anaerobic spirochete that has been implicated as a possible etiologic agent of chronic periodontitis and periimplantitis. Characteristic motility and morphology of the organism may be discerned by dark-field microscopy.

trial base: A device or material that represents the base of a removable dental prosthesis and usually has an attached wax rim. Used to record the maxillomandibular relationship for the purpose of setting denture teeth in their proper functional and esthetic location.

trial denture: Placement of teeth, usually in wax, to evaluate the proposed maxillomandibular relationships, esthetics, and function of the prosthesis.

trial-fit gauge: (syn): Implant try-in. Replica or near replica of the body of a specific dental implant configuration used for testing the size of the osteotomy.

trial flask closure: Preliminary closure of a dental prosthesis processing flask that ensures that the mold is completely filled with finishing material and allows excess material to be eliminated.

trial placement: A set-up of denture teeth (usually in wax) on a base material so that a try-in denture may be placed in the patient's mouth to verify esthetics and necessary records or to verify any other necessary steps before completion of the denture.

triamcinolone: An intraarticular, topical, and inhaled glucocorticoid with a long half-life. See: Glucocorticoid.

triangular mesh: A type of polygon mesh used in computer graphics. It comprises a set of triangles connected by their common edges or corners. This allows for 3D digital constructs and their ready manipulation.

tricalcium phosphate (TCP) ($Ca_3(PO_4)_2$): Biodegradable bone substitute that may be used as a carrier; the biodegradation profile is unpredictable. It is similar in composition to naturally occurring bone mineral, provides an osteoconductive matrix, and is resorbed through cellular activity.

trifurcation: Tooth root that is divided into three distinct individual roots, the area where a tooth divides into three distinct roots.

trigeminal: Concerning the fifth cranial nerve (trigeminal nerve).

tripodization: 1. An occlusal scheme characterized by a cusp to fossa relationship in which there are three points of contact about the cusp and opposing fossa with no contact on the cusp tip. 2. Placement of three dental implants using a staggered offset (i.e., not in a straight line) to increase resistance to nonaxial loading. See: Staggered offset.

trismus: Inability to open the mouth due to spasm of the muscles of mastication.

trismus appliance: An ancillary prosthesis that assists the patient in increasing the oral aperture width in order to eat and maintain oral hygiene. (syn): Dynamic bite opener,

interarch expansion device, occlusal device for mandibular trismus.

troche: A tablet with an active ingredient made to dissolve in the oral cavity, especially for medication of the throat.

trough, gingival: See: Gingival crevice.

try-in: Placement of a wax pattern for a tooth restoration, tooth arrangement, or any other tentative restoration in the mouth for jaw record verification, evaluation, and/or alteration prior to completion. Metal castings (e.g., single-tooth restorations, frameworks, copings, or attachments) can also be placed in the mouth for evaluation of fit prior to restoration completion. **T. of framework**: See: Framework. **T. of unglazed restoration**: Try-in of a ceramic or metal-ceramic restoration to evaluate contour, color, occlusion, and proximal contact tightness. The try-in is completed prior to the application of the final ceramic glaze to minimize the need for final adjustments and to create as optimal a restoration as possible.

try-in screw: Threaded component matching the abutment screw, used by the restorative dentist in clinical procedures. Its use avoids damaging the prosthetic screw which is reserved for the clinical insertion of the prosthesis.

tubercule: A small bony nodule or eminence commonly occurring on the palatal alveolar bone.

tuberosity: An osseous projection or protuberance, usually for the attachment of a muscle or tendon. **Maxillary t.**: The most distal protuberance of the posterior portion of the maxillary alveolar ridge that typically curves upward.

tuberosity reduction: The surgical excision of fibrous or bony tissue of the maxillary tuberosity. May be included as part of a distal wedge or osseous resective surgery.

tumefaction: A swelling; the state of being swollen or the act of swelling.

tunica mucosa: See: Mucosa

tunnel dissection: A surgical procedure in which the periosteum is dissected from bone through a small opening made by an incision;

access to the desired bone site is through a tunnel-like opening under the soft tissue.

tunnel preparation: A surgical procedure implemented on a multirooted tooth (usually mandibular molar) that results in a totally opened furcation. The procedure is performed to allow easier and complete access to the area between the roots for the purpose of oral hygiene and improved tissue health.

turgid: Swollen and distended or in a state of congestion.

turned implant surface: The surface texture of an implant as generated by milling machines used in manufacturing of the final implant shape. The surface is not altered subsequent to the machining process. Called also machined implant surface. Compare: Turned surface. See: Machined surface.

turnover: Rate at which biomolecules or cells are lost and/or regenerated through cell division.

twist drill: A rotary cutting instrument with several grooves in its body used to create or widen an osteotomy.

two-implant overdenture: See: Implant overdenture.

two-part implant: A dental implant in which the endosseous and transmucosal portions combine to present a joint surface to the tissues (i.e., implant-abutment junction). See: One-part implant.

two-piece abutment: An abutment that connects to a dental implant with the use of an abutment screw. See: One-piece abutment.

two-piece implant: Anchorage component and element of the prosthetic component manufactured as two separate pieces. Implant and transmucosal abutment are assembled as separate components or elements.

two-stage grafting procedures: These procedures are performed when the bone defect is too large for simultaneous implant placement and sufficient primary implant stability; implant placement is delayed. Compare: One-stage grafting procedures.

two-stage implant: (syn): Submergible implant. An endosseous dental implant designed to be placed according to a two-stage surgery protocol. It undergoes osseointegration while covered with soft tissue. See: One-stage implant.

two-stage implant placement: Protocol followed using two separate surgical procedures for implant placement. In the first stage, an osteotomy site is prepared, the implant is placed, and primary closure is accomplished. The second stage occurs after a specified healing period in which a soft tissue exposure is necessary to uncover the implant and allow connection to transmucosal components prior to definitive implant restoration.

two-stage surgery: A surgical protocol consisting of placing an endosseous root-form dental implant in the bone and leaving it covered with a flap. A second surgery is needed to expose the implant in order to create the prosthesis.

two-stage surgical approach: Category of surgical procedures that must be performed in two interventions. This group includes implant placement with submerged healing that requires a separate uncovering procedure or ridge augmentation procedures with secondary implant placement.

typodont: A model used in training dental students that represents the oral cavity. The model includes a replica of the natural dentition and alveolar mucosa and is set to average condylar movements. Also known as a typodent.

U

UCLA abutment: Prosthetic implant component developed as a plastic castable pattern that can be modified by adding wax for custom shape and dimensions. This is a foundation for creating a cast-to-custom option. The component is screw retained directly into the implant, which circumvents the attachment screw. See: Castable abutment.

UCLA abutment substand: An informal term used to describe a screw-retained dental crown that is screwed directly into the implant body without an intervening abutment.

ulcer, ulceration: A lesion on the surface of the skin or mucosa characterized by discontinuation of the epithelium, deeper than erosion; exhibits gradual tissue disintegration and necrosis, usually with inflammation.

ultimate strength: The maximum stress a material can withstand at its point of rupture. Also known as ultimate tensile strength.

ultrasonic bone surgery: See: Piezoelectric bone surgery.

ultrasonic scaler: An instrument vibrating in the ultrasonic range (approximately 25 000–30 000 cps) which, accompanied by a stream of water, can be used to remove adherent deposits from teeth.

ultrasound stimulation: Treatment modality traditionally used in physiotherapy to treat soft tissue disorders by deep heating tissues. It has been used with good results in treatment of fractures or delayed union and/or nonunions in extremities via a pulse sound wave at 1.5 MHz with an intensity of 30 mW per square cm. It does not seem to stimulate healing of either defects or vertical distraction of the mandible.

ultrastructure: The detailed structure of a biological specimen that is beyond the resolution power of the light microscope, e.g., it may be observable using electron microscopes or technologies that provide greater resolution.

ultraviolet: A wavelength of electromagnetic radiation that is shorter than the violet end of the visible spectrum but longer than that of X-rays. Normally, it refers to wavelengths <380 nm.

uncovery: Popular term for the act of surgically exposing a submerged dental implant, following healing from stage one surgery. See: Stage two surgery.

undercut: 1. The portion of the surface of an object that is below the height of contour in relationship to the path of placement. 2. The contour of a cross-sectional portion of a residual ridge or dental arch that prevents the insertion of a dental prosthesis. 3. Any irregularity in the wall of a prepared tooth that prevents the withdrawal or seating of a wax pattern or casting.

underwood cleft: See: Maxillary sinus septum.

underwood septum: See: Maxillary sinus septum, Septum.

undulate: Having an irregular, wavy border; used of a colony of microorganisms.

uniform color space: If a color space is perceptually uniform, it means a change of length x in any direction of the color space would be perceived by a human as the same or an equal change.

Glossary of Dental Implantology, First Edition. Khalid Almas, Fawad Javed and Steph Smith.
© 2018 John Wiley & Sons, Inc. Published 2018 by John Wiley & Sons, Inc.

unilateral: Confined or relating to only one side; one sided.

unilateral subperiosteal implant: An eposteal dental implant that provides for one or more abutments and that supports and/or retains a removable or fixed dental prosthesis on one side of a partially edentulous dental arch. See: Subperiosteal implant.

uninterrupted suture: See: Continuous suture.

unit load: The part of the total load on a bone, carried by a square unit of its cross-section or surface, that causes a corresponding strain and stress. It is arithmetically equal to the total load divided by the cross-section area of the bone carrying it. Also load calculated as being applied to an individual implant within a multiple-implant restoration. Also, part of the total load on bone imposed by an endosseous implant. Unit compression load usually equals the unit compression stress.

upright: The vertical or normal position of a tooth.

uprighting: Tipping inclined teeth to a more normal vertical axial inclination.

urticaria: A vascular reaction of the skin that presents with pale red, raised, and itchy bumps. Commonly referred to as hives and may be associated with the sensation of burning or stinging. It often occurs in response to an allergic reaction but it can be induced by nonallergic conditions. Allergic-induced reactions usually last less than 6 weeks and are called acute urticaria. Nonallergic reactions usually last longer than 6 weeks and are called chronic urticaria.

V

vacuum tube: See: X-ray tube.

Valsalva maneuver: Performed by attempting to forcibly exhale while keeping the mouth and nose closed. It is an assessment tool, used during surgery, to evaluate the loss of integrity of the Schneiderian membrane.

variance: Degree of dispersion of data about the mean. The square root of the variance is the standard deviation. For bell-shaped curves, the larger the variance, the flatter the distribution curve; the smaller the variance, the more peaked the curve. See: Standard deviation (SD).

Varicella zoster (shingles, herpes zoster): Caused by the herpetovirus (varicella zoster virus); a painful papular or vesicular eruption is seen usually unilaterally on the skin or oral mucosa following the path of the involved sensory nerve. The patient exhibits fever and malaise.

VAS (abbrev.): Visual analog scale.

vascular endothelial growth factor (VEGF): Peptide factor, existing in four forms with different lengths (i.e., 121, 165, 189, and 206 amino acids), that is mitogenic for vascular endothelial cells and promotes tissue vascularization. Its levels are elevated in hypoxia, and it is important in tumor angiogenesis.

vascular pain: A type of deep pain that develops when blood flow to a tissue, organ, or nerves is interrupted.

vascular supply: The source of blood to a tissue or organ.

vascularization: The process of infiltration by blood vessels; regarded as a critical support for the health and maintenance of living tissue or the healing of a graft. See: Angiogenesis.

vasoconstriction: A mechanism that results in a decrease in vessel lumen diameter, especially in arterioles, which in turn increases pressure within the vessel or creates a state of hemostasis.

vasoconstrictor: An agent that promotes decrease in blood vessel diameter. Used in dentistry to prolong anesthesia, and to reduce bleeding during surgical procedures.

vasodepressor: 1. Having the effect of lowering the blood pressure through reduction in peripheral resistance. 2. An agent that causes vasodepression.

vasodilation: The process of increasing the lumen diameter of a blood vessel, especially an arteriole.

vat: A large container used for storing or holding liquids, typically resins used in additive manufacturing processes.

VDO (abbrev.): Vertical dimension of occlusion.

VDR (abbrev.): Vitamin D receptor.

vector: Quantity described both in magnitude and in direction. A force vector is the application of force of a given magnitude in a given direction.

VEGF (abbrev.): Vascular endothelial growth factor.

Veillonella spp.: Gram-negative, nonmotile, anaerobic cocci found in supra- and subgingival plaque.

velum: A membranous structure that partly obscures an opening or covers another structure.

Glossary of Dental Implantology, First Edition. Khalid Almas, Fawad Javed and Steph Smith.
© 2018 John Wiley & Sons, Inc. Published 2018 by John Wiley & Sons, Inc.

veneer: Coating of predetermined thickness, usually resin or ceramic, attached to a crown restoration or pontic by bonding, cementation, or mechanical retention.

vent: An opening in the implant body that allows for tissue ingrowth for increased retention, stability, and antirotation.

verification cast: New cast made from the reassembled index of implants following the validation of fit. See: Verification index.

verification index: Assembled recording of the positional relationship of implants made on a cast or in the mouth for the interchangeable validation of fit. If the fit is incorrect, the index is sectioned and reassembled.

verification jig: (syn): Confirmation jig. An index of multiple implants fabricated on the master cast and tried in the mouth to check the accuracy of the master cast. If the jig does not fit in the mouth, it is cut and reconnected. A new cast or an alteration of the master cast is then made from the reconnected jig, which is called a verification cast. Also, a verification jig can be fabricated directly in the mouth, and a verification cast poured from that.

verification jig: See: Verification index.

vertex: The smallest component of a polygon model. It is simply a point in 3D space. By connecting multiple vertices together, a 3D polygon model can be created. These points can be manipulated to create the desired shape.

vertical alveolar distraction: Alveolar distraction in an apicocoronal direction. See: Alveolar distraction osteogenesis.

vertical bone height: Height of the mandible in the midsagittal plane measured from the inferior border of the edentulous mandible to the top of the crest of the alveolar ridge. This measurement may also be made on a panoramic radiograph. For the maxilla, a superior landmark is defined and the height is measured from there to the crest of the residual ridge.

vertical dimension: Available distance between the incisal and/or occlusal surfaces of the teeth or trial wax occlusion rims during directed acts of speech. Called also speaking space.

vertical dimension decrease: An obsolete term for a change in the teeth, denture base, soft tissue, or bony tissue that brings the maxillary and mandibular dental arches closer together while in occlusion.

vertical dimension increase: An obsolete term for a change in the teeth, denture base, soft tissue, or bony tissue that increases the distance between the maxillary and mandibular dental arches while in occlusion.

vertical dimension of occlusion (VDO): Measurement between facial reference marks when the teeth or wax occlusion rims are in contact. See: Occlusion. **Occlusal v.d.**: The vertical dimension of two designated points on the face when the teeth are in contact in centric occlusion. **Rest v.d.**: The vertical dimension of two designated points on the face when the mandible is in its postural position.

vertical dimension of speech: An alternative to the conventional vertical dimension technique. This distance is frequently measured while the patient is emitting an "s" sound.

vertical incision: A cut made in the soft tissue in the apicocoronal direction to allow elevation and mobilization of a flap.

vertical mattress suture: See: Mattress suture.

vertical opening: See: Vertical dimension.

vertical overlap: 1. The distance teeth lap over their antagonists as measured vertically, especially the distance the maxillary incisal edges extend below those of the mandibular teeth. It may also be used to describe the vertical relations of opposing cusps. 2. The vertical relationship of the incisal edges of the maxillary incisors to the mandibular incisors when the teeth are in maximum intercuspation.

verticentric: A record of the vertical dimension of occlusion with the jaws in centric relation. It is used in complete removable dental prosthesis fabrication.

vesicle: An elevation of the skin or mucous membrane containing a watery fluid and less than 5 mm in diameter. See: Bulla.

vestibular: Common reference to the trough or space between the lateral or buccal surfaces of the teeth or residual ridges and the lips and cheeks; may also refer to the trough or space between the lingual surfaces of the teeth or residual ridges and the tongue.

vestibular incision: Incision placed in the buccal mucosa of the vestibulum. See: Mucobuccal fold incision.

vestibule: 1. Any of various bony cavities, especially when serving as or resembling an entrance to another. 2. The portion of the oral cavity that is bounded on the medial side by the teeth, gingiva, and alveolar ridge or the residual ridge, and on the lateral side by the lips and cheeks.

vestibuloplasty: Plastic surgery of the vestibular region of the mouth designed to restore alveolar ridge height (deepen the vestibular trough) by lowering the muscles that attach to the buccal, labial, and lingual aspects of the jaws.

vibrating line: An imagined line across the posterior part of the maxillary palate marking the division between the mobile and nonmobile tissues of the palate that can be visualized when the mobile tissues are in function.

Vincent's angina: Painful membranous ulceration of the oropharynx, throat, or gums that may be caused by *Fusobacterium nucleatum* infection. It is usually associated with necrotizing ulcerative periodontitis and referred to as trench mouth. See: Bulla.

virology: The study of viruses – biosystems that require a host to replicate, are capable of being pathogenic and can be classified according to their nucleic acid genome (DNA or RNA).

virtual articulation: The process of simulating static and dynamic relationship of teeth in opposite arches using computer software.

virtual model: Digital 3D representation of a dental model created from an intraoral or desktop scan of an object.

virtual reality (VR): A term that applies to computer-simulated environments that can simulate a physical presence in places in the real world, as well as in imaginary worlds. Most current VR environments are primarily visual experiences, displayed either on a computer screen or through special stereoscopic displays. Some simulations include additional sensory information, such as sound through speakers or headphones.

virtual reality modeling language (VRML): Text file format where, for example, vertices and edges for a 3D polygon can be specified along with the surface color, UV-mapped textures, shininess, transparency, etc.

virtual surgical planning: Presurgical manipulation of 3D models of the surgical site to predict outcomes, design surgical guides, or develop options. Generally limited to surgery involving movement of bone, specifically in craniofacial, orthopedic surgery, dental implant placement, and heart and other soft tissue surgical planning.

virulence: The disease-producing potential of a microorganism. Often defined in terms of virulence factors, which are specific characteristics or abilities of the microorganism.

virus: One of a group of minute (15–300 nm) infectious agents characterized by a lack of independent metabolism and the ability to replicate only within living cells.

visceral pain: Deep somatic pain that results from the activation of nociceptors of the mucosal linings, walls of hollow viscera, parenchyma of organs, glands, dental pulps, and vascular structures. These visceral structures may not respond to stimuli that normally evoke pain, such as cutting or burning nuy are sensitive to distension (stretch), ischemia, and inflammation.

visible spectrum: The portion of the electromagnetic radiation spectrum detectable by the human eye. It is referred to as light or visible light and involves wavelengths from approximately 390 to 700 nm.

visual analog scale (VAS): Rating scale used to determine the degree of conditions or stimuli (i.e., pain) a patient is experiencing. Visual analog scales represent a line with clearly defined endpoints expressing on one side of the scale the absence of stimuli (i.e., no pain) while the opposite side represents the highest degree of stimuli (i.e., worst pain ever). The pain or stimuli perception is marked by making a point along the line.

vital biomechanics: Subfield of biomechanics that concerns the manner of biologic response to mechanical usage and loads as well as other physical stimuli.

vital bone content: The percentage of newly formed bone in a histological section obtained from a healed bone grafted site.

vitality test: See: Pulp vitality tests.

vitalometer: An instrument used in determining pulp vitality that measures a tooth's response to variable intensities of electrical stimulus.

vitamin D receptor (VDR): Member of the steroid hormone receptor superfamily through which vitamin D and its analogs exert their actions. Vitamin D is a potent modulator of the immune system and involved in regulating cell proliferation and differentiation.

vitreous carbon: Biomaterial with a glassy amorphous structure once used for the fabrication of endosseous implants or as an implant coating.

Volkmann's canals: Passages containing arteries. They run within the osteons perpendicular to the Haversian canals, interconnecting the latter with each other and the periosteum. See: Haversian canal.

voxel (volumetric pixel or volumetric picture element): Volume element, representing a value on a regular grid in 3D space. Isotropic is cube shaped (CBCT) and orthotropic is rectangular (CT).

VR (abbrev.): Virtual reality.

VRML (abbrev.): Virtual reality modeling language.

V-Y advancement flap: Flap designed to lengthen an area of soft tissue and/or assure primary coverage without tension following tissue removal. Incision is first made in the form of a V and then sutured in the form of a Y.

W

wandering abscess: A localized abscess formed by pus burrowing along fascial planes and forming finger-like projections that may discharge exudate at a distance from the primary focus of infection. Also known as a migrating abscess.

wash impression slang: See: Final impression.

wax: The process of contouring wax into a needed shape, such as making a wax base for a trial-fit denture.

wax pattern: A wax form that represents an item to be made.

wax trial prosthesis: Preliminary prosthetic restoration seated in the mouth for the evaluation of maxillomandibular records, fit, and appearance.

wax try-in: See: Trial placement.

wax-up: Wax and/or plastic pattern contoured to the desired form for a trial denture or castable framework.

waxing sleeve: A premade castable plastic pattern used to fabricate a custom abutment or the framework of a restoration. See: Castable abutment.

wedge procedure: A surgical procedure designed to reduce excessive soft tissue from an edentulous area such as the maxillary tuberosity. See: Distal wedge.

wet milling: Process of milling with diamond or carbide cutters, protected by a spray of cool liquid against overheating of the milled material. This kind of processing is necessary for all metals and glass ceramic material in order to avoid damage through heat development. "Wet" processing is recommended if zirconium oxide ceramic with a higher degree of presintering is employed for the milling process.

white blood cell: See: Leukocyte.

white-light scanner (WLS): A device for measuring the physical geometrical characteristics of an object using white-light interferometry. WLS systems capture intensity data at a series of positions along the vertical axis, determining where the surface is located by using the shape of the white-light interferogram, the localized phase of the interferogram, or a combination of both shape and phase. The white-light interferogram consists of the superposition of fringes generated by multiple wavelengths, obtaining peak fringe contrast as a function of scan position; the red portion of the object beam interferes with the red portion of the reference beam; the blue interferes with the blue, and so forth. A prodigious amount of data is available in a white-light interferogram.

whiting: Washed and ground pure white chalk (calcium carbonate) used for polishing dental materials.

wicking (effect): Bacterial colonization of a suture thread.

Wilcoxon rank sum test: See: Rank sum test.

wire splint: A dental appliance used to stabilize trauma-induced or periodontally involved teeth that are loose. The wire is attached to the mobile tooth (or teeth) and then also fixed to stable teeth on either or both sides of the mobile tooth (teeth).

WLS (abbrev.): White-light scanner.

Wolff's Law: Theory which states that a bone in a healthy person will develop or

Glossary of Dental Implantology, First Edition. Khalid Almas, Fawad Javed and Steph Smith.
© 2018 John Wiley & Sons, Inc. Published 2018 by John Wiley & Sons, Inc.

adjust to a shape or structure that is most suited to resist the loads (forces) being applied to it.

work: Force moved over a distance.

work authorization: A signed prescription that the dentist provides to the dental laboratory specifying the type of dental appliance or prosthesis to be made and the materials to be used for its construction.

working articulation: The points of occlusal contact of the teeth on the side toward which the mandible is moved.

working contacts: An obsolete term for the points of occlusal contact the opposing teeth make on the side toward which the mandible has been moved.

working model: The dental cast used to construct a dental appliance or prosthesis.

working occlusal surface: An obsolete term for the external area of a tooth or teeth on which mastication occurs.

working occlusion: An obsolete term referring to when the mandible is moved from its centric occlusal position; the occlusal contacts made on the side toward which the mandible is moved.

working side: When the mandible is moved from its centric occlusal relationship into a lateral excursion, it is the side toward which the mandible is moved. See: Occlusion. **W.s. condyle**: When the mandible is moved into a lateral excursion, it is the condylar process (the rounded protuberance at the superior end of the mandible that forms the articulation with the skull) on the side toward which the mandible is moved. **W.s. condyle path**: When the mandible is moved into a lateral excursion, it is the path the condyle travels on the working side. **W.s.contacts**: When the mandible is moved from its centric occlusal relationship into a lateral excursion, it is the point(s) of contact made by the teeth on the side toward which the mandible is moved.

wound: Any break in the continuity of a tissue.

wound closure: Flap approximation with sutures. See: Healing by first (primary) intention. **Sutures for w. c.**: Sutures that assist in keeping flap margins well adapted to each other without tension. Varying suturing techniques may be used.

wound dehiscence: Incomplete wound healing because of insufficient blood supply, excessive postsurgical edema, or compromised healing. See: Dehiscence. **Hyperbaric oxygen treatment for w. d.**: Use of hyperbaric oxygen in cases of severely compromised wound healing. See: Hyperbaric oxygen treatment (HBOT).

wound healing: Natural process of restoration of integrity to traumatized tissue in the body. It comprises a set of events that take place in a predictable fashion to repair the damage. These events overlap in time and are categorized into separate phases: inflammatory, proliferative, and maturation.

woven bone: Collagen fibrils oriented in a random or felt-like manner; primarily formed in embryos. In adults, it reappears when accelerated bone formation is required (i.e., healing bone). It has interlacing fibrils, numerous and large osteocytes, and a rather high mineral density. The mineralization process starts 1–3 days after osteoid formation. See: Osteogenesis.

wrench: Device or tool used to apply torsional force to an object, as in tightening or loosening a screw or bolt. See: Cylinder wrench, Open-ended wrench, Torque driver.

wrought: Shaped into a form by use of hands or tools.

X

xenogenic graft: Placement of a tissue obtained from an animal species over, or into, an affected area of another species. Also known as a heterologous graft.

xenograft: (syn): Heterogeneous graft, heterograft. Grafting material harvested from different species from that of the recipient.

xeroderma: Excessive dryness of the skin due to a slight increase of the horny layer and diminished cutaneous secretion.

xeroradiography: The dry photoelectric process by which an X-ray image is captured using metal plates coated with a semiconductor, such as selenium.

xerostomia: Dryness of the mouth due to lack of or inadequate secretions (e.g., inadequate salivary secretions).

X-ray: Limited part of the spectrum of electromagnetic radiation; a self-propagating transverse oscillating wave of electric and magnetic fields.

X-ray tube: Vacuum tube designed to produce X-ray photons. In the tube, there is a cathode to emit electrons into the vacuum and an anode to collect the electrons, where the X-rays are produced by bremsstrahlung.

Glossary of Dental Implantology, First Edition. Khalid Almas, Fawad Javed and Steph Smith.
© 2018 John Wiley & Sons, Inc. Published 2018 by John Wiley & Sons, Inc.

Y

yeast: Classified in the kingdom Fungi, these eukaryotic microorganisms are mostly unicellular but can become multicellular through the formation of pseudohyphae or strings of connected budding cells. Yeast can reproduce by mitosis, asymmetric division or budding. Yeast can become pathogenic in the body, including the oral cavity, especially in people who are immunocompromised through disease or drug therapy.

Young's modulus: Describes the rigidity or stiffness of a material, usually given the symbol E. It is a measure of elasticity equal to the ratio of the stress acting on a substance to the strain produced. A higher modulus (GPa, psi) signifies a greater rigidity or stiffness to the material. Also called modulus of elasticity.

Glossary of Dental Implantology, First Edition. Khalid Almas, Fawad Javed and Steph Smith.
© 2018 John Wiley & Sons, Inc. Published 2018 by John Wiley & Sons, Inc.

Z

zero-degree teeth: Posterior denture teeth having flat planes or zero-degree cusp angles relative to the horizontal occlusal surface of the tooth. See: Nonanatomic teeth.

zirconia: See: Zirconium (Zr), Zirconium dioxide (ZrO_2).

zirconia ceramic post: A ceramic post used instead of metal posts in the restoration of endodontically treated teeth. The ceramic material is preferred to the metal posts for esthetic reasons. Ceramic posts are usually used with a composite resin or compression ceramic to form the core.

zirconium (Zr): A steel-gray hard ductile metallic element with a high melting point that occurs widely in combined forms. It is highly resistant to corrosion, and is used especially in alloys and in refractories and ceramics.

zirconium dioxide (ZrO_2): (syn): Zirconia. White crystalline oxide of zirconium occurring in nature as the mineral baddeleyite. It is an amorphous, odorless, tasteless powder or crystalline solid, used as an opaquing agent for dental porcelain, and other ceramic processes. In implant dentistry, it is used for the fabrication of all-ceramic abutments, substructures of fixed partial dentures, crown copings, and dental implants.

zirconium oxide: Ceramic material used for implant components, with excellent mechanical properties. It is used in situations where esthetics are of primary importance and metal show-through of the tissues is a potential problem. Called also zirconia.

zoledronate: A very potent intravenous nitrogen-containing bisphosphonate used to prevent skeletal fractures in patients with cancers such as multiple myeloma and prostate cancer. It is also used to treat hypercalcemia caused by cancer.

Zr: Symbol: Zirconium.

zygoma: The area formed by the union of the zygomatic bone with the zygomatic processes of the temporal and maxillary bones.

zygomatic implant: A root-form dental implant that has its origin in the region of the former first maxillary molar. Its endpoint engages the zygomatic bone. The implant is directed in a lateral and upward direction with an angulation of approximately 45° from a vertical axis, following an intrasinusal trajectory.

zymogen: An inactive precursor that is converted to active enzyme by the action of another substance. Called also proenzyme.

Glossary of Dental Implantology, First Edition. Khalid Almas, Fawad Javed and Steph Smith.
© 2018 John Wiley & Sons, Inc. Published 2018 by John Wiley & Sons, Inc.

Appendix A   Digital Dental Terms

3D construction: The 3D merged image that is a combination of all individual elements and is suitable for additive or subtractive manufacturing.

3D file formats: File formats are used for creating and storing 3D data files. For example: ply, fbx, vrml, 3DMF, 3DML, 3DXML, obj, dxf, w3d, skp, fmz, s3d, m3g, vue, and STL are all 3D file formats. File formats must be consistent to share 3D datasets, and work within design and production platforms. There are more than 140 3D file formats. The STL file format is commonly used for many open platform dental scanning and design systems. Conversion between file formats can lead to data loss.

3D modeling: Process of developing a digital representation of any three-dimensional object surface (either inanimate or living) via specialized software. The 3D models describe the forms (geometry) of objects, but not their material properties or how they move.

3D printing: A general term describing additive manufacturing processes that build three-dimensional structures by depositing layers of material on top of each other until the final structure is achieved. 3D printing can produce objects made of single or multiple materials without being limited by undercuts or complexity.

3D rendering: Computer graphics process of automatically converting 3D wire frame models into 2D images with 3D photorealistic effects on a computer. Or, the process of converting digital information such as from a CBCT scan using modern 3D computer graphics processing into photorealistic images that can be visualized and manipulated on the computer screen.

3D scanner: A device that analyzes a real-world object to collect data on its shape and/or other attributes such as color or texture and transforms this data into a digital format that can be used with computer software for exportation to 3D printing or CAD CAM applications.

3D surface scanning: Surface mapping that allows for the surface geometry or shape of an object to be stored as a set of 3D points or vertices. The surface of the object is then stored as a series of polygons (or faces) that are constructed by indexing these vertices. The number of vertices the face may index can vary, though triangular faces with three vertices are common.

3D volume: Three-dimensional volume rendering, computed axial tomography (CAT), cone beam computed tomography (CBCT) which can be visualized and manipulated on the computer screen using specific software.

3D volumetric reconstruction: Three-dimensional volumetric reconstruction, Computed axial tomography (CAT), cone beam computed tomography (CBCT), which can be visualized and manipulated on the computer screen using specific software.

3MF: A 3D printing format that will allow design applications to send full-fidelity 3D models to a mix of other applications, platforms,

Glossary of Dental Implantology, First Edition. Khalid Almas, Fawad Javed and Steph Smith.
© 2018 John Wiley & Sons, Inc. Published 2018 by John Wiley & Sons, Inc.

services, and printers. The 3MF specification allows companies to focus on innovation, rather than on basic interoperability issues, and it is engineered to avoid the problems associated with other 3D file formats.

algorithmic dental occlusion (ADO): Computer algorithms used to establish virtual occlusion and movements. The algorithms encode physical motions and responses for each tooth and its respective antagonists and neighboring teeth. The advantage of ADO is that it allows for pursuing the goal of optimal occlusion – as defined by clinical standards – with the untiring effort of a computer.

beam hardening artifact: An imaging artifact that appears as streaks and shadows adjacent to areas of high density such as dense bones, shoulders, dental restoration, and hips.

billet: A length of metal/material that has a round or square cross-section. It is typically used to describe material disks used for milling.

CAD/CAM dentistry: Using computer technologies to design and produce different types of dental restorations, including crowns, veneers, inlays and onlays, fixed prostheses, dental implant restorations, and orthodontic appliances. See computer-aided design and drafting and computer-aided manufacturing.

calibration: A comparison between measurements – one of known magnitude or correctness made or set with one device and another measurement made as similar as possible with a second device. The device with the known or assigned correctness is called the standard. The second device is the unit under test, the test instrument, or any of several other names for the device being calibrated. Successful calibration has to be consistent and systematic. At the same time, the complexity of some instruments requires that only key functions be identified and calibrated. Under those conditions, a degree of randomness is needed to find unexpected deficiencies.

Cone beam computed tomography (CBCT): A medical imaging technique consisting of X-ray computed tomography where the X-rays are divergent, forming a cone. It allows for the collection, storage, and utilization of 3D radiographic data in the DICOM file format, utilizing the.dcm file extension. Machines are often classified as large volume (20 cm height and 15 cm diameter cylinder) and small volume/limited view ($40 \times 40\,mm^2$ or $60 \times 60\,mm^2$) based on the exposure area.

digital denture: A complete denture created by automation using CAD, CAM, and CAE in lieu of traditional processes. A digital denture is achieved when the final shape of the denture is manufactured through automation to ensure there are no conventional errors from pouring, investment casting, or injecting the material as done in traditional denture fabrication.

digital imaging: Computer-based digital technology allowing the dentist to create true-to-life photographs of the dentition, as if the recommended procedures had already been completed.

impression wand: Hand-held device used for intraoral digital scanning.

intraoral scanning: The process of scanning and capturing the intraoral cavity for translation into a digital file format, such as STL.

kinematic strain-free tooth movement: Virtual motion of a tooth among its antagonists and its neighboring teeth by treating the tooth as a rigid body (solid). Kinematic refers to the concept that a tooth is not allowed to interpenetrate another tooth and thus its motion is defined as part of a mechanism composed of its antagonists and neighbors and constraints of the occlusal surface and arch form. Strain-free refers to the concept that a tooth is not allowed to deform. Strain is caused by the deformation of a body (tooth) over part or all of its volume. Kinematic strain-free tooth movement is achieved by requiring the tooth to act as a rigid body, experiencing no deformation under motion. Used in some complete denture digital design software.

milling: The machining process of using rotary cutters (burs) to remove material from a workpiece by advancing (or feeding) in a direction at an angle with the axis of the tool. It covers a wide variety of different operations and machines, on scales from small individual parts to large, heavy-duty milling operations. It is one of the most commonly used processes to fabricate dental restorations with high precision. Mills have multiple axes (e.g., 3-axis, 4-axis, 5-axis) that determine the ability of the milling process to create final detail and complex geometries with undercuts, concave contours, and holes.

pixel: Abbreviation of picture element: the smallest possible element of a picture. A digital image is defined by a discrete number of pixels arranged in a 2D grid or mosaic. Many very small pixels blend together in the human eye and brain to give the illusion of a continuous, unbroken image.

radiodensity: The relatively opaque white appearance of dense materials or substances on radiographic imaging studies.

ring artifact: Phenomenon that occurs due to inaccurate calibration or failure of one or more detector elements in a CT scanner. They occur close to the isocenter of the scan, and are usually visible on multiple slices at the same location. They are a common problem in cranial CT and CBCT.

virtual articulation: The process of simulating static and dynamic relationship of teeth in opposite arches using computer software.

virtual model: Digital 3D representation of a dental model created from an intraoral or desktop scan of an object.

virtual surgical planning: Presurgical manipulation of 3D models of the surgical site to predict outcomes, design surgical guides, or develop options. Generally limited to surgery involving movement of bone, specifically in craniofacial, orthopedic surgery, dental implant placement, and heart and other soft tissue surgical planning.

Appendix B   Useful Websites

AB Dental USA
www.ab-dentusa.com

A. Titan Instruments, Inc
www.atitan.com

Accelerated Practice Concepts, Inc
www.apcdental.com

Accurate Manufacturing, Inc
www.accurategelpacks.com

ACE Surgical Supply Company
www.acesurgical.com

ACTEON North America
www.acteonusa.com

AD Surgical
www.ad-surgical.com

Adin Implants
www.adin-implants.com

Aegis Communications LLC
www.aegiscomm.com

Almitech Inc.
www.almitechimplants.com

AlphaDent
www.alphadent.com

Alpine Pharmaceuticals
www.alpinepharm.com

American Dental Society of Anesthesiology
www.adsahome.org

Anatomage
www.anatomage.com

Aseptico, Inc
www.aseptico.com

Astra Tech Inc.
www.astratechdental.com

Atec Dental GmbH
www.atec-dental.de

Atlantis Components
www.atlantiscomp.com

Benco Dental Company
www.benco.com

Beutlich Pharmaceuticals, LLC
www.beutlich.com

Bicon Dental Implants
www.bicon.com

Bicortical Implant Inc.
www.bicorticalimplant.com

Bident International
www.bident.com

Bien-Air Dental
www.bienair.com

BioHorizons
www.biohorizons.com

BIOLASE
www.biolase.net

Biomet 3i
www.biomet3i.com

Bioplant Inc.
www.bioplanthtr.com

Glossary of Dental Implantology, First Edition. Khalid Almas, Fawad Javed and Steph Smith.
© 2018 John Wiley & Sons, Inc. Published 2018 by John Wiley & Sons, Inc.

BQ Ergonomics LLC
www.BQE-USA.com

Brasseler USA
www.brasslerusa.com

BTI of North America
www.bti-implant.com

Cain, Watters & Associates, PLLC
www.cainwatters.com

Camlog Biotechnologies
www.camlogimplants.com

CareCredit
www.carecredit.com

Carestream Dental
www.carestreamdental.com

CeraRoot zirconia dental implants
www.ceraroot.com

Colgate
www.colgateprofessional.com

Collagen Matrix Dental
www.collagenmatrixdental.com

Community Tissue Services-Maxxeus
www.maxxeus.com

Consult Pro
www.consult-pro.com

Crescent Products
www.crescentproducts.com

Crest Oral-B
www.dentalcare.com

Curasan, Inc
www.curasaninc.com

DCIDS Tissue Bank
www.dcids.org

DecisionBase, Inc
www.decisionbase.com

Dental Tribune
www.dentaltribune.com

Dental USA, Inc.
www.mydentalusa.com

Dentalfone
www.dentalfone.com

DentalVibe
www.dentalvibe.com

Dentatus USA Ltd
www.dentatus.com

Dentis USA
www.dentis.co.kr

Dentium USA
www.dentiumUSA.com

DENTSPLY Implants
www.dentsplyimplants.com

DENTSPLY Professional Division
www.dentsply.com

Dentsply Sirona USA
www.corporate.dentsplysirona.com

Designs for Vision, Inc
www.designsforvision.com

DEXIS Digital X-Ray
www.dexis.com

3D Diagnostix, Inc
www.3ddx.com

Doctor.com
www.doctor.com

Dowell Dental Products, Inc
www.dowelldentalproducts.com

Dr. Fuji/Acigi Relaxation
www.fujichair.com

DSN Software, Inc
www.perioexec.com

Duo-dent Dental Implant systems LLC
www.duodent.com

Dyna Dental engineering b.v.
www.dynadental.com

Enova Illumination
www.enovaillumination.com

Enovative Technologies
www.enovativetech.com

Euro Dental Implant/euroteknica USA
www.Euroteknica.com

Exactech, Inc
www.exac.com

Froncare Inc
www.froncare.com

Geistlich Biomaterials
www.geistlich-na.com

Gendex/NOMAD/SOREDEX/Instrumentarium
www.genex.com

GIDE Institute
www.gidedental.com

Global Surgical Corporation
www.globalsurgical.com

Glustitch, Inc
www.glustitch.com

Guided Surgery Solutions LLC
www.guidedsurgerysolutions.com

Gumchucks at Oralwise, Inc
www.gumchucks.com

H & H Company
htmlreview.com/hhco-store.com.html

Hamilton Capital Management
www.hamiltoncapital.com

Handpiece Solutions, Inc
www.handpiecesolutions.com

Hartzell & Son, G.
www.ghartzellandson.com

Harvest Technologies Corp.
www.harvesttech.com

Hawaiian Moon
www.aloecream.biz

HealthFirst
www.healthfirstcorp.com

Hearst Media Services
www.hearstmediaservices.com

Henry Schein Dental
www.henryschein.com

Hi Tec Implants
www.dentalimplanttech.com

Hiossen, Inc
www.hiossen.com

HUBERMED, INC
www.hubermed.com

Hu-Friedy Manufacturing Company, LLC
www.hufriedy.com

i-CAT Imaging Sciences
www.i-cat.com

IDEA Interdisciplinary Dental Education Academy
www.ideausa.net

ids/Megagen USA, Inc
www.megagen.us

Impladent, Ltd
www.impladentltd.com

Implant Direct International
www.sybronimplants.com

Implant Direct LLC
www.implantdirect.com

Implants Diffusion International
www.idisystem.fr

Infinite Therapeutics
www.infinitetherapeutics.com

Institute for Advanced Laser Dentistry
www.theiald.com

Intra-Lock International
www.intra-lock.com

J. Morita USA, Inc
www.global.morita.com/usa

Kalbirth MedicalCorp
www.cphi-online.com/kalbirth-medical-corp-comp247442.html

Keystone Dental, Inc
www.keystonedental.com

Kilgore International, Inc
www.kilgoreinternational.com

KLS Martin
www.klsmartinnorthamerican.com

Laschal Surgical Instruments, Inc
www.laschaldental.com

Lasers4Dentistry Products, Fotona
www.dentalproductshopper.com/manufacturer/technology4medicine-llc

LED Dental, Inc
www.velscope.com

Lester A. Dine, Inc
www.dinecorp.com

Lexi Comp Publishing
www.lexi.com

LightScalpel
www.LightScalpel.com

Look/Surgical Specialties
www.angiotech.com

LumaDent, Inc
www.LumaDent.com

Mectron Dental
www.dental.mectron.com

Medical Protective
www.medpro.com

Medtronic
www.medtronic.com

Microsurgery Instruments, Inc
www.microsurgeryusa.com

Millennium Dental Technologies
www.LANAP.com

Miltex, An Integra Company
www.integralife.com/integramiltex

MIS Implants Technologies, Inc
www.misimplants.com

My Dental Hub – Practice MarketingTools
www.mydentalhub.com/mdh/login.php

Neodent USA, Inc
www.neodentusa.com

Neoss
www.neoss.com

Nobel Biocare
www.nobelbiocare.com

NSK Dental, LLC
www.nskdental.us

OCO Biomedical
www.ocobiomedical.com

Officite
www.officite.com

OMNIA, LLC
www.omniaspa.us

Oral IceBerg, LLC
www.ceraroot.com

Oraltronics Dental Implant Technology GmbH
www.oraltronics.com

OraPharma, Inc
www.orapharma.com

Orascoptic
www.orascoptic.com

Osada, Inc
www.osadausa.com

Osseous Technologies of America
www.osseoustech.com

Osstell, Inc.
www.osstell.com

OsteoCare implant System Limited
www.osteocare.uk.com

Osteogenics Biomedical
www.osteogenics.com

Osteohealth
www.osteohealth.com

Osteo-Ti
www.osteo-ti.com

Otto Trading Inc
www.irestmassager.com

Pallisades Dental
www.palisadesdental-llc.com

Panda Perio
www.pandaperio.com

Patient Marketing Specialist
www.patientmarketingspecialists.com

Patterson Dental Supply, Inc
www.pattersondental.com

PBHS Web Site Design & Marketing
www.pbhs.com

PDT, Inc
www.pdtdental.com

PeriOptix, Inc
www.perioptix.com

Perioscopy, Inc/Danville Materials LLC
www.danvillematerials.com

Phase II Associates
www.phasetwoassociates.com

Philips Sonicare and Zoom Whitening
www.philipsoralhealthcare.com

PhotoMed
www.photomed.net

Piezosurgery, Inc
www.piezosurgery.us

Pinhole Academy
www.pinholeacademy.com

Planmeca USA, Inc
www.planmecausa.com

PREAT Corporation
www.preat.com

Progressive Dental Marketing
www.progressivedentalmarketing.com

Prophy Perfect/Phb
www.prohpyperfect.com

ProphyMagic
www.prophymagic.com

ProSites
www.prosites.com

Quality Aspirators/Q-Optics
www.q-optics.com

Quintessence Publishing Company, Inc
www.quintpub.com

Renew Biocare Est
www.renewbiocare.us/re-mark

Reputation
www.reputation.com

Reputation.com | Reputation Management
www.reputation.com/dentists

Reuter Systems GmbH
www.reutersystems.de/en/contact

RGP Dental, Inc
www.rgpergo.com

Rx Honing (Sharpening) Machine
www.rxhoning.com

Sabra Dental: Dental Supplies and Surgical
Tools
www.sabradent.com

Salvin Dental Specialties, Inc
www.salvin.com

Schumacher Dental Instruments
www.karlschumacher.com

Sirona Dental
www.sironausa.com

Snap On Optics
www.snaponoptics.com

Snoasis Medical
www.snoasismedical.com

Solutionreach
www.solutionreach.com

Southern Anesthesia + Surgical, Inc
www.southernanesthesia.com

Springstone Patient Financing
www.springstoneplan.com

Steiner Laboratories
www.steinerlabs.com

STMD Corporation
www.stmdmedical.com

Straumann
www.straumannusa.com

Sunstar Americas, Inc
www.gumbrand.com

SurgiTel/General Scientific Corp
www.surgitel.com

Sybron Implant Solutions
www.sybronimplants.com

SW Gloves
www.swgloves.com

TePe Oral Health Care, Inc
www.tepeusa.com

Thommen Medical USA
www.thommenmedical.com

Treloar & Heisel, Inc
www.th-online.net

Trinon titanium GmbH Q-Implant
www.Trinon.com

UltraLight Optics
www.ultalightoptics.com

Unicare Biomedical, Inc
www.unicarebiomedical.com

USHIO America, Inc
www.ushio.com

Vatech America
vatechamerica.com

W&H IMPEX, Inc
www.wh.com/na

WaterPik, Inc
www.waterpik.com

Xemax Surgical Products, Inc
www.xemax.com

Yodle
www.yodle.com

Young's Dental
www.youngsdental.com

Zest Anchors, LLC
www.zestanchors.com

Zimmer Dental
www.zimmerdental.com

Zoll-Dental
www.zolldental.com

Appendix C   Recommended Reading

Academy of Prosthodontics. (2017) The glossary of prosthodontic terms, 9th edn. *J Prosthet Dent*, 117, issue 5S.

ADA Guidelines for Teaching Pain Control and Sedation to Dentists and Dental Students. www.ada.org/~/media/ADA/Member%20Center/FIles/anxiety_guidelines.ashx

Aibinu AM, Salami MJE, Shafie AA, Najeeb AR. (2008) MRI reconstruction using discrete fourier transform: A tutorial. World Academy of Science Engineering and Technology. *IJCIT*, 2(6), 1852–1858.

Alama T, Katayama H, Hirai S, et al. (2016) Enhanced oral delivery of alendronate by sucrose fatty acids esters in rats and their absorption-enhancing mechanisms. *Int J Pharm*, 515(1-2), 476–489.

Alexander PC. (1957) Orthodontic procedures in periodontal therapy. *J Periodontol*, 28(1), 46–48.

Allen EP, Bayne SC, Brodine AH, et al. (2003) Annual review of selected dental literature: Report of the committee on scientific investigation of the American academy of restorative dentistry. *J Prosthet Dent*, 90(1), 50–80.

Al-Nawas B, Wagner W. (2011) Materials in dental implantology. In: Comprehensive Biomaterials, Elsevier, Amsterdam, 341–377.

American Academy of Implant Dentistry (AAID). JOI Glossary of Terms. AAID, Chicago, 2016.

American Academy of Periodontology: www.perio.org

American Academy of Periodontology. (2001) Glossary of Periodontal Terms, 4th edn. American Academy of Periodontology, Chicago.

American Academy of Periodontology Task Force Report on the Update to the 1999 Classification of Periodontal Diseases and Conditions. (2015). *J Periodontol*, 86, 835–838.

American Dental Association. (1984) Classification system for cast alloys. *J Am Dent Assoc*, 109, 766.

Andreasen JO. (2012) Pulp and periodontal tissue repair – regeneration or tissue metaplasia after dental trauma. A review. *Dent Traumatol*, 28(1), 19–24.

Anitua E, Sánchez M, Nurden AT, Nurden P, Orive G, Andía I. (2006) New insights into and novel applications for platelet-rich fibrin therapies. *Trends Biotechnol*, 24(5), 227–34.

Aparicio C, Rangert B, Sennerby L. (2003) Immediate/early loading of dental implants: a report from the Sociedad Espanola de Implantes World Congress Consensus Meeting in Barcelona, Spain, 2002. *Clin Implant Dent Related Res*, 5, 57–60.

Apostolakis D, Brown JE. (2011) The anterior loop of the inferior alveolar nerve: prevalence, measurement of its length and a recommendation for interforaminal implant installation based on cone beam CT imaging. *Clin Oral Implants Res*, 23(9), 1022–1030.

Aravind NKS, Reddy S, Manjunath C, Reddy R. (2012) Rationale for orthodontic treatment in the deciduous and early mixed dentition – a review. *Ann Ess Dent*, 4(3), 60–62.

Glossary of Dental Implantology, First Edition. Khalid Almas, Fawad Javed and Steph Smith.
© 2018 John Wiley & Sons, Inc. Published 2018 by John Wiley & Sons, Inc.

Ash MM Jr. (1993) Wheeler's Dental Anatomy, Physiology and Occlusion, 7th edn. WB Saunders, Philadelphia.

Athanasiou KA, Zhu C, Lanctot DR, Agrawal CM, Wang X. (2000) Fundamentals of biomechanics in tissue engineering of bone. *Tissue Eng*, 6(4), 361–381.

Babu RR, Nayar SV. (2007) Occlusion indicators: a review. *J Indian Prosthodont Soc*, 7(4), 170–174.

Barazanchi A, Li KC, Al-Amleh B, Lyons K, Waddell JN. (2017) Additive technology: update on current materials and applications in dentistry. *J Prosthodont*, 26, 156–163.

Barker TS, Cueva MA, Rivera-Hidalgo F, et al. (2011) A comparative study of root coverage using acellular dermal matrix (Alloderm) versus (Puros Dermis). *J Periodontol*, 81(11), 1596–1603.

Bergendal B. (2014) Orodental manifestations in ectodermal dysplasia – a review. *Am J Med Genet A*, 164A(10), 2465–2471.

Bhanot S, Alex JC. (2002) Current applications of platelet gels in facial plastic surgery. *Facial Plast Surg*, 18(1), 27–33.

Bilgin E, Yasasever V, Soydinc HO, Yasasever CT, Ozturk N, Duranyildiz D. (2012) Markers of bone metastases in breast and lung cancers. *Asian Pac J Cancer Prev*, 13(9), 4331–4334.

Binon PP. (2000) Implants and components: entering into the new millennium. *Int J Oral Maxillofac Implants*, 15, 76–94.

Boucher CO. (1953) Occlusion in prosthodontics. *J Prosthet Dent*, 3, 633–656.

Brunski JB. (1988) Biomaterials and biomechanics in dental implant design. *Int J Oral Maxillofac Implants*, 3, 85–97.

Brunski JB, Puerto DA, Nanci A. (2000) Biomaterials and biomechanics of oral and maxillofacial implants: current status and future developments. *Int J Oral Maxillofac Implants*, 15, 15–46.

Buser D, Belser UC, Lang NP. (1998) The original one-stage dental implant system and its clinical application. *Periodontol 2000*, 17, 106–118.

Casko JS, Vaden JL, Kokich VG, et al. (1998) Objective grading system for dental casts and panoramic radiographs. *Am J Orthod Dentofacial Orthop*, 114(5), 589–599.

Caton JG, Greenwell H, Mahanonda R, et al. (1999) Consensus report: dental plaque-induced gingival diseases *Ann Periodontol*, 4(1), 18–19.

Caton JG, Rees T, Pack A, et al. (1999) Consensus report: non-plaque-induced gingival lesions. *Ann Periodontol*, 4(1), 30–31.

Choumerianou DM, Dimitriou H, Perdikogianni C, Martimianaki G, Riminucci M, Kalmanti M (2008) Study of oncogenic transformation in ex vivo expanded mesenchymal cells, from paediatric bone marrow. *Cell Prolif*, 41(6), 909–922.

Cochran DL.(1996) Implant therapy I. *Ann Periodontol*, 1, 701–791.

Cohen ES. (2007) Atlas of Cosmetic and Reconstructive Periodontal Surgery, 3rd edn. BC Decker, Ontario.

Consolo U, Travaglini D, Todisco M, Trisi P, Galli S. (2013) Histologic and biomechanical evaluation of the effects of implant insertion torque on peri-implant bone healing. *J Craniofac Surg*, 24(3), 860–865.

Cope JB, Samchukov ML. (2001) Mineralization dynamics of regenerate bone during mandibular osteodistraction. *Int J Oral Maxillofac Surg*, 30(3), 234–242.

Costello EJ, Angold A. (2010) Developmental transitions to psychopathology: are there prodromes of substance use disorders? *J Child Psychol Psychiatry*, 51(4), 526–532.

Craig RG, Powers JM, Wataha JC. (2004) Dental Materials Properties and Manipulation, 8th edn. Mosby, St Louis.

Cranin N. (2003) Glossary of implant terms. *J Oral Implant*, 29, 29–40.

Crismani AG, Bernhart T, Schwarz K, Celar AG, Bantleon HP, Watzek G. (2006) Ninety percent success in palatal implants loaded 1 week after placement: a clinical evaluation by resonance frequency analysis. *Clin Oral Implants Res*, 17(4), 445–450.

Da MX, Wu Z, Tian HW. (2008) Tumor lymphangiogenesis and lymphangiogenic growth factors. *Arch Med Res*, 39(4), 365–372.

Daood U, Bandey N, Qasim SB, Omar H, Khan SA. (2011) Surface characterization analysis of failed dental implants using scanning electron microscopy. *Acta Odontol Scand*, 69(6), 367–373.

Daskalogiannakis J.(2000) Glossary of Orthodontic Terms. Quintessence Publishing, Chicago.

Davies JE. (2000) Bone Engineering. Em Squared, Toronto.

den Hartog L, Raghoebar GM, Stellingsma K, Vissink A, Meijer HJ. (2011) Immediate non-occlusal loading of single implants in the aesthetic zone: a randomized clinical trial: Immediate loading of anterior single implants. *J Clin Periodontol*, 38(2), 186–194.

Drago C. (2014) Implant Restorations. A Step by Step Guide, 3rd edn. Wiley-Blackwell, Ames, Iowa.

Eliades G, Eliades T, Brantley WA, Watts DC. (2003) Dental Materials in Vivo Aging and Related Phenomena. Quintessence Publishing, Chicago.

English CE. (1990) Critical A-P spread. *Implant Soc*, 1(1), 2–3.

Esposito M, Hirsch JM, Lekholm U, Thomsen P. (1998) Biological factors contributing to failures of osseointegrated oral implants (I). Success criteria and epidemiology. *Eur J Oral Sci*, 106(1), 527–551.

Esposito M, Hirsch JM, Lekholm U, Thomsen P. (1998) Biological factors contributing to failures of osseointegrated oral implants (II). Etiopathogenesis. *Eur J Oral Sci*, 106, 721–764.

Esposito M, Hirsch J, Lekholm U, Thomsen P. (1999) Differential diagnosis and treatment strategies for biologic complications and failing oral implants: a review of the literature. *Int J Oral Maxillofac Implants*, 14, 473–490.

Filippi A, Pohl Y, von Arx T. (2001) Decoronation of an ankylosed tooth for preservation of alveolar bone prior to implant placement. *Dent Traumatol*, 17(2), 93–95.

Fiorellini JP, Engebretson SP, Donath K, Weber HP. (1998) Guided bone regeneration utilizing expanded polytetrafluoroethylene membranes in combination with submerged and non-submerged dental implants in beagle dogs. *J Periodontol*, 69(5), 528–535.

Frost HM. (1997) Indirect way to estimate peak joint loads in life and in skeletal remains (insights from a new paradigm). *Anat Rec*, 248(3), 475–483.

Frost HM. (1999) Joint anatomy, design, and arthroses: insights of the Utah paradigm. *Anat Rec*, 255(2), 162–174.

Frost HM. (2001) From Wolff's law to the Utah paradigm: insights about bone physiology and its clinical applications. *Anat Rec*, 262(4), 398–419.

Galindo-Moreno P, Avila G, Fernández-Barbero JE, et al. (2007) Evaluation of sinus floor elevation using a composite bone graft mixture. *Clin Oral Implants Res*, 18(3), 376–382.

Gamoh S, Nakashima Y, Akiyama H, et al. (2014) Fibrosarcoma of the temporomandibular joint area: benefits of magnetic resonance imaging and computed tomography. *Oral Surg Oral Med Oral Pathol Oral Radiol*, 118(3), 262–266.

Gargiulo AW, Wentz FM, Orban B. (1961) Dimensions and relations of the dentogingival junction in humans. *J Periodontol*, 32, 261–267.

Gräber HG, Conrads G, Wilharm J, Lampert F. (1999) Role of interactions between integrins and extracellular matrix components in healthy epithelial tissue and establishment of a long junctional epithelium during periodontal wound healing: a review. *J Periodontol*, 70(12), 1511–1522.

Grant GT, Campbell SD, Masri RM, Andersen MR, American College of Prosthodontists Digital Dentistry Glossary Development Task Force. (2016) Glossary of digital dental terms. *J Prosthodont*, 25, S2–S9.

Griffiths HJ, Parantainen H, Olsen P. (1993) Alcohol and bone disorders. *Alcohol Health Res World*, 17(3), 299–304.

Gutknecht N. (2007) Proceedings of the First International Workshop of Evidence Based Dentistry on Lasers in Dentistry. Quintessence Publishing, London.

Habibi A, Sedaghat MR, Habibi M, Mellati E. (2008) Silent sinus syndrome: report of a case. *Oral Surg Oral Med Oral Pathol Oral Radiol Endod*, 105(3), e32–35.

Hall SS, Thomas HV. (1938) Spontaneous hemorrhage into the maxillary sinus. *Arch Otolaryngol*, 28(3), 371–375.

Hardy DK, Cubas YP, Orellana MF. (2012) Prevalence of angle class III malocclusion: a systematic review and meta-analysis. *OJEpi*, 2, 75–82.

Harris RJ. (1992) The connective tissue and partial thickness double pedicle graft: a predictable method of obtaining root coverage. *J Periodontol*, 63(5), 477–486.

Hauschka PV, Wians FH Jr. (1989) Osteocalcin-hydroxyapatite interaction in the extracellular organic matrix of bone. *Anat Rec*, 224(2), 180–188.

Heasman P, McCracken G (eds). (2007) Harty's Dental Dictionary, 3rd edn. Churchill Livingstone, Edinburgh.

Hickey JC, Boucher CO, Hughes GA. (1968) Glossary of prosthodontics terms. The nomenclature committee academy of denture prosthetics. *J Prosthet Dent*, 20, 443–480.

Hoefert S, Hoefert CS, Albert M, et al. (2015) Zoledronate but not denosumab suppresses macrophagic differentiation of THP-1 cells. An aetiologic model of bisphosphonate-related osteonecrosis of the jaw (BRONJ). *Clin Oral Investig*, 19(6), 1307–1318.

Holland EA. (1989) Osteoporosis: impact on the elderly, societal concerns, and the role of radiology. *Curr Probl Diagn Radiol*, 18(2), 44–61.

Hürzeler MB, Zuhr O, Schupbach P, Rebele SF, Emmanouilidis N, Fickl S. (2010) The socket-shield technique: a proof-of-principle report. *J Clin Periodontol*, 37, 855–862.

Irokawa D, Takeuchi T, Noda K, et al. (2017) Clinical outcome of periodontal regenerative therapy using collagen membrane and deproteinized bovine bone mineral: a 2.5-year follow-up study. *BMC Research Notes*, 10, 102.

Ison TG. (2009) Intraoral nerve blocks for orofacial anesthesia. *Clin Pediatr Emerg Med*, 1(4), 270–275.

Jackson A, Lemke R, Hatch J, Salome N, Gakunga P, Cochran D. (2008) A comparison of stability between delayed versus immediately loaded orthodontic palatal implants. *J Esthet Restor Dent*, 20(3), 174–184.

Jacobs R, van Steenberghe D. (2006) From osseoperception to implant-mediated sensory-motor interactions and related clinical implications. *J Oral Rehabil*, 33(4), 282–292.

Jambhekar S, Kernen F, Bidra AS. (2015) Clinical and histologic outcomes of socket grafting after flapless tooth extraction: a systematic review of randomized controlled clinical trials. *J Prosthet Dent*, 113(5), 371–382.

Jauhiainen L, Korhonen HT. (2005) Optimal behaviour sampling and autocorrelation curve: modelling data of farmed foxes. *Acta Ethologica*, 8(1), 13–21.

Jee WS, Ma YF. (1997) The in vivo anabolic actions of prostaglandins in bone. *Bone*, 21(4), 297–304.

Jensen OT. (2002) Alveolar Distraction Osteogenesis. Quintessence Publishing, Chicago.

Jensen OT. (2006) The Sinus Bone Graft, 2nd edn. Quintessence Publishing, Chicago.

Jensen OT, Shulman LB, Block MS, Iacono VJ. (1998) Report of the sinus consensus conference of 1996. *Int J Oral Maxillofac Implants*, 13(Suppl), 11–45.

Jokstad A.(2009) *Osseointegration and Dental Implants*. Wiley-Blackwell, Chichester.

Jokstad A, Braegger U, Brunski JB, Carr AB, Naert I, Wennerberg A. (2003) Quality of dental implants. *Int Dent J*, 53, 409–443.

Jordan BA, Hughes AN. (1978) A review of the factors affecting the design, specification and material selection of screws for use in orthopaedic surgery. *Engineer Med*, 7(2), 114–123.

Kalb S, Mahan MA, Elhadi AM, et al. (2013) Pharmacophysiology of bone and spinal fusion. *Spine J*, 13(10), 1359–1369.

Kang Q, Sun MH, Cheng H, et al. (2004) Characterization of the distinct orthotopic bone-forming activity of 14 BMPs using recombinant adenovirus-mediated gene delivery. *Gene Ther*, 11(17), 1312–1320.

Kara C. (2008) Evaluation of patient perceptions of frenectomy: a comparison of Nd:YAG laser and conventional techniques. *Photomed Laser Surg*, 26(2), 147–152.

Kemp K, Mallam E, Scolding N, Wilkins A. (2010) Stem cells in genetic myelin disorders. *Regen Med*, 5(3), 425–439.

Khan MM, Darwish HH, Zaher WA. (2010) Perforation of the inferior alveolar nerve by the maxillary artery: an anatomical study. *Br J Oral Maxillofac Surg*, 48(8), 645–647.

Komine F, Gerds T, Witkowski S, Strub JR. (2005) Influence of framework configuration on the marginal adaptation of zirconium dioxide ceramic anterior four-unit frameworks. *Acta Odontol Scand*, 63(6), 361–366.

Kraus KH, Kirker-Head C. (2006) Mesenchymal stem cells and bone regeneration. *Vet Surg*, 35(3), 232–242.

Kunert-Keil C, Scholz F, Gedrange T, Gredes T. (2015) Comparative study of biphasic calcium phosphate with beta-tricalcium phosphate in rat cranial defects – a molecular-biological and histological study. *Ann Anat*, 199, 79–84.

Laidler P. (1994) Neuromuscular plasticity. In: Stroke Rehabilitation. Springer, Boston.

Laney WR. (2007) Glossary of Oral and Maxillofacial Implants. Quintessence Publishing, Berlin.

Lang NP, Karring T. (1994) Proceedings of the First European Workshop on Periodontology. Quintessence Publishing, London, pp. 296–365.

Lang NP, Karring T, Lindhe J. (1999) Proceedings of the 3rd European Workshop on Periodontology and Implant Dentistry. Quintessence Publishing, London.

Last JM. (2001) A Dictionary of Epidemiology, 4th edn. Oxford University Press, New York.

Lee A, Brown D, Wang HL. (2009) Sandwich bone augmentation for predictable horizontal bone augmentation. *Implant Dent*, 18(4), 282–290.

Lee JE, Jin SH, Ko Y, Park JB. (2014) Evaluation of anatomical considerations in the posterior maxillae for sinus augmentation. *World J Clin Cases*, 2(11), 683–688.

LeMoon K. (2008) Terminology used in fascia research. *J Bodyw Mov Ther*, 12(3), 204–212.

Liew A, Barry F, O'Brien T. (2006) Endothelial progenitor cells: diagnostic and therapeutic considerations. *Bioessays*, 28(3), 261–270.

Lin LM, Rosenberg PA. (2011) Repair and regeneration in endodontics: repair and regeneration in endodontics. *Int Endod J*, 44(10), 889–906.

Lindhe J, Lang NP, Karring T. (2008) Clinical Periodontology and Implant Dentistry, 5th edn. Blackwell Munksgaard, Oxford.

Lynch SE, Marx RE, Nevins M, Wisner-Lynch LA. (2008) Tissue Engineering: Applications in Oral and Maxillofacial Surgery and Periodontics, 2nd edn. Quintessence Publishing, Chicago.

Man D, Plosker H, Winland-Brown JE. (2001) The use of autologous platelet-rich plasma (platelet gel) and autologous platelet- poor plasma (fibrin glue) in cosmetic surgery. *Plast Reconstr Surg*, 107(1), 229–237.

Mangano F, Mangano C, Ricci M, Sammons RL, Shibli JA, Piattelli A. (2011) Single-tooth Morse taper connection implants placed in fresh extraction sockets of the anterior maxilla: an aesthetic evaluation. *Clin Oral Implants Res*, 23(11), 1302–1307.

Mangano FG, Tettamanti L, Sammons RL, et al. (2013) Maxillary sinus augmentation with adult mesenchymal stem cells: a review of the current literature. *Oral Surg Oral Med Oral Pathol Oral Radiol*, 115(6), 717–723.

Maurice CG. (1968) An annotated glossary of terms used in endodontics. *Oral Surg Oral Med Oral Pathol*, 25(3), 491–512.

McCord JF, Grant AA. (2000) Registration: Stage I – Creating and outlining the form of the upper denture. *Br Dent J*, 188(10), 529–536.

Mersel A. (2002) Immediate or transitional complete dentures: gerodontic considerations. *Int Dent J*, 52(4), 298–303.

Metgud SC. (2008) Primary cutaneous actinomycosis: a rare soft tissue infection. (Case Report). *Indian J Med Microbiol*, 26(2), 184–186.

Misch CE. (2005) Dental Implant Prosthodontics. Mosby, St Louis.

Misch CE. (2008) Contemporary Implant Dentistry, 3rd edn. Mosby, St Louis.

Misch CE. (2015) Dental Implant Prosthetics, 2nd edn. Mosby/Elsevier, St Louis.

Misch CE, Misch CM. (1992) Generic terminology for endosseous implant prosthodontics. *J Prosthet Dent*, 68, 809–812.

Mishra N, Singh BP, Rao J, Rastogi P. (2010) Improving prosthetic prognosis by connective tissue ridge augmentation of alveolar ridge. *Indian J Dent Res*, 21(1), 129–131.

Mombelli A, Casagni F, Madianos PN. (2002) Can presence or absence of periodontal pathogens distinguish between subjects with chronic and aggressive periodontitis? A systematic review. *J Clin Periodontol*, 29(Suppl 3), 10–21.

Naito M, Kato T, Fujii W, et al. (2010) Effects of dental treatment on the quality of life and activities of daily living in institutionalized elderly in Japan. *Arch Gerontol Geriatr*, 50(1), 65–68.

Nanci A. (1999) Content and distribution of noncollagenous matrix proteins in bone and cementum: relationship to speed of formation and collagen packing density. *J Struct Biol*, 126(3), 256–269.

Newman MG, Takei H, Klokkevold PR, Carranza FA. (2015) Carranza's Clinical Periodontology, 12th edn. Elsevier Saunders, St Louis.

Niamtu III J. (2008) Local anesthetic blocks of the head and neck. In: Shiffman M, Mirrafati S, Lam S, Cueteaux C (eds). Simplified Facial Rejuvenation. Springer, Berlin.

Nilsson O, Wängberg B, Kölby L, Schultz GS, Ahlman H. (1995) Expression of transforming growth factor alpha and its receptor in human neuroendocrine tumours. *IJC*, 60(5), 645–651.

O'Brien WJ. (2002) Dental Materials and their Selection. Quintessence Publishing, Chicago.

Okeson JP. (2009) Management of Temporomandibular Disorders and Occlusion, 4th edn. Elsevier, St Louis, pp. 180–182.

Osawa S, Rhoton AL Jr, Seker A, Shimizu S, Fujii K, Kassam AB. (2009) Microsurgical and endoscopic anatomy of the vidian canal. *Neurosurgery*, 64(5 Suppl 2), 385–411.

Pachore NJ, Patel JR, Sethuraman R, Naveen YG (2014) A comparative analysis of the effect of three types of denture adhesives on the retention of maxillary denture bases: an in vivo study. *J Indian Prosthodont Soc*, 14(4), 369–375.

Patel K, Mardas N, Donos N. (2013) Radiographic and clinical outcomes of implants placed in ridge preserved sites: a 12-month post-loading follow-up. *Clin Oral Implants Res*, 24(6), 599–605.

Pathak C, Salil P, Gupta A, Meenu G, Aditi GP. (2015) Andrews A bridge for anterior ridge defect – a case report. *Clin Dent*, 9(2), 21–27.

Patras M, Naka O, Doukoudakis S, Pissiotis A. (2012) Management of provisional restorations' deficiencies: a literature review. *J Esthet Restor Dent*, 24(1), 26–38.

Payne A, Walton J, Alsabeeha N, Worthington HV, Esposito M. (2009) Interventions for replacing missing teeth: attachment systems for implant overdentures in edentulous jaws. *Cochrane Database Syst Rev*, 4, CD008001.

Phabphal K, Geater A. (2013) The association between BsmI polymorphism and risk factors for atherosclerosis in patients with epilepsy taking valproate. *Seizure*, 22(9), 692–697.

Pipko DJ. (2011) Endosseous dental implant torquing continuum. *Implant Dent*, 20(3), 180–181.

Porwal A, Sasaki K. (2013) Current status of the neutral zone: a literature review. *J Prosthet Dent*, 109(2), 129–134.

Quick Study for Medical Terminology (2006) Bar Charts Inc., Florida.

Quirynen M, Herrera D, Teughels W, Sanz M (eds). (2014) Implant surgery – 40 years of experience. *Periodontology 2000*, 66, 7–12.

Raimundo LB, Orsi IA, Kuri SE, Rovere CA, Busquim TP, Borie E. (2015) Effects of peracetic acid on the corrosion resistance of commercially pure titanium (grade 4). *Braz Dent J*, 26(6), 660–666.

Rathoure AK. (2014) Microbial biomass production. *Microb Biotechnol*, 279–296.

Rickert D, Slater JJ, Meijer HJ, Vissink A, Raghoebar GM. (2012) Maxillary sinus lift with solely autogenous bone compared to a combination of autogenous bone and growth factors or (solely) bone substitutes. A systematic review. *Int J Oral Maxillofac Surg*, 41(2), 160–167.

Rodella LF, Buffoli B, Labanca M, Rezzani R. (2012) A review of the mandibular and maxillary nerve supplies and their clinical relevance. *Arch Oral Biol*, 57(4), 323–334.

Romanos GE. (2012) Advanced Immediate Loading. Quintessence Publishing, Chicago.

Rompen E, Domken O, Degidi M, Pontes AE, Piattelli A. (2006) The effect of material characteristics, of surface topography and of implant components and connections on soft tissue integration: a literature review. *Clin Oral Implants Res*, 17(Suppl 2), 55–67.

Rozen A. (2006) Effect of cadmium on life-history parameters in Dendrobaena octaedra (Lumbricidae: Oligochaeta) populations originating from forests differently polluted with heavy metals. *Soil Biol Biochem*, 38(3), 489–503.

Ryhänen J, Kallioinen M, Tuukkanen J, et al. (1999) Bone modeling and cell-material interface responses induced by nickel-titanium shape memory alloy after periosteal implantation. *Biomaterials*, 20(14), 1309–1317.

Saadoun AP. (2013) Esthetic Soft Tissue Management of Teeth and Implants. Elsevier, Amsterdam.

Samchukov ML, Cope JB, Harper RP, Ross JD. (1998) Biomechanical considerations of mandibular lengthening and widening by gradual distraction using a computer model. *J Oral Maxillofac Surg*, 56(1), 51–59.

Scarano A, Degidi M, Perrotti V, Piattelli A, Iezzi G. (2011) Sinus augmentation with phycogene hydroxyapatite: histological and histomorphometrical results after 6 months in humans. A case series. *Oral Maxillofac Surg*, 16(1), 41–45.

Scharf DR, Tarnow DP. (1993) Success rates of osseointegration for implants placed under sterile versus clean conditions. *J Periodontol*, 64(10), 954–956.

Schneider RL. (1987) Significance of abutment tooth angle of gingival convergence on removable partial denture retention. *J Prosthet Dent*, 58, 194–196.

Schopper C, Moser D, Sabbas A, et al. (2003) The fluorohydroxyapatite (FHA) FRIOSR AlgiporeR is a suitable biomaterial for the reconstruction of severely atrophic human maxillae. *Clin Oral Implants Res*, 14(6), 743–749.

Sendhilnathan D, Sivagami G. (2008) Stabilization of interocclusal records during programming of the semiadjustable articulator. *J Indian Prosthodont Soc*, 8, 42–43.

Sethi A, Kaus T. (2012) Practical Implant Dentistry. The Science and Art, 2nd edn. Quintessence Publishing, Chicago.

Shannon J, Shannon J, Modelevsky S, Grippo AA. (2011) Bisphosphonates and osteonecrosis of the jaw. *J Am Geriatr Soc*, 59(12), 2350–2355.

Shillingburg HT, Hobo S, Whitsett LD, Jacobi R, Brackett SE. (1997) Fundamentals of Fixed Prosthodontics, 3rd edn. Quintessence Publishing, Chicago.

Siddiqi A, Payne AG, Zafar S. (2009) Bisphosphonate-induced osteonecrosis of the jaw: a medical enigma? *Oral Surg Oral Med Oral Pathol Oral Radiol Endod*, 108(3), e1–8.

Simon H, Yanase RT. (2003) Terminology for implant prostheses. *Int J Oral Maxillofac Implants*, 18, 539–543.

Snyder R, Jerrold L. (2007) Black, white, or gray: finding commonality on how orthodontists describe the areas between Angle's molar classifications. *Am J Orthod Dentofacial Orthop*, 132(3), 302–306.

Sowmya S, Bumgardener JD, Chennazhi KP, Nair SV, Jayakumar R. (2013) Role of nanostructured biopolymers and bioceramics in enamel, dentin and periodontal tissue regeneration. *Progr Polymer Sci*, 38(10-11), 1748–1772.

Srinivasan B, Kailasam V, Chitharanjan A, Ramalingam A. (2013) Relationship between crown-root angulation (collum angle) of maxillary central incisors in Class II, division 2 malocclusion and lower lip line. *Orthodontics*, 14(1), e66–74.

Staubli P, Bagley D. (2008) Attachments and Implants Reference Manual, 8th edn. Attachments International, San Mateo.

Stedman's Plastic Surgery ENT/Dentistry Words, 2nd edn. (2003) Lippincott Williams and Wilkins, Baltimore.

Steigenga J, Al-Shammari K, Misch C, Nociti FH, Wang HL. (2004) Effects of implant thread geometry on percentage of osseointegration and resistance to reverse torque in the tibia of rabbits. *J Periodontol*, 75(9), 1233–1241.

Stelzle F, Rohde M. (2014) Elevation forces and resilience of the sinus membrane during sinus floor elevation: preliminary measurements using a balloon method on ex vivo pig heads. *Int J Oral Maxillofac Implants*, 29(3), 550–557.

Sujin K, Rasmussen E. (2008) Characteristics of tissue-centric biomedical researchers using a survey and cluster analysis. *J Assoc Inf Sci Technol*, 59(8), 1210–1223.

Sumner-Smith G, Fackelman GE. (2002) Bone in Clinical Orthopedics, 2nd edn. Thieme Medical Publishing, New York.

Sykaras N, Iacopino AM, Marker VA, Triplett RG, Woody RD. (2002) Implant materials, designs, and surface topographies: their effect on osseointegration. A literature review. *Int J Oral Maxfac Implants*, 15, 675–690.

Szulc P. (2012) The role of bone turnover markers in monitoring treatment in postmenopausal osteoporosis. *Clin Biochem*, 45(12), 907–919.

Tabesh H, Amoabediny G, Nik NS, et al. (2009) The role of biodegradable engineered scaffolds seeded with Schwann cells for spinal cord regeneration. *Neurochem Int*, 54(2), 73–83.

Taylor TD, Agar JR. (2002) Twenty years of progress in implant prosthodontics. *J Prosthet Dent*, 88, 89–95.

Temmerman A, Hertelé S, Teughels W, Dekeyser C, Jacobs R, Quirynen M. (2011) Are panoramic images reliable in planning sinus augmentation procedures? Reliability of panoramic images. *Clin Oral Implants Res*, 22(2), 189–194.

Termeie DA.(2013) Periodontal Review. A Study Guide. Quintessence Publishing, Chicago.

Tuuminen R, Loukovaara S. (2016) Statin medication in patients with epiretinal membrane is associated with low intravitreal EPO, TGF-beta-1, and VEGF levels. *Clin Ophthalmol*, 10, 921–928.

Ueta C, Iwamoto M, Kanatani N, et al. (2001) Skeletal malformations caused by overexpression of Cbfa1 or its dominant negative form in chondrocytes. *J Cell Biol*, 153(1), 87–100.

Van Waas MAJ, Geertman ME, Spanjaards SG, Boerrigter EM. (1997) Construction of a clinical implant performance scale for implant systems with overdentures with the delphi method. *J Prosthet Dent*, 77(5), 503–509.

Vandersall DC. (2007) Concise Encyclopedia of Periodontology. Blackwell, Ames.

Visser A, Geertman ME, Meijer HJ, et al. (2002) Five years of aftercare of implant-retained mandibular overdentures and conventional dentures. *J Oral Rehabil*, 29(2), 113–120.

von Arx T, Lozanoff S. (2017) Clinical Oral Anatomy. A Comprehensive Review for Dental Practitioners and Researchers. Springer, Berlin.

Vrielinck L, Politis C, Schepers S, Pauwels M, Naert I. (2003) Image-based planning and clinical validation of zygoma and pterygoid implant placement in patients with severe bone atrophy using customized drill guides. Preliminary results from a prospective clinical follow-up study. *Int J Oral Maxillofac Surg*, 32(1), 7–14.

Wang HL, Misch C, Neiva RF. (2004) "Sandwich" bone augmentation technique: rationale and report of pilot cases. *Int J Periodontics Restorative Dent*, 24, 232–245.

Wang HL, Ormianer Z, Palti A, Perel ML, Trisi P, Sammartino G. (2006) Consensus conference on immediate loading: the single tooth and partial edentulous areas. *Implant Dent*, 15(4), 324–333.

Werner H, Katz J. (2004) The emerging role of the insulin-like growth factors in oral biology. *J Dent Res*, 83(11), 832–836.

Wieland M, Textor M, Chehroudi B, Brunette DM. (2005) Synergistic interaction of topographic features in the production of bone-like nodules on Ti surfaces by rat osteoblasts. *Biomaterials*, 26(10), 1119–1130.

Wilson TG. (2015) Complications associated with flapless surgery. In: Froum SJ (ed.), Dental Implant Complications: Etiology, Prevention, and Treatment, 2nd edn. John Wiley & Sons, Hoboken.

Wilson TG Jr, Kornman KS. (2003) Fundamentals of Periodontics, 2nd edn. Quintessence Publishing, Chicago.

Xynos ID, Hukkanen MV, Batten JJ, Buttery LD, Hench LL, Polak JM. (2000) Bioglass ®45S5 stimulates osteoblast turnover and enhances bone formation in vitro: implications and applications for bone tissue engineering. *Calcif Tissue Int*, 67(4), 321–329.

Yamanishi Y, Yamaguchi S, Imazato S, Nakano T, Yatani H. (2012) Influences of implant neck design and implant abutment joint type on peri-implant bone stress and abutment micromovement: three-dimensional finite element analysis. *Dent Mater*, 28(11), 1126–1133.

Yin Y, Huang L, Zhao X, et al. (2007) AMD3100 mobilizes endothelial progenitor cells in mice, but inhibits its biological functions by blocking an autocrine/paracrine regulatory loop of stromal cell derived factor-1 in vitro. *J Cardiovasc Pharmacol*, 50(1), 61–67.

Zaizen T, Sato I. (2014) A morphological study of the multi infraorbital canals of the maxilla in the Japanese macaque by cone-beam computed tomography. *Anat Sci Int*, 89(3), 171–182.

Zangrando MSR, Veronesi GF, Cardoso MV, et al. (2017) Altered active and passive eruption: a modified classification. *Clin Adv Periodontics*, 7(1), 51–56.

Zinman EJ. (2015) Medicolegal REFIIDs related to implant complications. In: Froum SJ (ed.), Dental Implant Complications: Etiology, Prevention, and Treatment, 2nd edn. John Wiley & Sons, Hoboken.

Zinner ID, Panno FV, Small SA, Landa LS. (2004) Implant Dentistry: From Failure to Success. Quintessence Publishing, Chicago.

Zorlutuna P, Annabi N, Camci-Unal G, et al. (2012) Microfabricated biomaterials for engineering 3D tissues. *Adv Mater*, 24(14), 1782–1804.

Zucchelli G, Mounssif I. (2015) Periodontal plastic surgery. *Periodontology 2000*, 68(1), 333–368.

Zwemer TJ, Fehrenbach MJ, Emmons M, Tiedemann MA. (2004) Mosby's Dental Dictionary. Mosby, St Louis.

Internet sources

www.Juniordentist.com
www.Pocketdentistry.com
www.perio.org
www.Scribd.com
www.Saudident.com
www.mercksource.com
www.4dent.net
www.humanhealth.idea.org
www.endoexperience.com
www.dictionary.reference.com
www.wizliq.com
www.orthomagic.com
www.medical-dictionary.thefreedictionary.com
www.Science.gov
www.resources.usahealthstore.com
www.aae.org
www.jcdr.net
www.thinkthroughmath.com
www.bethesda.med.navy.mil
www.quintpub.com
www.elabscience.com
www.aopublishing.org
www.onlinelibrary.wiley.com
www.pathway2curis.com
www.freepattentsonline.com
www.bentham.org
www.ptei.org
www.removpros.dentistry.dal.ca
www.cdc.org
www.ncbi.nlm.nih.gov
www.periopeak.com
www.neomarkers.com
www.phsioclinic.net
www.studyblue.com
www.cellapplications.com
www.ada.org
www.faculty.ksu.edu.sa
www.sld.cu
www.iti.org

www.authorstream.com
www.cialisdefinition.com
www.slideshare.net
www.media.proquest.com
www.merriam-webster.com
www.rooksheathscience.com
www.icmis.net
www.docslide.us
www.kosmix.com
www.origin-dictionary.reference.com
www.wmo.int
www.ivythesis.typepad.com
www.dental.pitt.edu
www.ukessays.com
www.medschool.slu.edu
www.ehealthinitiative.org
www.ats.studysphere.com
www.righthealth.com
www.google.com
www.aadc.org
www.techopedia.com
www.aaomembers.org
www.cirem.org.uk
www.pages.nxtbook.com
www.eletsonline.com
www.rootcanalcentr.com
www.unr.edu
www.cmf.globalmednet.com
www.botany.ubc.ca
www.jenndeluca.com
www.studystack.com
www.superhealthcenter.com
www.scitechnol.com
www.cancerci.com
www.ordainhealth.com
www.careerdrive.co.ind
www.sdm.buffalo.edu
www.distraction.net
www.sld.cu
www.sign-a-rama.co.za
www.dentalintranet.com
www.sparkboom.org
www.jokstad.no
www.guaranteedplans.com
www.ejbjs.org
www.uwo.ca
www.docs.uwo.ca
www.docs.ksu.edu.sa
www.monash.edu.au

www.britannica.co.uk
www.cda.org
www.bd.com
www.dentalqna.com
www.dentalimplantssf.com
www.dictionary.rare-cancer.org
www.todaysthv.com
www.wellsphere.com
www.etd.lib.metu.edu.tr
www.cbtrf.org
www.content.health.msn.com
www.documents.ms
www.jeffreydikken.nl
www.healthscout.com
www.thefreedictionary.com
www.reference.com
www.labs.library.gvsu.edu
www.docslide.us
www.theoncologist.aplhamedpress.org
www.sti.nasa.gov
www.dl4a.org
www.drugline.org
www.criany.org
www.up.4dent.net
www.irjponline.com
www.kmle.com
www.worlddental.org
www.dhs.state.ri.us
www.answers.com
www.arachnoidcyst.org
www.db.uth.tmc.edu
www.oralhealthgroup.com
www.allenlee.com
www.msrdc.ac.in
www.consilient-health.com
www.evs.nci.nih.gov
www.libertydentaloceanside.com
www.medbib.com
www.studystack.com
www.wrongdiagnosis.com
www.regenerativeupdate.com
www.iticu.edu.tr
www.kmc.co.nz
www.biolab.com.cn
www.ptei.org
www.archive.org
www.namrata.co
www.wwhotv.com
www.dentalarticles.com

www.velocityincome.com

www.agd.org

www.retterdentalcare.com

www.absolutegeometries.com

www.videodoc.ncca-kaliningrad.ru

www.keystonedental.com

www.ashm.org.au

www.anchorsemi.com

www.prosth.net

www.erpublications.com

www.joethedentist.com

www.ukessays.com

www.health.nsw.gov.au

www.goodrichortho.com

www.my.webmed.com

www.dentistrytoday.com

www.intechopen.com

www.painhealth.com

www.dentaleduindia.com

www.jhc.org

www.dolforums.com.au

www.microdental.com

www.4drs.org

www.finedentistry.ca

www.journalagent.com

www.civilengineeringcompanies.org

www.ru.ac.za

www.dictionary.reference.com

www.chiroaccess.com

www.dental-webinars.com

www.virtualtrial.com

www.curehunter.com

www.ndif.org

www.cellmontage.cbrc.jp

www.sciencepub.net

www.cfpub.epa.gov

www.cylex-review.co.uk

www.healthexpertguide.org

www.bookrags.com

www.composite.tqn.com

www.docstoc.com

www.flashcardmachine.com

www.digitalartsguild.com

www.tisseelengineering.com

www.prohealthsys.com

www.fda.gov

www.ejgd.org

www.cdphe.state.co.us

www.coursehero.com

www.labs.library.gvsu.edu

www.nap.edu

www.patientsacademy.edu

www.intranet.tdmu.edu.ua

www.ash.confex.com

www.radiographics.rsna.org

www.emb.lib.ulg.ac.be

www.jisikworld.com

www.galaxyofhealth.com

www.justmedic.net

www.sifem-project.eu

www.dentaldecks.com

www.topics.sciencedirect.com

www.acoustic-glossary.co.uk

www.parkridgehospital.org

www.dentalreference.com

www.biochem.wisc.edu

www.dentatususa.com

www.nbihealth.com

www.todsmeeting.com

www.cdphe.state.co.us

www.de.dict.md

www.adha.org

www.gumsurgery.com

www.biomedcentral.com

www.healthexpertguide.org

www.esciencecentral.org

www.nou.edu.ng

www.blog.tcu.edu.tw

www.drotterholt.com

www.glucose.sextreffnorge.com

www.myhealthyspeak.co.in

www.berkeleybob.org

www.cglearn.com

www.ukessays.com

www.issuu.com

www.sprojects.mmi.mcgill.ca

www.medicalartprosthetics.com

www.iust.edu.sy

www.studystack.com

www.sickgums.com

www.freebase.com

www.kijob.or.kr

www.implantologiaitalia.it

www.medpro.smiletrain.org

www.antiquusmorbus.com

www.cincinnatichildrensblog.org

www.adha.org

www.statemaster.com

www.freshens.com
www.physrev.physiology.org
www.ndif.org
www.apps.elsevier.es
www.lib.bioinfo.pl
www.iera.org
www.geneontology.org
www.drstuartfroum.com
www.healthfoundation.eu
www.dimensionsofdentalhygiene.com
www.annalsofdentalspecialty.net.in
www.koldental.com.pl
www.incedental.com
www.thieme-connect.de
www.sustainableminds.com
www.endoexperience.com
www.auif.utcluj.ro
www.naun.org
www.radiopedia.org
www.primateportal.org
www.sld.cu
www.imagamegeek.co.uk
www.citaexam.com
www.jisponline.com
www.dr.library.brcku.ca
www.swissnf.com
www.slovarionline.ru
www.princeton.edu
www.annualreport.straumann.com
www.quizlet.com
www.sbdmj.com
www.scitechnol.com
www.themunnsreport.com
www.etraxx.com
www.absoluteastronomy.com
www.tankonyvtar.hu
www.coursehero.com
www.qataronlinedirectory.com
www.berkeleybob.org

www.unidoicamt.org
www.alligatordental.com
www.lymphedemapeople.com
www.articles.mums.ac.ir
www.authorstream.com
www.cscmpindy.com
www.allbusiness.com
www.musc.edu (www3)
www.baiviet.net
www.kitaosaka-implant.com
www.lookfordiagnosis.com
www.nzgg.org.nz
www.cueflash.com
www.cga.ct.gov
www.hmma.com
www.upcphills.org
www.harvest.co.kr
www.sdgmag.com
www.accessibilit.com
www.aje.oxfordjournals.org
www.ijcem.com
www.nature.com
www.expertwitness.com
www.avu.org
www.pricklessandgoo.com
www.html-live.ru
www.against-the-day.pynchonwiki.com
www.medgle.com
www.sdgmag.com
www.accessibilit.com
www.ijcem.com
www.mouthhealthy.org
www.researchgate.net
www.opensourcemachine.com
www.cdn.intechopen.com
www.blackwellpublishing.com
www.content.nhiondemand.com
www.en.wikipedia.org
www.sustainableminds.com